Praise for *A Return to Healing*

"This book dives deep into the history of how health care in the United States has evolved both scientifically and culturally to where it is today. Drs. Lazris and Roth take the reader from the roots of modern medical training based on understanding illness to our current market-driven profit driven health care delivery that has failed to meet its mandate of providing the care our communities need. There are solutions founded in a primary care-based model that the authors bring forth that need to be explored if we hope to repair health care delivery in our country. A must read for health care leaders seeking to make this change happen."

Michael Tuggy, MD, Family Physician, Converging Health

"Andy Lazris and Alan Roth's book offers profound insights into modern health care, blending clinical expertise with practical wisdom. From the outset, American medicine veered onto the wrong path, following the Flexner Report's emphasis on scientific rigor while neglecting William Osler's relationship-centered and expert clinician-focused approach. The authors challenge these historical missteps, advocating for patient-centered care, transparency, and a focus on lifestyle and emotional well-being. I strongly recommend this timely and transformative book for those interested in healing health care."

Scott Conard, MD, Co-Founder and Partner, Converging Health and Professor Emeritus, UT Southwestern Dallas

A Return to Healing

FLEXNER, OSLER, AND HOW
AMERICAN MEDICINE
WENT ASTRAY

Andy Lazris, MD, and Alan Roth, DO

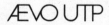

Aevo UTP
An imprint of University of Toronto Press
Toronto Buffalo London
utorontopress.com

ISBN 978-1-4875-6286-1 (cloth)   ISBN 978-1-4875-6288-5 (EPUB)
                                  ISBN 978-1-4875-6287-8 (PDF)

Library and Archives Canada Cataloguing in Publication

Title: A return to healing : Flexner, Osler, and how American medicine went
    astray / Andy Lazris, MD, and Alan Roth, DO.
Names: Lazris, Andrew, author | Roth, Alan (Alan R.), author.
Description: Includes bibliographical references and index.
Identifiers: Canadiana (print) 20240533747 | Canadiana (ebook) 20240533771 |
    ISBN 9781487562861 (paper) | ISBN 9781487562885 (EPUB) |
    ISBN 9781487562878 (PDF)
Subjects: LCSH: Medical care – United States. | LCSH: Medical care – United States –
    Decision making. | LCSH: Health care reform – United States. |
    LCSH: Flexner, Abraham, 1866–1959. | LCSH: Osler, William, Sir, 1849–1919.
Classification: LCC RA395.A3 L39 2025 | DDC 362.10973 – dc23

Printed in Canada

Cover design: Kathleen Lynch
Cover images: iStock.com/CCaetano

We wish to acknowledge the land on which the University of Toronto Press
operates. This land is the traditional territory of the Wendat, the Anishnaabeg, the
Haudenosaunee, the Métis, and the Mississaugas of the Credit First Nation.

University of Toronto Press acknowledges the financial support of the Government of
Canada, the Canada Council for the Arts, and the Ontario Arts Council, an agency of
the Government of Ontario, for its publishing activities.

 Canada Council **Conseil des Arts**
for the Arts **du Canada**

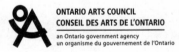 ONTARIO ARTS COUNCIL
CONSEIL DES ARTS DE L'ONTARIO
an Ontario government agency
un organisme du gouvernement de l'Ontario

Funded by the   Financé par le
Government   gouvernement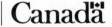
of Canada   du Canada

Andy: In memory of my dad, who taught us the value of assuring that everything we do is motivated by intelligence, respect, and an eye toward helping others. Thank you, dad, for making me the man I am. To my amazing children, Michael, David, and Rachel, who are my best friends, my unflappable support network, my inspiration, and the joy of my life. Thank you for being you.

Alan: In loving memory of my mom Lilly, who never stopped believing in me and who gave me the gift of dreams and the ability to realize them. In dedication to my wife Nelly, who has been the most profound inspiration of my life and has taught me about what matters most to me in life – I love you more.

Contents

PART TWO: THE COGS OF THE FLEXNERIAN MEDICAL-INDUSTRIAL COMPLEX

Preface

We wrote this book to expose the seeds of American health care's flaws so that we as a nation can work together to establish a patient-centric system based on science, humanism, and common sense. We have been practicing medicine for a combined 60 years and have both been immersed in and studied our health care system through a primary care lens. When we explored all that is wrong with our model of care and all that can be right, we realized that a decision made in Baltimore more than 100 years ago triggered a cascade of events that has damaged and offers the solution to what ails medical care in the United States.

There was a fork in the road, and we took the wrong one. It is our job to explain why, and how to get us back on course.

This book is written for patients and policymakers in a pragmatic way to offer advice about how to be a better-informed patient and how to institute meaningful reforms.

As we were finishing the book, COVID-19 struck our shores. Both of us treated hundreds of patients with the virus; we were consumed by it for its entire course; we were in the trenches and also studying it. We have deliberately kept COVID-19 out of this book; our next book will address it exclusively. But the lessons we provide here could have helped us craft a better response to the pandemic, and we trust that all readers will see that fact clearly.

A note of explanation. We typically write the book in the first-person singular, but every chapter is written by both of us, and the patient stories we relay are both Andy's and Alan's. The "I" is often "we."

We believe that we have uncovered a flaw in our health care system that has been long neglected, and by discussing it we hope to open some eyes as to what is wrong, why it happened, and how to fix it.

In the end, by shifting course and getting back on the right road, we hope this book offers everyone a beacon of hope for the future of our wellness and our health care system.

Andy and Alan

Acknowledgments

Andy: I thank David Lazris, whose hard work compiling data about and incorporating into our book the racial ramifications of the Flexner Report led to chapter 25, which he took charge of writing.

To all those who helped us to compile data and to our patients, who are our lifeblood.

Thank you to Brenda Copeland, who helped us in our initial editing of the manuscript and in paring down our very long initial draft into something cogent and readable, and to Alan, who throughout this long project kept me sane.

Alan: With extreme gratitude to those who have meant the most to me in life.

To Bruce Flanz and Mounir Doss for always being there for me through the good and bad years at Jamaica Hospital. To my Jamaica friends and colleagues, Bill, Sabiha, Gino, Fred, James, Gina, Robert, Sally, Cameron, Zharia, and Shania, thank you all.

To the Kew Gardens team and Lauren, who keeps me going daily in the pursuit of the health of our patients.

To the mentors in my career who have guided me and helped me become the clinician, teacher, and person I have become: Ed Bope, Larry Bauer, Dave Weissman, Michal Fine, and Wayne Jonas, who truly taught me about what matters most in life.

And of course, to my loving family, who have always been there for me, for giving me the love and guidance to pursue my lifelong dreams: Nelly, Jonathon, Elona, Noah, Jude, Nate, Eva, Allison, Jim, and my grandchildren Shiloh and Liam. A special shout out to my brothers Steven and Mitchell for sticking with me in the good and bad times, with additional kudos to Mitch for all he has done for us in making this book a reality.

Last, to my friend and writing partner Andy, without your support and collaboration, the success of this book would not be a reality; thank you, my friend!!

Introduction

JD is a 70-year-old man who in 2015, after retiring, worked hard to support a system of universal health care in the United States. A high school teacher, he knew little about health and heath care beyond what his army of doctors – and the newspapers and TV news shows he consumed voraciously – told him, but he knew enough to realize that our wonderful system saved his life many times over, and now he wanted that gift to be shared with everyone because so many Americans lacked access to the nation's medical sanctuary.

He had been seeing an array of doctors since age 40, getting annual exams and screening, lab tests, and even yearly stress tests by his cardiologist, who believed that it was best to keep an eye on things with copious testing – some people get sick without symptoms. Until a few years ago he bicycled 10 miles a day, swam, and tried to eat well, but knew that was not enough. And so, when his cholesterol popped up a bit, he went on high-dose statins, another medicine called Zetia, and yet another called Repatha, all of which together cost thousands of dollars a year but were all paid for by Medicare, as were his medical visits and tests. He also treated his prediabetes with two drugs, one of which helped with weight loss, while taking more drugs for keeping his blood thin, keeping his blood pressure low, and treating his big prostate and bone-density loss. He took a half dozen supplements, including high-dose vitamin D and a multivitamin, on top of his 15 prescription pills.

The results spoke for themselves. His LDL cholesterol remained under 70 mg/dl, the magical number below which his cardiologist believed to be lifesaving, and his A1c (a measure of diabetes control) remained under 6 percent, the goal of his endocrinologist. He rarely had a systolic blood pressure reading over 110, which pleased his kidney doctor and his other providers. His weight had dropped from his medicines, which was good because soon after consuming this buffet of lifesaving pills his legs became weaker and he was always tired, and thus he stopped exercising. His doctor sent him to several specialists to determine the cause of his weakness, but after tens of thousands of dollars of tests showed nothing, they attributed it to his advanced age.

Despite all his good health care, one day in 2018 a routine stress test showed that he had slow blood flow to one of his heart blood vessels. He went for a cardiac catheterization and developed a large hematoma (bleed) in his groin that never went away, but they found two 70 percent blockages in his heart, showing how important that routine test truly was. That is when his doctors saved his life again, inserting two metal tubes called stents into his blocked arteries. During the procedure he developed a brief heart rhythm called atrial fibrillation (afib), but his doctors fixed that and put him on a blood thinner called Eliquis. Now on three blood thinners, he developed anemia, went through inconclusive tests from a hematologist, and had both an upper and lower endoscopy from his gastroenterologist before starting a regimen of lifelong iron, which constipated him, leading to a lifetime of laxatives.

He could barely walk; sometimes he had to use a wheelchair. Often he slept much of the day. But he was grateful for having his life saved and went on to work for the campaign of US senator Bernie Sanders (I-VT), hoping to help him become president and allow all Americans to have access to the extraordinary health care that he enjoyed. He was furious that some insurance companies would not pay for all the drugs and tests, for everyone, that he had been allowed under Medicare, and even angrier that some people lacked health insurance at all. He knew that Senator Sanders could change that.

Did his stents really save his life, as his doctors promised?

In the United States, more than a million stents are placed in heart arteries every year at a total cost of more than $35 billion, a far greater cost than anywhere else in the world. A typical stent costs the patient $35,000 or more in the United States, but in Europe the cost is closer to $5,000. What's more, most stents are used to open arteries in people who have blockages and no symptoms, often based on results of routine stress tests, as was the case with JD. Such stents have been definitively shown to prevent no heart attacks and to save no lives.[1] Worse, this "just in case" intervention can instigate strokes, bleeding, and other severe complications, such as JD's hematoma. We will discuss many of JD's other interventions throughout this book, showing how the myth of their lifesaving prowess is not only harming and deceiving people, but also fueling a behemoth medical-industrial complex that feeds money into many players in the health care landscape, even as it bankrupts the country and prevents many people from receiving sensible care.

In October 2019, JD's candidate, Bernie Sanders, had his own experience with the health care system as he campaigned in Las

Vegas for the Democratic presidential nomination. Nothing epitomized Senator Sanders's campaign pledge more than "Medicare for All," the very issue that drew JD to his campaign. Such a promise flew in the face of powerful lobbying groups, including the American Medical Association (AMA), which believed that the cost of care was simply too high for such a plan to be feasible. Sanders contested that it could work. Like it or not, he said, "the United States will join every other major country on earth and guarantee healthcare to all people as a right."[2]

And then, in Las Vegas at a grassroots event calling for universal health care, among other things, Sanders developed chest pain. He was taken to urgent care and then to the hospital, where tests showed that he was in the throes of a heart attack. To prevent damage, doctors inserted two stents into his blocked artery, immediately averting the attack. Within days the senator was back on the campaign trail.

Sanders's campaign and the press were slow to release details of what had happened. No one knew. Did he have a heart attack? Would he be all right? Because of his age, and the vulnerability any medical issues might lay upon his campaign, there was a general hush. When the truth did creep out three days after the event, Sanders said that he was fine, that the doctors had saved his life, and that he was ready to campaign again.

What a missed opportunity for Sanders, and all those who advocate universal health care, to point out the promises and perils of our US health care system. Sanders's stent in the setting of a heart attack is likely beneficial, but its prolific use in people without sudden blood vessel closures, as with JD's (to open blockages, in other words), its excessive cost, and the abundance of medical care consumed by JD and so many others – care that often causes more harm than good, even if the unwary consumer is led to believe their life has been saved – are the very reasons why we can't afford universal health care in this country. Until we have a sensible health care system whose aim is to prevent and mitigate illness in a rational and patient-centric way, rather than the number-fixing drug-obsessed medical-industrial complex in which we live now that rewards providers of care as it harms consumers, Medicare for All is a distant illusion.

Why don't those who seek to expand our health care system point out its flaws, and why instead do they support and repeat the medical myths that have provided an illusion of better health, even as they tear our country's health to shreds?

The reason is simple. Since the publication of the Flexner Report in 1911, US health care has followed a dangerous, high-cost trajectory that has won the hearts and minds of most Americans, including, apparently, Senator Sanders and JD. With the Flexner Report, doctors were implored to repair every abnormality they could find, whether it needed to be corrected or not, pushing aside a more integrative patient-centered approach in which doctors treat the patient, not just the measurable numerical abnormalities. Is it any wonder that we have a bloated health care system viewed as lifesaving, even by those who promise to fix it, while it costs more and has worse outcomes than virtually everywhere else in the world?

To understand the *Zeitgeist* of the US health care system – why both doctors and their patients have bought into a model of care that is expensive, ineffective, and deceptive – we must look back to the Flexner Report, which inaugurated how we practice medicine today. During that singular moment, we had a choice of two roads to take, one that was paved by Abraham Flexner and the AMA, the other that was designed and constructed by William Osler and his experimental medical school at Johns Hopkins University in Baltimore.

This book is an analysis of the present, but it peeks back at the roots of the current mess, arguing that only by taking that other road, the one that Osler so brilliantly defined, can we regain what we lost. And thus, in this introduction, we will look at Osler, Flexner, and the report, opening a window that evades health care experts, such as Bernie Sanders, and consumers of health, such as JD, and prevents them from understanding why we have such a detrimental health care system and how we can get back on track. The system has only become more dysfunctional since 1911 – with health insurance and drug company/academic marriages twisting the provision of care into a drive for profit, something we will discuss throughout the book – but the moment of 1911 is a watershed that must be understood if we are to ever fix the mess that we have normalized. So let's take a quick look back at Baltimore where Flexner and arguably the nation's most influential doctor – pathologist William Welch, the founder and leader of Johns Hopkins Hospital, former AMA president, and noted eugenicist – came to an agreement that launched us into the very abyss that has thrown a blindfold over JD and Senator Sanders while assuring that their dream will never come to be.

It was a chilly day in Baltimore, and Abraham Flexner was preparing for his meeting. Tightening his wide tie over his dark black suit, he went to the kitchen for a cup of coffee, absorbed in his own thoughts. At just over six feet tall, with small wire spectacles outlining his tiny black eyes, Flexner seemed to exist in a space all his own. As his friends and enemies often said, he lived within his own perception of reality. In a mere year, this former minor educator had vaulted himself to fame and prominence, taking the medical world by storm. He understood the significance of his accomplishments, and today hoped to transform them into something big.

Flexner's hotel sat just outside the Johns Hopkins medical campus, in a tidy area of east Baltimore well beyond the stench of its more industrial harbor. Here there was a mix of poverty and wealth, and the Johns Hopkins Hospital – an innovative leader in medical education – catered to both. Flexner himself had graduated from Johns Hopkins many years ago with a degree in education. He obtained his diploma in just two years, and moved to Indiana to establish a school. His brother, Simon, himself a prominent doctor on staff, had achieved his own notoriety by discovering a bacterial infection that still bears his name. But Abraham Flexner was contemplating a far broader matter than mere scientific discovery.

One year earlier, in 1910, Abraham Flexner had authored a comprehensive report sponsored by the Carnegie Foundation. More than just scrutinizing all of the nation's medical schools, this report selected the winners and losers among them. For Flexner and his allies, the report that would ultimately bear his name was the first step in professionalizing and standardizing not only medical education but the entire field of health care in the United States. This was the culmination of work by the AMA, an organization that had been fighting for half a century to gain hegemony over the training and practice of doctors. Now, with Flexner's report, the AMA had given itself the power to determine a school's worthiness in graduating "credentialed" physicians. Many did not make the cut. Many doctors – including Black and female physicians, alternative practitioners, and those without certified education – lost their ability to practice medicine altogether. The entire medical landscape changed in an instant.

On that day in 1911, a well-groomed and stern-faced Flexner walked through Baltimore armed with a blueprint for change and a $1 million grant from the Rockefeller Foundation, intending to drive in the first stake of a grand new program of reform, and he would do it with William Henry Welch, president of Johns

Hopkins Hospital. Together, Flexner and Welch would transform Johns Hopkins from a clinical institution that taught students how to care for patients into the nation's most prominent research facility, replacing clinical staff with full-time scientists and instituting a standardized curriculum that emphasized pure science. It was a program that every credentialed school would ultimately be compelled to follow, one that has remained largely intact today.

One of the "Big Four" founders of the hospital, Welch had become the most powerful upon the retirement of his rival, Sir William Osler. Osler had helped create and lead the new medical school in 1882. Essentially, he built the school from scratch, designing a curriculum based on his primary dictate: that students learn through immersion in direct patient care. From the day they entered the medical school, students interacted with patients, an act that became their only forum of learning in the third and fourth year. To further students' clinical proficiency, Osler invented the residency, whereby new doctors would take apprenticeships for several years before going off to practice on their own.

Believing that medicine "is learned by the bedside and not in the classroom," Osler had established a program of clinical instruction at Hopkins in which practicing physicians – not scientists – trained medical students. Osler not only transformed Hopkins into a premier medical institution through his patient-centric approach to teaching, but he did it with part-time instructors: practicing doctors who made their living seeing patients in the community. Although he valued research and teaching, Osler believed that both were subservient to a real-world education that could only be obtained by working with real patients. "He who studies medicine without books sails an uncharted sea," he said. "But he who studies medicine without patients does not go to sea at all."

Osler had held sway at Hopkins, but with his retirement, Welch drove out Osler's hand-picked clinical colleagues, replacing them with scientists. With Flexner's money and new educational template, Welch had the means to expunge Osler's stamp from Hopkins. Students now received their education in the class, in labs, and on the wards – not in the offices of community physicians. What's more, they were taught by doctors who did not practice medicine themselves, but who merely read and researched it.

On that cold Baltimore day, Flexner and Welch shook hands and consummated a deal that would push US health care off the road of scientific pragmatism and compassion that William Osler hoped to pave and onto the road built with the bricks of the Flexner Report. The report's basic premise was that from now on, only schools sanctioned by the AMA that used a basic-science lab-based curriculum under the tutelage of full-time faculty would be able to graduate licensed physicians. Students would be taught that medicine was a science in which the measurements of abnormalities trumped the subjective and often unnecessary interaction between doctor and patient. Doctors would be expected to follow this credo into their careers, and their salaries and credentials, all monitored by the AMA, would be contingent on their obedience. Finally, all of it would be paid for by large corporate foundations that would willingly withdraw funding from any institutions that verged from the very specific rules and regulations elucidated in Flexner's report.

As Flexner and Welch sat in a warm office on the campus of Johns Hopkins, Welch accepted corporate money to transform his institution into Flexner's scientific laboratory and thus affected the direction of health care across the nation. Thus began the wedding among corporate interests, a medical establishment focused on control of its doctors, and a philosophy of care that put numbers over patients, a marriage with us even today.

Medical care in the United States was in a precarious position through the latter part of the nineteenth century. Both Osler and Flexner understood this sordid fact. Without any agreed-upon standards or skills to which doctors had to adhere, charlatans and patent doctors were free to push snake oil on unsuspecting patients. And because a great number of these practitioners lacked even the most rudimentary scientific knowledge and acumen, many harmful treatments were dispensed: untested pills, bleeding, and even surgeries conducted without sterile technique.

Most medical schools were diploma mills, and only students who could pay were able to obtain a degree. Hundreds of such schools were scattered across the country, producing far more doctors than necessary.[3] Educated people typically eschewed the medical field. A survey in 1851 showed that 26 percent of graduates from top colleges became clergymen and lawyers, and only 8 percent became doctors. Doctor salaries were low and the competition for patients fierce, a situation that remained intact at least until the twentieth century.[4]

In an attempt to counter the beleaguered state of health care, a group of physicians started a small organization called the AMA. Meeting in New York City in 1846, these doctors orchestrated a national organization whose goals were to raise and standardize medical degrees with the aim of improving the caliber of practice, decreasing the physician pool, and increasing doctor salaries. Throughout the century, the AMA met only once a year and remained small, exerting most of its influence on state medical societies. The AMA gained members and exerted influence by helping these societies gain control over licensing and setting standards of practice.[5] This went a long way toward creating a set of licensed doctors who could distinguish themselves from the mass of untrained practitioners dotting the medical landscape of the United States.

At this point, the AMA was essentially a trade association, imposing laws and restrictions favorable to its members. Only in 1900 did it begin to see the advantage of "touting itself as a promotor of scientific education" to advance its agenda.[6] And advance that agenda it did. In 1906, for example, the AMA promoted a pharmaceutical policy that, on the surface, sought to remove sham drugs from the market, but in reality promoted a regulatory system to "withhold information from consumers and re-channel drug purchasing through physicians." The intent of the AMA was not to improve the drug market, but to make sure that doctors had control over it.[7]

In addition to these sorts of policy mandates, the AMA sought to improve its status and that of its licensed physician members by exercising firm control of medical education. As long as medical schools remained unregulated, as long as they could spit out poorly trained snake oil salesmen who had an MD degree, American doctors could not achieve the status, money, and exclusiveness they desired. The AMA sought to cultivate a landscape with fewer schools training fewer doctors, all of which would be directly controlled by its own regulatory system. To that end, in 1904 the organization established a council of medical education, formulating standards to be implemented in all medical schools. In 1906, it inspected all 160 medical schools and made judgments about which ones (82 in all) met minimal standards. But it kept its findings secret, fearful that any verdict it imposed would be viewed as self-serving,[8] which of course it was.

To appear more objective, the AMA commissioned the Carnegie Foundation to essentially repeat its survey so as to get "independent and presumably disinterested support for its efforts."[9] The Carnegie Foundation, led by Henry Pritchett, had similar concerns about medical education as the AMA, so their collaboration made sense. It's important to realize that by 1908, when the AMA sanctioned this second survey, medical education had already been improving on its own as a result of state regulations and a natural disintegration of poor schools from high operating costs. The 450 schools training doctors in the late 1800s had been whittled down to 150. Many were already undergoing reforms to improve themselves, but not all. Numerous marginal schools remained, without lab equipment or hospital affiliations. Some had sparse curricula; others were situated in private homes. Sixty percent of schools did not have requirements for admission, an eighth of the schools required two years of college, and many remained for-profit institutions.[10]

The Carnegie Foundation, like the AMA, touted the German model of medical education as the template upon which any changes should be based. Drawn to a hard-science curriculum, Carnegie and the AMA wanted to graduate students well versed in chemistry, physics, biology, and physiology; clinical experience was far less important. The goal was to stamp the Germanic system upon every US medical school without variation.[11] To orchestrate and implement the "new" survey of medical schools, Pritchett chose a relatively unknown former educator, a man with no medical training or background. ✗

So why Flexner?

According to one source, the hiring of Flexner was "one of the strangest appointments in education history." But Pritchett was counting on the AMA to lead the actual effort, with Flexner being more of a figurehead who would follow the road map set out for him.[12] Flexner, however, was not the type to be directed. As someone who had himself lived in Germany, who had graduated from Johns Hopkins, and had experience in education, Flexner had established ideas about what he hoped to achieve with his survey. He made many profound decisions about schools by spending only a few hours studying them. LOL

Flexner's report made front-page news across the country. The *New York Times* announced that medical school "Factories for the Making of Ignorant Doctors" were going to disappear thanks to the Carnegie report.[13] The report, it was believed, represented a milestone in medical care, a turning point whereby the country's health care delivery system would be purged of its most corrupt and loathsome elements. The response was uniform adulation.

All doctors henceforth trained and credentialed in the United States would be scientifically oriented and experts in research. They would be taught by full-time researchers, not clinicians. And they would follow a science-based premedical and medical curriculum uniform in structure. Flexner hoped that Johns Hopkins would be the nidus of his new educational reforms, but to do that he had to first bulldoze over what William Osler, whose legacy was the soul of Johns Hopkins Medical School, had created.

Osler and others fought back as best they could. He wrote to Welch and to his clinical colleagues asking them to repudiate the report and not move Hopkins and the entire medical educational establishment in a direction he knew to be deleterious to the field. At Harvard, Francis Peabody, another clinician who was trying to inculcate medical education with real-life experiences, similarly assailed the Flexner Report. Peabody, who famously stated that "the secret of the care of the patient is in caring for the patient," felt that Flexner's approach "weakened the soul of the clinic."[14] Like Osler, he believed that Flexner's report "fossilized medical education into following a standardized format" that moved so far away from patients as to be useless in training competent physicians. "Osler and Peabody recognized the danger of reducing the patient to simply a pathophysiology characterized by laboratory tests" while fearing that such a parochial focus blinds doctors from "the broader contextual issues that so often play a crucial function in disease," said one author.[15]

But there were more powerful forces afloat than merely a few men who fought over medicine's direction. Despite the experience, status, and wisdom of men such as Osler and Peabody, their words evaporated in the report's wave of acclamation. Not only did the AMA gain power by grabbing the reins of medical education and licensing, but other corporate philanthropic groups, such as the Carnegie Foundation, which sponsored Flexner's study, and the Rockefeller Foundation, where Flexner worked for much of his subsequent life, had carefully crafted the report to construct a medical system in the United States that met their needs and expectations.

For the next 15 years of his life, Flexner worked at the Rockefeller Foundation on the general education board, dictating which schools would receive foundation money and which would not: "During that time, he approved the donation of half a billion dollars to schools that met all the rigid criteria of his report and in the process profoundly altered the medical education landscape." The schools that did not follow Flexner's script received no money and could not afford to stay afloat, failing to be granted requisite accreditation by the AMA.[16] One author states, "Money was power, and contributors to medical education knew that."[17]

What was the agenda of groups such as the Rockefeller Foundation, and why did they buy into Flexner's model? Essentially, their hope was to create great bastions of medical research, whereby medical institutions could engage in scientific study that matched that of Europe and achieve breakthroughs that would advance the medical industry and, undoubtedly, generate financial gain and a boost in reputation for the foundations and their parent corporations. These foundations had very specific agendas for the many schools they sponsored, and their donations were tied to the realization of those agendas, which typically required moving the schools from a clinical direction to one that was purely scientific and lab-based.[18] This instigated bitter struggles between old-line clinical teachers, such as Osler, and the newer research scientists who were now taking over. Full-time faculty could only exist if the schools were subsidized, and these large foundations were happy to pay the schools so long as the schools adhered to their rules.[19]

The foundation leaders – who were in fact agents of the large corporations who funneled money to them – then dictated to these schools the forms of research they desired. This began a cycle in US medicine in which clinical skills fell prey to basic science, and in which corporate entities dictated the direction of medical education, medical research, and medical practice. Within years, the clinical institutions that Osler always envisioned, ones in which patients and clinicians taught students, and in which students would leave the school with both a scientific and a humanistic knowledge of disease and treatment, vanished from the medical landscape. Osler's name remained well known and respected, but Flexner's ideas won the day. All this occurred because the corporate boards gained enough power to influence the direction in which medicine would flow. Wrote one author, "Though the board represented itself as a purely neutral force responding to the dictates of science and the wishes of the medical schools, its staff actively sought to impose a model of medical education more closely wedded to research than to medical practice. These policies determined not so much which institutions would survive as which would dominate, how they would be run, and what ideals would prevail."[20]

Within a decade, all medical schools fell in line: "Many have argued that this was a mistake. They would have preferred to see only a few schools like Johns Hopkins training scientists and specialists, while the rest, with more modest programs, turned out general practitioners to take care of the everyday ills that make up the greater part of medical work. But this was not the course that American medical education followed."[21]

The other winner in the battle for medicine's soul was the AMA. After the codification of Flexner's report, "the AMA would largely control medical school accreditation which would become bureaucratized and sclerotic. It also became the officially recognized entity authorized to speak on behalf of all physicians."[22] Flexner himself believed that medical education and practice would change and grow as times changed: "The flexibility and freedom to change – indeed the mandate to do so – was part of the system's mission from the very beginning. Contrary to popular myth, the system was always intended to evolve."[23] Unfortunately, groups such as the Rockefeller Foundation and the AMA were not interested in these changes.

Today, medical schools, and the entire health care network in this country, reflect the legacy of Flexner: "The practice of medicine was seen as a rigorist science with clear answers to defined questions, the foibles of patients being the province not of the laboratory-trained physicians but of clergymen and social workers."[24] The medical system would now focus on "disease organically defined, not on the system of health care or on society's health more generally." Patient-centered care, prevention, and the nuances of disease all were dismissed as being soft science, now made subservient to an absolutist creed of basic science, which, if studied rigorously, could unlock the mysteries of the human body and provide the key to both diagnosis and cure.[25] Using a narrow set of courses in chemistry, physics, and biology to determine which students best qualified to be physicians, and then teaching students the science of human health through a rigid science-based classroom curriculum that today is nearly identical to the one recommended by Flexner, medical schools have moved far away from the vision of Osler. Humanistic qualities, critical thinking, and a patient-focused approach to care have lost their role both in the selection of students and in their training: "Isn't it astonishing that the medical school curriculum structure has remained unchanged for more than 100 years? And if we omit the 'dynamic sociological encounter between patient and physician' [as Osler advocated], is it any wonder a health care crisis would emerge?"[26]

The legacy of Flexner's report and the rise of the AMA has left many scars with which we are living today. On the positive side for physicians, many charlatan practices have disappeared, and physician competency and income have increased considerably. In 1900, the average doctor earned $750 to $1,500 a year, but by 1928, the average rose to $6,354, with salary escalating continually because of a deliberately low physician supply and strong advocacy by the AMA.[27] But, however, the field became dependent on a scripted formula of practice to achieve success. The increased cost of medical education, required to help defray costs for full-time faculty and research facilities, eliminated all but the wealthy from the ranks of medical students. And Flexner's report and its ramifications triggered deliberate policies of discrimination against women, African Americans, and Jews.[28] Only two African American medical schools remained after the report decimated the rest, and the Black doctor only endured in the profession through the diligent and tireless efforts of the newly created National Medical Association, which sponsored a parallel Black medical system that sidestepped the pervasive bigotry sewn into the AMA and the medical system it helped to create.

We are indeed in a health care crisis. In our country we spend a trillion health care dollars for interventions that have been shown to be ineffective or even dangerous. Almost 50 percent of all we do as doctors is considered low value. Despite all we spend on health care, we rank among the worst in outcomes among all industrial countries. We are a nation of specialists who advance high-tech medical interventions and excessive drug use to ameliorate number-based diseases that are generically defined. Virtually all research is financed and controlled by industry and is conducted within medical schools whose research faculty are dependent on industry to survive and thrive, thus sullying medical science with a raw self-interest that has led it to reach often gravely misleading conclusions. Patients feel frustrated, and their needs often fall prey to generic protocols and an emphasis on rigid scientific dogma. Medical students continue to be trained as scientists, and not as physicians. Said one historian, "The Flexner Report ... has taught us the danger of establishing a confining (and ultimately damaging) standard" in medical education and practice.[29]

Can our health care delivery system ever change? To do so, we first must understand why it has moved so far off the rails of common sense and medical sanity. Today, more than 100 years after the Flexner Report and Osler's death, we should ask why we have not changed yet. Are there too many people and organizations benefiting from the current system? Do medical thought leaders believe that Flexner's formula is still the best one for our health care delivery system? Or is it perhaps inertia and a lack of understanding of what needs to be fixed? Certainly, if we are ever to transcend the health care mess in which we are embroiled, we must understand and embrace Osler and finally acknowledge the flaw of Flexner's errant road.

Relevant Reading

Arrington, Jasmine. "The Flexner Report and the African-American Health Experience: Black Collective Memory and Identity as Shaped by Afro-Cultural Trauma and Re-Membering." *Vanderbilt Undergraduate Research Journal* 10 (2015). https://doi.org/10.15695/vurj.v10i0.4063.

Bliss, Michael. *William Osler: A Life in Medicine*. New York: Oxford University Press, 2007.

Bonner, Thomas Neville. *Iconoclast: Abraham Flexner and a Life in Learning.* Baltimore: Johns Hopkins University Press, 2002.

Bryan, Charles S. *Osler: Inspirations from a Great Physician*. New York: Oxford University Press, 2010.

Duffy, Thomas. "The Flexner Report – 100 Years Later." *Yale Journal of Biology and Medicine* 84, no. 3 (2011): 269–76. PMID: 21966046; PMCID: PMC3178858.

Flexner, Abraham. *Medical Education in the United States and Canada: A Report to the Carnegie Foundation for the Advancement of Teaching*. Washington, DC: Science & Health Publications, 1978.

Ludmerer, Kenneth M. *Time to Heal: American Medical Education in the 20th Century*. New York: Oxford University Press, 1999.

Nevins, Michael A. *Abraham Flexner: A Flawed American Icon*. New York: iUniverse Inc., 2010.

Osler, William. *The Principles and Practice of Medicine*. New York: D. Appleton and Co., 1911.

Osler, William. *The Quotable Osler*. Edited by Mark E. Silverman, T. Jock Murray, and Charles S. Bryan. Philadelphia: American College of Physicians, 2008.

Page, Douglas, and Adrian Baranchuk. "The Flexner Report: 100 Years Later." *International Journal of Medical Education* 1 (2010): 74–5. https://doi.org/10.5116/ijme.4cb4.85c8.

Starr, Paul. *The Social Transformation of American Medicine: The Rise of a Sovereign Profession & the Making of a Vast Industry*. New York: Basic Books, 2017.

PART ONE

The Philosophy of Flexnerian Medical Care

CHAPTER ONE

Born from the Womb of Eugenics

In these days of aggressive self-assertion, when the stress of competition is so keen and the desire to make the most of oneself so universal, it may seem a little old-fashioned to preach the necessity of this virtue, but I insist for its own sake, and for the sake of what it brings, that a due humility should take the place of honor on the list.

– William Osler[1]

Flexner and Osler lived in an America where virtually anyone could buy or steal a medical degree. A world in which medical interventions and medications were more likely to kill and maim than to cure, one in which patients' misplaced faith in their doctors often led to tragic repercussions. And they both believed that science was the bedrock upon which medical society could rebuild its army of doctors.

Scientific theories abounded in the first few decades of the twentieth century, many of which claimed to unlock the mysteries of not just nature, but humanity. From social Darwinism to biological causes of poverty to marginalist economic theory,

these ideas were quantified by mathematical formulas and statistics to generate a singular truth. To the progressive thinkers
of Flexner's era, measurements, diagnoses, and strictly defined
immutable remedies paved the path to salvation. This was the
era of the IQ test (developed in 1905) and the SAT (invented in
1923), allegedly objective assessments that set out to measure a
person's innate intelligence distinct from cultural or social determinants. The notion that a test could unlock the mysteries of the
body and mind in ways that were scientific and indisputable
embedded itself in the field of medicine after the 1911 Flexner
Report.

This intellectual philosophy emanated from Germany and was
built upon the bricks of prevailing scientific notions, the use of
math and numerical constructs to prove a theory, rigid obedience
to prevailing norms and to authority figures, and a dismissal of
nuance and creativity as being subjective and thus prone to error.
At that time, German thought stressed that for every problem
there was a single, immutable answer that solved it. Once that
answer was discovered, no further investigation was needed.[2]
Albert Einstein actually renounced his German citizenship early
in his career, not because of antisemitism, as many believe, but
because of his disdain for the German intellectual tradition. He
believed that the one-right-answer philosophy was rigid and
uncreative, that it encouraged rote memorization of useless facts
and created a paradigm of education by which students were
expected to submit to whatever the all-knowing teacher determined to be correct. "A foolish faith in authority is the worst
enemy of truth," he would later say.[3]

Like Osler, Einstein believed that to get to the truth we need to
keep searching, keep studying, keep questioning. Unfortunately,
when Flexner imported German educational and intellectual
ideals into the medical realm, he did just the opposite. Medicine

became a study of unassailable facts and truths that did not vary from person to person.

Nothing captures the ethos of this era more than eugenics, a movement that grew in parallel with and fed into the same Germanic seeds as Flexnerism. Eugenicists were all about numbers and data: "columns of numbers, pages of numbers, mountains of numbers," author Daniel Okrent says.[4] Many spent their lives collecting data about such things as head dimension, nose width, arm length, and ear size. Multiple-choice assessments were administered to test students' acceptance of "unassailable scientifically derived truths." Armed with this culturally and linguistically rigged data, eugenic scientists set out to prove that certain races were inferior to others, that everything – from strength to intelligence to worth – could be measured, and that we could improve our society through selective breeding. Eugenicists hailed from the most prestigious universities. Some were among the most respected politicians and journalists of the day. Who could doubt them or their sincerity, especially since everything they preached was anchored by the indisputable weight of science?

Robert Yerkes, a Harvard psychologist and advocate of eugenics, was asked to devise an intelligence test to identify potential officers among the US soldiers being prepared to be deployed to France in World War I. Yerkes made a statement that applied to Flexnerian science as much as to eugenics: "Theoretically man is just as measurable as a bar of steel." His multiple-choice test – based on information that would clearly favor established Americans over new immigrants – revealed that about 50 percent of all army recruits were "morons," most of whom came from Jewish and southern European bloodlines. To Yerkes and his eugenic colleagues, such scientific proof was beyond challengeable.

Others in the eugenics movement made statements echoing the mantra of contemporaneous policymakers. Future president Calvin Coolidge proclaimed that "biologic science" must shape the country's immigration policy. Charles Davenport, perhaps the most academic and well respected of the eugenicists, believed that prostitutes possessed measurable genetic and biological abnormalities that led them to a life on the streets. Never mind complex socioeconomic and cultural factors. Humans acted as they did because of biology, and thus measurements and data could reveal who was most likely to become a prostitute.

Eugenic scientists such as Harry Laughlin and Francis Galton could manipulate data to establish any result they were asked to derive. According to historians of eugenics, they piled so much data (some of it clearly bogus) into their reports that few people ever sought to refute their conclusions. Data, whether real or not, proved to be the fuel that created a general belief that what they were saying was true.[5] It was his scientific work that was cited in the near-unanimous US Supreme Court case of *Buck v. Bell* (1927), a case that allowed states to sterilize individuals declared "defective" and that led to as many as 70,000 forced sterilizations.[6] Like Flexner, Laughlin was a failed educator before becoming a respected scientific leader. And like Flexner, he worked for the Carnegie Foundation. Laughlin himself believed that about 10 percent of the population fit into the "defective" category. His position, much like Flexnerian physicians of his era and of ours, derived not from his opinion but from the bedrock of science.

The eugenics mantra is the very heart and soul of Flexnerian science, even today. It is striking to note that William Welch, the Johns Hopkins founder who was instrumental in inspiring and implementing the Flexner Report, and who was an avowed enemy of William Osler and all he stood for, was a devoted eugenicist.[7] He, like many founders of our current health care structure and ethos, participated in prominent eugenic groups as enthusiastically as he imprinted a eugenic-style health care system upon our national soil.

As with eugenics, the Flexner system advocates achieving human improvement by measuring, labeling, and fixing numerical surrogates of health. Everything that plagues a person is measurable. Since it is measurable, it is fixable. The adherence by eugenicists to science as being the singular, irrefutable bridge to progress and their dehumanization of people as a collection of numbers – all of this thinking was incorporated into the reforms that Flexner and his cronies sought to inculcate into medical society. The only difference was that the eugenics movement was thoroughly debunked and reversed, but Flexnerian medicine is thriving, in the United States and beyond.

Vinayak Prasad and Adam Cifu, in *Ending Medical Reversals*, cite an editorial by Dr. Arthur Stutsky titled "The Seduction of Physiology." Medical students, under the Flexnerian system, are immersed in basic science from their undergraduate years through medical school. They are taught, much like the eugenicists of Flexner's day, that science is immutable and universally applicable and that understanding basic science opens the door to understanding every living person by breaking that person down into measurable and fixable numbers, what Stutsky refers to as "physiology." Say Prasad and Cifu, "Stutsky understood that doctors like interventions that cause improvements in vital measures like blood pressure and oxygenation. We know these numbers are important, are objective, and correspond to improvements in physiology that we understand. It is reasonable to assume that if we can improve these measures ... we can improve survival. Therein lies the false seduction of physiology. Many times, we have found that interventions that improve these measures do nothing to improve the survival of the patient. Improving physiological measures is comforting, but it does not always affect outcomes."[8]

Flexnerian students – most of whom are trained in hard science during their undergraduate years – sit in the classroom during those first years of medical school memorizing scientific "facts" and only venture into the patient realm once their mastery of science is deemed to be adequate. They are tested by standardized multiple-choice exams where there is one right answer. Patients – their wants, needs, particular circumstances, complex and intertwined bodies – are largely irrelevant to this calculus. Why spend time with patients when everything derives from measurements?

The mantra of Flexner is simple. There are certain absolute truths about human physiology, they do not vary from person to person or from one era to the next, and once they are discovered to be abnormal, they can be labeled as diseases and thus fixed. Osler's cautious view of uncertainty and nuance with which he approached health care had no role in this scientific epiphany. The mantra is "Test, diagnose the numbers, fix." It doesn't get easier than that.

As a resident at the hospital at the University of Virginia, I was lucky enough to meet several doctors who bucked the number and diagnosis certitude of Flexnerian scientists, something rare in my career. As young doctors, we are taught by Flexnerians who feed us unalterable facts and protocols that we are expected to swallow unquestioningly and to regurgitate back in exams and on rounds. So, to me, these Oslerian doctors saved my medical life.

I remember how one of my physician-teachers in residency challenged the primacy of testing in medical diagnosis. A young woman had come in with some mild shortness of breath. She was very anxious because of multiple life changes, something we only learned later after Dr. B talked with her during rounds; we had never thought to delve so deeply into her life because we were taught to focus on her medical problems and tests. In the emergency room they ran a test called a V/Q scan (ventilation/perfusion), which determines if a person has a clot in the lung called a pulmonary embolism (PE), one of the causes of shortness of breath. Hers came back positive, so we admitted her with a PE and put her on strong blood thinners.

"Do you really think that she has a PE?" Dr. B asked us at rounds. "She had no risk factors, no swelling of her legs, no symptoms, and she is very anxious. This looks more like a panic attack."

"But the test was positive," one of the residents said.

"How accurate is the test?" Dr. B asked.

Everyone shrugged. We just assumed that all tests were accurate enough.

"Let's say the test is right 95 percent of the time, which is pretty good, right?" he said. Then he started drawing on the board. He came up with a calculation that changed my life. He showed that even if a test is very accurate, a positive result is very unreliable when a person does not have a high clinical likelihood of having the disease for which the test is looking. In other words, when a doctor who actually speaks with and examines her patient determines that it is not likely the patient is suffering from a certain condition, then a test for that condition becomes increasingly inaccurate.

"Once you have a sense that your patient does not have a clot to her lungs, you shouldn't do the test, because any test is likely to be a false positive, even if that test is accurate for the average person." "In this case," he said, after making the calculations, "even with a positive test, there is about a 10 percent chance she has a PE. Doing tests on people not likely to have the disease is considered bad medicine. Now all of you have given this poor young woman a diagnosis that will commit her to at least six months of dangerous blood thinners and will forever color her medical records, likely making it harder for her to get health insurance, perhaps even a job, for the rest of her life."

Dr. B's well-argued scientific wisdom influenced my thinking for the rest of my career. I still converse with him today. He was a rare bird among those who taught us. Even rarer was Dr. H, one of the few "real doctors" who taught me.

Dr. H was a burly, vivacious man with a deep Southern drawl who hailed from the Virginia hinterlands in a town called Grundy, where he had been a general practitioner, treating patients from birth to death, and becoming an intimate friend and healer to all those lucky enough to be under his care. Later in his life he became certified in hematology, the study of blood cells, and gained a faculty position at University of Virginia. But Dr. H was not willing to follow the standard script, even after entering academics and being handed the Flexnerian Bible. He delved into his patients' lives, provided unorthodox treatments (or got them off their more orthodox treatments), and helped more people (many of whom worshiped him) than any of the more standard Flexnerians who flooded academia.

As a first-year resident on the neurology service, I helped care for a nice man named Mr. G, a high school principal in West Virginia. "You should come out and practice in our town when you're done," he and his wife told me. "There's not a single traffic light in the whole county, and everyone loves their doctor." It certainly sounded appealing.

Mr. G had been transported to the University of Virginia because of rapid muscular deterioration, whose cause no one could identify. Now he would be put in the hands of the best and brightest. Mr. G's new doctors repeated all the tests that had already been completed, sorting through numbers and pictures in search of an answer. Every specialist had a theory, but each refused to commit to anything until the tests and labs showed them what was going on. There was not a test this man did not have. Some were conducted multiple times. All along, he continued to deteriorate.

"We have faith," his wife told me.

His doctors did not. As they scratched their heads and ran more and more tests, Mr. G was moved to the intensive care unit and put on a breathing machine. His lungs stopped functioning. I remember one day his neurologist wrote an order in the chart describing how he wanted the autopsy done on the patient's brain stem when he died, which the neurologist presumed would be within a few days.

Enter Dr. H.

I don't remember who called Dr. H. It may have been Mr. G's primary care physician, who later told me, "Yeah, when I can't figure out what's going on sometimes I call Dr. H, because he has an instinct that no one else seems to have." I remember him coming in, scouring the chart, spending a great deal of time with Mr. G's wife, and shaking his head.

He called the team together. "All these tests don't tell us shit," he proclaimed. "This guy has got some kind of inflammation tearing apart his body and we got to stop it now or he's not going to walk out."

The head resident, who was a snarky know-it-all, pushed back with a smug smile. "I don't think so," she told Dr. H. "We ran tests for inflammation, and that's not what's going on."

"To hell with the damned tests," he yelled back at her. "I don't give a shit about tests. I know what's going on. And we got to load this man up with steroids and do it now."

The resident laughed. "I don't think so," she said to the doctor, whom she regarded as a hick who knew nothing about modern medicine. "Steroids will only make things worse if he has an infection. Too many side effects. And we have no diagnosis or indication for their use."

"I don't give a crap," Dr. H said. "Your antibiotics didn't help a damned thing. So, there ain't no infection. Let me tell you something I learned in my medical life, sometimes the hard way. You don't ever let anyone die without first giving them a shitload of steroids. That's what we're going to do."

Mrs. G acceded to Dr. H's plan to give huge doses of intravenous steroids, and we started them that day. The resident was upset. The neurologist was irate, believing that the steroids would sully the autopsy results. But Mrs. G had a great deal of faith in Dr. H; when she talked about him, she had tears in her eyes. He had touched her.

There was no need for an autopsy.

Three days later Mr. G. was pulled off the breathing machine. A week later he was up and walking. Two weeks later he left the hospital. He and Mrs. G gave me a big hug, thanking me profusely, even though, at least in my eyes, I did nothing. It was all Dr. H. It was his ability to rely on intuition and experience, to not be swayed by copious tests that told him nothing, or a need to label his patient with a precise diagnosis before we could treat him. No one gave him credit, not the resident, not the neurologist, not the other specialist doctors. But I knew what he had done was amazing. So did Mr. and Mrs. G.

The happy couple came back to visit the hospital a year later, bringing gifts to the doctors and nurses. They went to dinner with Dr. H, and once again implored me to come out to their county. "We still have no stoplights," Mrs. G said.

Months later, passing him in the hall, I asked Dr. H what disease he believed to be responsible for Mr. G's decline.

"Hell if I know," he laughed. "And I don't give a crap. All I care about is that he is back in that town teaching those kids a little bit of discipline. Kids today need a man like that in their lives."

Science to Dr. H was not staid facts, not measuring and fixing, not labeling people with diseases and conditions. It was, rather, a very human experience; it was knowledge mixed with humanism and humility. It encapsulated everything that William Osler preached.

Journalist Meghan O'Rourke, in *The Invisible Kingdom*, reminds us that Flexnerian medicine not only injures the well by ascribing to them numerical illnesses and assaulting them with fear, cost, and an arsenal of often feckless and injurious medical interventions, but it also injures the sick by denying their illness in the wake of "normal" numbers.[9] If a medically ill person does not fit into the norm of Flexner's discrete numerical abnormalities and diagnoses, if her aliments cannot be explained through the lens of rigidly defined science, as was the case with Mr. G, then the myopic doctors trained in their Flexnerian haze often ascribe that person's illness to malingering, mental disease, or simply the unknown, often failing to help them because they know no cure but that of number-fixing.

Today I saw a patient who could have used Dr. B's understanding and Dr. H's insight. Mr. C was a big, active guy in his late 70s who regularly saw a cardiologist to monitor his pacemaker. He had undergone a lot of stress tests and echocardiograms at the cardiologist's request, tests that Medicare paid for and that Mr. C believed to be necessary. One day Mr. C started feeling dizzy, kind of like vertigo. We discussed possible causes, including medicines, his very low blood pressure, and some life stressors. The next day he stood up and fainted. His wife called 911, and Mr. C was whisked to the hospital.

What struck the hospital doctors were two abnormal findings having nothing to do with his dizziness. First, his blood pressure was too high. Whose wouldn't be under those circumstances? Still, the doctors were worried and changed around his blood pressure medicines. Second, one of his blood tests – a troponin test that tells you if you are having a heart attack – was mildly abnormal.[10] Could he be having a heart attack, they asked? He had no symptoms of a heart attack. His electrocardiogram was normal. He was just dizzy, a fact that the doctors no longer even addressed. But the doctors couldn't just dismiss a blood test like that. In reality, that test is often abnormal in patients who are elderly and have some kidney disease, as Mr. C did. Still, the doctors pressed the panic button just because of that one irrelevant blood test that should never have been ordered. They called in a cardiologist, and Mr. C's rocky ride through hell began.

The cardiologist performed a catheterization on his heart, a test with a 1 percent risk of causing a stroke and a higher risk of putting someone like Mr. C into kidney failure.[11] Luckily, none of that happened. He had plaque all over his blood vessels, something we had already ascertained based on his multiple risk factors. That was why he was on a statin (used to lower cholesterol, a lipid-lowering class of drugs that reduces inflammation of heart blood vessels), the only proven treatment to prevent heart attacks in people with plaque. They also found that one of his arteries had an 80 percent blockage. They threw him in an ambulance and sent him to a nearby university hospital where he could have a stent placed. "Find a blockage, fix a blockage." Flexner would be proud!

No one considered what had brought Mr. C to the hospital or even if their "fix" was medically helpful. But they put in a stent, bumped up his cholesterol medicine, added new blood thinner medicines, and increased his blood pressure pills. When he saw me after discharge, he was still dizzy – that had never been addressed! Predictably, he felt worse on all those medicines, which I promptly reduced. Now he was stuck with a piece of metal wedged into his heart and was given a frightening diagnosis that he presumed would kill him. No one discussed weight loss or other lifestyle changes. No one ever does in the Flexnerian universe.

When doctors are trained to use scientific measurements as proxies for a person's health, when those numbers take on a life of their own, when fixing those numbers to preordained levels is the only goal of a doctor, then we have the dysfunctional health care system with which we all contend today. Mr. C. was worse off than he had been before. And no one took care of the medical problem that sent him to the hospital or the medical risk factors that were most potentially harmful to him.

Ironically, by focusing on number-fixing, we have returned to the nonscientific health care system that both Flexner and Osler disparaged. We are training doctors taught and encouraged to disregard scientific subjectivity in lieu of numerical absolutism and emphasizing a form of simplistic science that is not relevant to the complex human beings for whom we care. It's comforting to think that if we find and fix all the errant values in our body, if we test ourselves before we are sick and identify problems early, then we can control our own medical destiny. We as humans do not like uncertainty. We want to think we can alter our destiny without working so hard at it. Flexnerian medicine, couched in a faux science and validated by white-garbed and well-meaning scientist-doctors, gives us the illusion of certainty and the illusion of control. But it is not science. It's medical deception. It's snake oil.

CHAPTER TWO

The Road Taken: Flexner's Legacy in the Modern World

One element must always be taken into account in the prognosis and that is the personal equation of the patient. No two cases of the same disease are ever alike; the constitution of the person, his individuality, stamps each with certain peculiarities.

– William Osler[1]

On June 6, 2019, I attended a lecture by Dr. Paul Rothman, dean of the Johns Hopkins Medical School faculty. Commemorating the 100th anniversary of William Osler's death, the lecture – held fittingly in Osler Hall – sought to demonstrate Osler's enduring legacy in American health care, especially at Hopkins, the school he helped to found. As I listened to the lecture, I could only shake my head at how far Johns Hopkins and virtually every other medical school in this country has veered away from Osler's vision. A man in the audience asked why, with all of health care's advances over the past 20 years, the cost of care in this country had escalated from $600 billion a year in 1995 to $4 trillion in 2016, with a decline in longevity during that stretch. The lecturer had no good response.

That's because even as Dr. Rothman extolled Osler's vision, he was actually talking about the legacy not of Osler but of Flexner. Like most of those in the medical profession, he did not comprehend the hold that Flexner's ideas have over all of us in health care. He likely didn't know.

What Osler preached was the very antithesis of Flexnerian thinking. "Gentlemen, if you want a profession in which everything is certain, you had better give up medicine," he said. Osler understood that people want quick fixes. That was, after all, the problem with health care in his day and why so many flocked to patent-medicine doctors who concocted potions that had no scientific validity. Knowing that "man has an inborn craving for medicine," he sought to train doctors to be broad, critical thinkers whose goal was to care for patients, not diseases.

To Flexner and his scientific colleagues at Hopkins, medical science was just as certain and absolute as physics. Flexner may have inveighed against patent-medicine doctors who lacked a scientific basis for what they peddled, but even so he believed in handing out potions if they fixed some measurable number: in other words, an abnormality that could be found and fixed through testing. Such thinking is blessed with the comforting allure of certainty, a certainty dressed in a veil of science.

So, when we see an ad on TV for a new diabetic drug called Ozempic, we can taste a palpable dose of Flexnerian philosophy. "Oh," the happy actors say, using the "O" from the drug to proclaim their joy at its scientifically wondrous properties. "Oh, I can lower my A1c below 7." Which means, with this drug, they can fix their high sugar number (A1c is a measure of sugar level, important for diabetics), which seems to be the one endpoint that the drug and its commercial target. The only studies done on Ozempic were financed and conducted by Novo Nordisk (and their academic medicine doctors who carried out the drug-company-directed protocols) and were short-lived enough to assure that no serious side effects or adverse outcomes could occur. The drug proved to dramatically lower A1c only, and that bought its passage through a Food and Drug Administration (FDA) drug approval process entirely funded by the pharmaceutical industry, and onto the shelves of doctors, who prescribed it profusely.

In the first half of 2019, Ozempic earned $500 million for Novo Nordisk, the company that makes it. Those numbers increased as its number-fixing prowess was touted by academic doctors, the press, and the never-ending Ozempic ads. Soon, though, it was found that the drug could drop another number: BMI (body mass index). It could help people lose weight. This further escalated sales; projected sales in 2023 are $12.5 billion.[2]

Novo Nordisk does not write prescriptions for Ozempic. Doctors do. Then we must ask, Why are doctors writing $12.5 billion of Ozempic prescriptions, a drug with no track record, a drug shown only to lower sugar and weight (and no one knows how the weight loss is achieved or if it will be sustained and lead to health benefits or possibly risks)? Certainly, doctors have no financial gain for doing this. Most of them are not compensated by Novo Nordisk to prescribe the drug for their patients, nor do they get paid more or earn extra income by prescribing this drug. The only reason they are doing it is because they think that it works.

"Oh, it gets my A1c under 7! And, oh, I will lose weight!"

Ozempic fixes measurable numbers. To Flexnerians, that is the job of doctors: measure and fix numbers. But does it help people feel better, live longer, or become healthier? Do we know that lowering the A1c below 7 is a valuable goal? Do other drugs that accomplish that Flexnerian achievement consistently prevent poor outcomes? The answer to both questions is no. Studies show that aggressive lowering of A1c can in fact be very danger-ous, especially to the often older patients to whom this drug is prescribed, and many drugs that lower A1c have increased the rate of heart attacks and death, let alone mental decline, fatigue, falls, and debility.[3] And what about lowering weight, is that a beneficial outcome? Many weight-loss drugs do so by damag-ing parts of the body, such as the liver. Maybe Ozempic causes weight loss by destroying muscles, by damaging the body, by making us sicker. We can't possibly know because the drug com-pany studies touting its numerical benefits fail to consider all these possibilities.

But what is most disturbing is how many doctors are writ-ing prescriptions for a drug that may well kill and maim, even if it does lower a few numbers. This is Flexnerian thinking in a nutshell. Measure a number, equate that number to a diagno-sis, and then fix the number. Patient variability and real-world health outcomes are never considered by doctors who view their patients through so myopic a lens.

Numbers can be manipulated. What number defines who is diabetic? Studies indicate that the A1c should be far higher than 7 to qualify as diabetic. But by lowering the threshold of diabetes to an A1c of 6.5, and then creating a new diagnosis of prediabe-tes for anyone with an A1c over 5.5, we have in effect labeled a large part of the population as having diabetes – we have created a diabetes epidemic – which now has to be aggressively treated with expensive drugs.[4] Once the number is fixed, then the patient is cured. That is the ethos of Flexnerian medicine, and for many patients it has led to an increase in disability and death at a very high cost to society and with copious profits for many who live in our medical universe.

Ms. L went to her cardiologist to get an annual echocardio-gram and stress test, just to make sure her heart was all right.

When the test was over, the cardiologist explained that he saw some minor abnormalities that could indicate blockages of the right coronary artery. He would recheck it in six months and, if still abnormal, perform a catheterization to determine the precise degree of blockage. "We can open it with a stent if it's more than 70 percent blocked," he told her.

Ms. L was pleased with the precise and important information her doctor's test had uncovered, and now she told her friends that she had a dangerous diagnosis of coronary artery disease and that her thorough cardiologist would monitor it with regular testing and treat it if necessary to avert an inevitable medical catastrophe. "He saved my life," she told her friends.

But Ms. L had no symptoms of heart disease, such as chest pain or shortness of breath. Her doctor also had her taking a statin for high cholesterol, with an LDL number he insisted be lowered to below 70, based on new guidelines. Unfortunately, even in focusing his gaze on test results and the possibility of a procedure down the line, the doctor ignored the obvious. Ms. L is obese and doesn't exercise, both of which can lead to many diseases down the road, including heart disease and diabetes. She also had significant leg pain from the high-dose statins, and this even limited how much she could walk. But her heart doctor did not discuss this, emphasizing instead the results of a stress test that provides little value.[5] Stress tests don't save lives. They don't prevent heart attacks. If Ms. L's doctor puts in a stent, he may cause her more harm than good, as every study has demonstrated. And yet, his approach sounds much more appealing than saying, "We really need to talk about your diet and get you on an exercise program and probably lower your statin dose because the level of LDL is far less important than your being able to walk and stay active."

Such a myopic approach to health care deceives the patient into thinking she is being helped, ignores the true determinants that affect her health, and is also very expensive. In fact, despite an increase in stress tests and echocardiograms in the last quarter century, heart attack rates haven't declined and people aren't living longer – just the opposite, in fact. But a lot of blocked arteries and "abnormal" numbers are being "fixed" at extraordinarily high cost.

If diabetes and coronary artery disease are both measurable diagnoses correlated with numerical abnormalities (we will discuss scores of increasing expansive numerical illnesses that our medical system targets and treats with very poor results) and thus demonstrate how Flexnerian thinking now dominates health care delivery, atrial fibrillation (afib) reveals another dark side of Flexner's legacy: that of dogmatic absolutism and one-right-answer thinking. Afib is a multibillion-dollar industry, one almost religiously embraced by doctors and the public, and one that the American College of Cardiology says is underdiagnosed and undertreated. It's hard to turn on the TV these days without seeing an ad for Eliquis or Xarelto or various other expensive drugs for a condition that has taken on a mythical aura described in a classic Flexnerian binary language: dangerous if left untreated, treatment being both necessary and safe.

In afib, the heart's pacemaker starts to beat irregularly, and one of the heart's chambers begins to quiver, leading to a chance that blood clots can attach to the heart wall. If those clots dislodge, a patient can suffer from a stroke. Thus, if doctors detect any afib, they will insist on prescribing blood-thinning drugs, such as Eliquis, to assure that clots don't appear, and they will perform an array of tests to assure that the afib is controlled and is not associated with other cardiac conditions. Like all robotic Flexnerian formulas, this one is precise and seemingly beneficial. But is it?

Ms. P is a 78-year-old woman who is overall healthy and typically gets good reports from her heart doctor, whom she sees just to make sure she's okay. But then one day, despite years of normal testing and reassuring exams, Ms. P received some bad news: she had a heart condition called afib. The abnormal heart rhythm may well have been there for years, fluctuating based on her level of pain or stress, or maybe it appeared briefly now by chance. "You have a very serious condition," said her cardiologist. "Luckily we caught it just in the nick of time. You could have had a stroke any day."

Even though her afib had resolved, the cardiologist insisted that she take the newest and most expensive blood thinner (Eliquis) to prevent her otherwise inevitable stroke. Her cardiologist proclaimed that this new blood thinner would cut her risk of stroke by 50 percent and cause less bleeding than an older blood thinner (Coumadin) that is cheaper but "more dangerous." The doctor plugged a few numbers into a calculator and told her, "Based on your risks, you have an 8.4 percent risk of having a stroke this year if you don't take the drug. That risk will multiply every year, so in five years your risk of stroke will be about 50 percent unless you get on Eliquis immediately."

The doctor's calculator, so precise and frightening, convinced Ms. P that she had better start the Eliquis now, even though she could barely afford it. The doctor and his calculator did not explain any alternatives or risks and did not delve into Ms. P's particular circumstances that could potentially make Eliquis dangerous or even ineffective. My patient was irrelevant to his calculus; she just as easily could have been any generic human being in his office. When she asked if it was really necessary, he simply said, "Yes, you have no other choice."

This is an example of Flexnerian one-right-answer absolutism that we will run into throughout this book, and it has led to the proliferation of drugs and procedures that often cause more harm than good.

Most studies on afib are being conducted by pharmaceutical companies anxious to demonstrate the large benefit of taking the medicines. So, rather than focusing on how many clinically meaningful strokes these drugs prevent (strokes that leave patients with noticeable weakness or other symptoms), they count all strokes, even strokes about which patients are not aware. Most strokes that these drugs prevent are small blips on a CT scan, not something that triggers any symptoms at all. The patient has no idea they even occur. In fact, though the doctor's calculator may have correctly stated that Ms. P's stroke risk was 8 percent without treatment, and maybe 4 percent with treatment (thus a 50 percent reduction from the drug), the actual reduction in disabling strokes is closer to 0.5 percent, something his drug-company-programmed calculator, and his Flexnerian mind, failed to even consider. In other words, 99.5 percent of people don't benefit from taking a drug that Ms. P's doctor insisted would cut her stroke risk by 50 percent.[6]

But the faulty thinking doesn't end there. About the same number of people (0.5 percent) who take these drugs bleed in their brain or die from the drugs themselves. That risk is even higher for Ms. P, who is elderly, who bleeds, and who falls. Another 4 percent of people on these drugs have other life-threatening bleeds (15 percent of frail elders, by a recent study cited in footnote 6, "Safety of Switching"). Such people are typically excluded from Eliquis studies because they make the outcomes look bad, yet they are the primary people put on these drugs. Thus, people such as Ms. P are not included in the calculations the doctor used to define the benefits of this drug to Ms. P and that failed to acknowledge any risk.

Osler's assessment would have been much different than Ms. P's Flexnerian cardiologist. He would have known the clinically relevant risks and benefits – and the nuance and uncertainty – of treatment as it applied to Ms. P. "There is no right answer," he might have said. "No study has really been done in your age group, but we know that the drug is risky for you. It does help avoid a few strokes, but it can kill you and has a larger chance of causing a stroke than of preventing one. You have to decide which direction to go. Either way, we can change our minds down the road."

Ms. P had her own humorous response when I told her about the drug's risks. "Well," she said. "My heart doctor seems to think I'll die if I don't take the drug, and you seem to think I'll die if I take it, so I'm going to just take half the dose and get you both angry!"

The bottom line is that tens of billions of dollars a year are being paid to find, treat, and monitor afib. Our Flexnerian health care system has elevated this disease into an epidemic, one that is easily identified and treated through testing. Cardiology societies believe that virtually everyone with the condition must be treated lest disaster ensue, and they minimize the risk and variability of treatment.

As I am writing this, Johnson and Johnson, which makes a drug like Eliquis called Xarelto, just settled a lawsuit for $775 million based on the fact that patients were not adequately warned about the bleeding risk. Pradaxa was hit with a $650 million settlement in 2014, and it's likely that more such lawsuits and settlements are upcoming. But Johnson and Johnson is not that upset. In 2018 alone, Xarelto brought in $2.5 billion for the company. Other blood thinners also generate huge profits; Eliquis earned $2.7 billion for Bristol Myers Squibb in 2017. That we as a country are spending $5.2 billion a year on two drugs that have minimal benefit and equal or greater harm shows how deeply Flexnerian philosophy has infiltrated our health care system and its doctors. When there is only one right answer, and when that answer is defined by drug company data and presented in a skewed way that makes it look precise and scientific, doctors and patients alike don't see the nuance and often go down a very dangerous and expensive road that they insist is "necessary and lifesaving."

The American Medical Association (AMA) recently assailed pharmaceutical ads for forcing doctors into prescribing medicines that don't work. When it voted to curtail drug ads in 2015, AMA board chair-elect Patrice Harris said, "Today's vote in support of an advertising ban reflects concerns among physicians about the negative impact of commercially-driven promotions, and the role that marketing costs play in fueling escalating drug prices. Direct-to-consumer advertising also inflates demand for new and more expensive drugs, even when these drugs may not be appropriate."

But the AMA is missing the point.

These ads, and their drugs, appeal directly to the Flexnerian instincts of the doctors who prescribe them. A good Oslerian would welcome the ads and would learn about the products advertised. (Let's not forget that these drugs are products.) But Oslerian doctors would be innately skeptical about new drugs, would dig deeper than what they read in a drug-sponsored study, and would be thrilled to discuss all of this with their patients. Flexnerian doctors are not so scientifically vigilant. If a drug fixes something, then they embrace it. That the AMA seeks to curb drug ads is merely an admission of how deep into the Flexnerian hole doctors have fallen.

There are a few basic principles of Flexnerian philosophy that germinated on the campus of Johns Hopkins in 1911 and that still penetrate deeply into the psyche of the country's doctors and patients today. Many of these ideals directed how we as a nation confronted COVID-19, and they are certainly responsible for the high-cost, low-value health care delivery system that we have

accepted as being normal. We will delve into all of these principles and ideals throughout this book. Our goal is to demonstrate
that if we seek a better health care system, if we hope to create
universal care that is beneficial to all, then we must acknowledge
and repair the stain that Flexner left in Baltimore more than 100
years ago, and embrace Osler.

CHAPTER THREE

Why So Much Medical Science Is Not Reliable

Far too large a section of the treatment of disease is today controlled by the big manufacturing pharmacists, who have enslaved us in a plausible pseudo-science.

– William Osler[1]

Today's doctors rely on published science to justify their leap into aggressive medical care. The prolific use of drugs for dementia and for cholesterol, prescribed by our physicians to the tune of tens of billions of dollars a year, shows how published data that are put into protocols and clinical recommendations sway prescribing practices of doctors. But what happens when science is deceptive, misleading, or just dead wrong? What if its objective is to sell products and procedures rather than attain scientific knowledge to help humankind? What if the vast majority of funding for medical research flows from industry to academic centers, and those companies can design and interpret the studies in ways that most benefit them?[2]

Studies are easy to manipulate. Some look at endpoints called "surrogate markers" (measurable numbers) that are not clinically relevant. Others recruit carefully selected subjects to minimize bad outcomes. Almost always, the academic scientists who orchestrate and author the study (at the behest of industry sponsors) twist the data to make a conclusion look more profound, and less harmful, than it really is. And this is one of the building blocks of our health care system.

Stanford professor John Ioannidis has shown that medical research is hampered by copious biases needed for their academic authors and their industry patrons to succeed. "Our incentive is to publish papers, to get promoted, to get more funding," he says about academic researchers. Evidence-based medicine is "splendidly serving vested interests" by validating what the pharmaceutical funders seek to show. Academic physicians need money to conduct clinical research, and it's up to the drug companies to pick and choose who will direct their next big study. Thus, medical researchers must do what their industry funders ask, something their academic institution both expects and demands of them. "The most dangerous tool of evidence-based medicine has become physicians," Ioannidis says.[3]

Ioannidis and others contend that many doctors accept today's research – and its ramifications – blindly. They, like their patients, perceive health care through a lens of scientific certainty. We assume that what doctors and medical societies tell us is carved out of the bedrock of absolute proof. Doctors cite detailed evidence. They quote from articles and guidelines, use scientifically precise calculators, and tell us things we may have read ourselves or have heard from our friends. How could it possibly be misleading?

Ioannidis makes a few recurring points throughout his lectures – for example, that about half of all clinical reviews published by reliable organizations are based on evidence that is either manipulated by the study designers or not relevant to a great deal of the patients to whom the research is geared. Most research publications are not transparent, and few present enough data to determine if the conclusions reached are justified based on actual findings. Not only do most research publications lack transparency, but 40 percent of clinical studies are refuted or reversed within a few years. That's hardly surprising. "The only way to get published is to say something extravagant," Ioannidis says.

How can we believe in a system in which 97 percent of the results of published studies are not only funded by a drug manufacturer but designed by that manufacturer to show a benefit of the drug being studied? How can we rely on studies that utilize a highly selected group of patients, most of whom have been screened to achieve maximum benefit and minimum risk from the studied drug? How can we rely on studies conducted in a time frame that is optimal for their objectives? And how can we rely on the system when those who conduct our studies – the pharmaceutical companies that fund them – only publish results that are in accordance with their goals?

Examples of this abound. For instance, virtually every study on dementia medicines ends at a year, when placebo starts to overtake the studied drug in efficacy. This is also true of bone-density-medicine studies, which typically end after four years, because at five years the fracture rate in people taking the drug is higher than in those taking placebo. The Centers for Disease Control and Prevention (CDC) mandates the use of Tamiflu (an antiviral drug) when influenza outbreaks strike nursing homes, and yet no randomized studies demonstrate any benefit of the drug, while many unpublished studies show that the risk outweighs any potential benefit.[4]

Medical research is far more subjective and engineered than most people realize. If randomized controlled studies are financed and designed by pharmaceutical companies trying to prove that their drug or device is effective, it really doesn't matter that they were conducted at Harvard or by renowned scientists or involve a large number of people. They are by nature biased and thus their outcomes are suspect.

It's not just Ioannidis who has noticed this. Vinayak Prasad and Adam Cifu, in their insightful book *Ending Medical Reversals*, reveal how "despite tremendous advances in the clinical, genomic, and surgical sciences, doctors continue to use medical practices, sometimes for decades, that are later shown to be of no benefit to their patients." These authors show that biased research lulls doctors and patients into espousing ineffective treatments, "that a sizable proportion of what doctors have done has turned out to be wrong – not wrong in retrospect but unfounded when they were doing it. We also argue that much of what doctors still do is wrong."

Flexnerian doctors who rely on such "science" in the absence of critical thinking, not to mention a thorough knowledge of the patient sitting in front of them, can be easily swayed into a scientific haze. Blindly accepting medical science as dogma, they rarely customize it to their own patients or acknowledge its limitations. Doctors also pick and choose those studies that substantiate their actions. If they want to put in a stent, they'll find a study to back them up, ignoring the many other studies that question their position. Medical societies and advocacy groups do the same, cherry-picking studies that support what is supposedly best for their doctors or patients, twisting data in ways that validate their positions. Amid this deluge of scientific certainty and generic absolutism, common sense and patient-centered critical thinking fade away.

Researchers and their pharmaceutical company financers use many tricks that make a certain intervention seem better than it really is. It is crucial that we understand these because they are very frequently used to justify the buffet of tests and treatments that flow from what is declared to be scientific certainty.

One is the use of surrogate endpoints, which the US Congress has authorized the FDA to allow as a marker for a drug's efficacy. What is a surrogate? Let's say that being more than six feet tall is something that basketball coaches use as a recruiting tool to pick players. That height is considered a surrogate for a good basketball player. It is a way of achieving a desired outcome, in this case recruiting people able to play quality basketball, without having to go through all the trouble of holding tryouts or going to tournaments and digging into a player's skills. If coaches simply chose from a pool of players of six-feet-plus without caring how well they played basketball, then you'd have a team built upon the bricks of a single surrogate marker.

Of course, coaches would never do that because many tall people do not play well, and many shorter people do, even if most players are taller than six feet. In the world of health care, we have constructed similar surrogates. Unlike coaches, however, doctors use them as unassailable markers of disease, and researchers gear their drugs to targeting them. Thus, if a drug lowers cholesterol, it is considered to be effective in preventing heart attacks since cholesterol is a surrogate for heart attacks. If a drug improves bone density, then it is considered to be effective in preventing fractures since low bone density is a surrogate for fractures.

It is far more difficult to design and run a study that demonstrates the true benefit of a drug over time than to show it improves a surrogate. And thus, as is the wont of physicians who see the human body as a series of numbers and measurements, we use surrogates across the medical landscape to prove that many medical interventions are effective.

A second trick is that of observational studies. The ideal study is randomized. One group receives a drug or other intervention and another group receives a placebo. Over time the outcomes of the two groups are compared in terms of how well they improve a defined endpoint – which, we'd hope, isn't a surrogate. Both groups must be similar in every important medical and demographic characteristic for the studies to be valid.

Observational studies take a short cut. They look backward and compare two groups. For instance, if educators want to see which kids are most disruptive, they may gather a bunch of data about every kid who went through the school in the past 10 years. Then they may look at various traits – hair color, height, eye color, shoe size, nose length – and see if any one of those traits is more common in disruptive kids. If there is one, then they can declare, for instance, that long-nosed kids tend to be more of a problem in school than those with shorter noses.

Observational studies pollute the entire medical landscape. They are ubiquitous because they are so easy to conduct and can often find something useful for the researchers to print. But they prove a correlation that likely is not a cause-and-effect relationship. Recently, an observational study linked the use of an acid-reducing drug called a proton pump inhibitor (PPI) to kidney disease. I contacted the researcher, who quite honestly told me that he just threw a bunch of data into the computer and this finding emerged, so he printed it. He acknowledged that it didn't prove that these drugs cause kidney disease, and he even agreed – as I postulated to him – that people with kidney disease may be more likely to have acidic stomachs and thus are more likely to take these drugs.[5] But the newspapers all reported that PPIs *cause* kidney disease, and the calls from patients to my office that day were unending.

Observational studies are inherently inaccurate because they look backward and do not control for any variables, often comparing groups that are not similar. They can also be manipulated to create a desired outcome. If an observational study shows that people with high cholesterol have more heart attacks, that cannot be interpreted as proving that high cholesterol causes more heart attacks. There is a connection but not necessarily a cause and effect. Maybe people with high cholesterol also are more likely to smoke and be obese, which are more important factors. It certainly doesn't prove that lowering cholesterol leads to fewer heart attacks, which many such studies falsely presume.

Another trick is to magnify the benefit of the intervention through statistical trickery, simultaneously minimizing any untoward effects. A study by Ioannides and others found that only 9 percent of clinical trials of drugs demonstrate a very large treatment effect, and that 90 percent of those benefits are shown to be much smaller in follow-up studies that explore the same drugs years later. Similarly, many studies discount or do not discuss the negative consequences of drugs (see note 3).

As with the dementia and bone-density drugs, many studies are terminated prematurely because the intervention seems to be working too well to justify continuing the study. This is another trick used by researchers to amplify the benefits of the drug while concealing any downsides of its prolonged use. Prasad and Cifu use the analogy of a free throw shooter in basketball. If someone is asked to shoot nine free throws and makes the first three, you cannot ask him to stop there and make the assumption that he will make all the others. When studies are terminated too quickly, they miss what may happen later. In fact, almost 30 percent of trials of interventions shown to have no benefit would have demonstrated a benefit if stopped early.

If a study does not reach the conclusion that the industry sponsors desire, that study may not be published. This is especially true of smaller studies, thus tilting the available literature toward showing a benefit of interventions, even if many (unpublished) studies have disputed that benefit. When medical researchers conduct a meta-analysis of interventions – gathering all the available studies that they consider worthy and pooling them together to reach a broad conclusion – they are only able to utilize published studies, and thus often reach a conclusion that an intervention is more efficacious than it actually is because many negative studies are never published.

Prasad and Cifu conclude, "There is great temptation to create bias when the very companies that develop the drugs, devices, and infusions also design the studies that test whether these products work ... Each year we discover new ways that bias has been introduced, new ways that we have been fooled – reasons why trials we believed were accurate were, in fact, not."

A good window into the devolution and duplicity of medical research at the hands of the pharmaceutical companies can be seen by looking at the career of noted cardiologist Eugene Braunwald.[6] In his early years, Braunwald spearheaded landmark studies that altered the landscape of cardiac care, a legacy from which we still benefit today. But, as commercial interests metastasized into the academic realm, as self-serving corporations held the financial cards as to which institutions and physicians would be able to conduct meaningful clinical research, Braunwald – like so many of his colleagues – slid down a dangerous slope. At a certain point, he allied with pharmaceutical companies to help prove that their products were effective and superior. Much of his work after this time has not persevered; some in fact has been found to be specious and even fraudulent.

As a medical resident, I lived in an exciting time for cardiology. The death rate of people presenting to the hospital with heart attacks had been 35 percent, but it was precipitously dropping into the single digits. The reason for this was a clot-busting medicine containing an enzyme called tissue plasminogen activator (TPA), which, if given correctly, could open a blocked artery and reverse a heart attack. I was thrilled to be part of this revolution, one among many during my residency. I never doubted the efficacy and lifesaving results generated by TPA, especially because the cardiologists told me that it was based on undisputed research.

But beneath the apparent miracle that TPA wrought lay a darker side of the drug and the research that promoted it, much of it having been orchestrated by Braunwald and the pharmaceutical company he worked with. TPA's efficacy was based on a surrogate marker (increased blood flow through a blocked artery), not a meaningful outcome, such as how many lives were saved, how many heart attacks were prevented, and how well people did subsequently. It used a highly selected population of people not likely to bleed, ignoring the fact that TPA can trigger massive bleeding, including bleeding in the brain, and even death.

What about the amazing reduction in heart attack deaths from TPA that I and others witnessed? No study demonstrated cause and effect between TPA and death reduction. During this time, new sensitive tests were being introduced to detect very tiny heart attacks that may not even be clinically relevant, the very tests we discussed earlier including troponin. So, Jeanne Lenzer demonstrates in her book *The Danger within Us*, let's say that in the old days, out of 100 people who presented to the hospital with classic heart attacks – chest pain, shortness of breath, EKG changes – 35 of them died. Now let's say that we have new testing that can pick up minor heart attacks, ones that are not likely to kill or maim anyone and may have no symptoms as all. Because of this testing, now 400 people present to the hospital with heart attacks, and let's say that 35 people still die. In the old days, the death rate from heart attacks was 35 percent. But today, the death rate drops to 8 percent, not because fewer people are dying, but rather because more people are being diagnosed with nonlethal heart attacks as a result of new supersensitive testing. ✗

Even today, an elderly patient can go to the emergency department with a cold, and the physicians, based on hospital protocol, will order a troponin test and tell the patient that he or she has had or is having a heart attack. Certainly, in the absence of any signs or symptoms of heart disease, it is very unlikely that the patient is really having a heart attack. Maybe the cold itself caused a bump in the troponin level, maybe the patient has kidney disease and always has a high level because poorly functioning kidneys do elevate troponins, especially in the elderly. Any doctor who speaks with and examines the patient in an Oslerian way would know that this patient has a likely respiratory illness and will not order a test for troponin, which even if positive is likely not indicative of any impending heart disease. But in a Flexnerian world in which test results trump a patient's presentation, patients are labeled with a diagnosis of a heart attack, and sometimes given stents and other medicines to "fix" them. Such people are counted among today's heart attack survivors. All this is based on surrogate markers rather than clinical reality.

Even when subsequent research debunks what a deceptive study shows, the old deceptive research has become so ingrained into our health care psyche that its conclusions remain gospel. We now know, for example, that stents that open heart arteries when people aren't having a heart attack do not help people live longer. Newer research shows that stents don't even stop heart pain.[7] Nevertheless, tens of billions of dollars of unhelpful stents are still placed, and patients still believe their lives have been saved, often "just in the nick of time."

Osler emphasized the importance of medical research in pushing health care out of the dark ages. To him, the ideal researcher was a pure scientist devoted to truth and not swayed by money. Osler said, "Fortunately, the medical profession can never be wholly given over to commercialism, and perhaps this work of which we do so much, and for which we get so little – often not even thanks – is the leaven against its corroding influence."

Virtually every defect of medical research can be tied to the marriage between industry and academia born in the era of Flexner, which has given birth to a plethora of expensive and often ineffective drugs, tests, procedures, and devices by academic scientists whose careers are tied to their ability to produce results acceptable to their corporate sponsors. Osler assailed snake oil salesmen and corporate incursion into medical care. If only he knew just how pervasive both have become.

CHAPTER FOUR

Why Patients (and Doctors) Are Enticed by Flexnerian Logic

Our work is an incessant collection of evidence, weighing of evidence, and judging from the evidence, and we have to learn early to make allowances for our own frailty, and still larger for the weaknesses, often involuntary, of our patients.

– William Osler[1]

While on vacation recently, I overheard a woman talking about her husband, who was quietly enjoying a stack of pancakes and syrup, with a side order of bacon and a big glass of orange juice. The wife, a nurse, relayed to another couple how she had saved her husband's life by pushing his doctor to do something about his shortness of breath. "They kept telling us that he can't breathe because he's overweight," she said, "but I knew that it was more than that." Finally, she persuaded a cardiologist friend to give him a stress test. "Sure enough, that showed a blockage in his heart, and he was whisked off for an emergency stent," she declared. "Because I was persistent, I saved his life."

The man was morbidly obese. Later that morning I saw him smoking. These factors were still impairing his breathing, despite his opened heart artery. Likely they had been the culprit from the start, just as his doctors told him. But, in her mind, his wife had saved his life by insisting on a procedure that opened a quarter inch of a blocked blood vessel in his heart, even as the rest of his body continued to be pummeled by his poor health choices. His blockage was found, it was fixed, and his life was saved. Nothing else seemed to matter.

We as human animals are vulnerable to faulty thinking. We believe what we want to believe, even when overwhelming evidence exists to the contrary. This sort of inconsistency is called "cognitive dissonance," a concept by which we believe in something that we think *should* be true, even if it is actually *not* true. Cognitive dissonance encourages us to explain a situation in a way that makes it more comfortable to live with, or to reject information that is not consistent with our beliefs. For instance, the stented man's wife believed that something other than obesity and smoking triggered her husband's breathing problems. She also believed that if the doctors could find and fix that one problem, then her husband would be cured. Finally, she accepted as dogma that if an artery is blocked, then opening that artery will make things better. The fact that his breathing problem did not improve after the stent in no way deterred her from announcing that the stent saved his life.

Osler understood cognitive dissonance, even if he didn't label it as such. He often warned doctors of the allure of quick fixes, of our brain's ability to fool us into doing more than we should. He, after all, lived in the era of quack medical care, and spent his entire life assailing it. And he understood the need to embrace uncertainty in medical care and to treat every patient as a complex individual, not as a series of numbers. Unfortunately, we are right back to the very culture of snake oils that Osler so feared. We can thank cognitive dissonance and reliance on Flexner's enticing elixir for that.

When applied to health care decision-making, cognitive biases help to explain why Flexnerian medicine has taken such deep root. Here are a few biases:[2]

- **Anchoring bias:** We tend to stick to our preconceived notions and are not willing to change. "I have always believed that food high in cholesterol causes heart attacks, so I am not eating eggs."
- **Confirmation bias:** We favor information that conforms to what makes sense to us even if science shows it not to be true. "Since blood vessels get blocked by cholesterol, I better take medicines to bring my cholesterol down or I will get a heart attack."
- **Availability bias:** If we know someone who had a certain outcome with an intervention, then we will believe that the intervention makes sense. "My friend had a stent placed in his heart and he didn't have a heart attack, so the stent must have worked."
- **Gambler's fallacy:** We have a hard time understanding statistics that deal with uncertainty and usually err on the side of avoiding bad outcomes. "Better to take a statin to avoid a heart attack even if it hurts my muscles and prevents me from running."

These biases allow us to believe that our health is controllable, that we don't have to do all the hard stuff, such as changing our lifestyles, and we don't have to wallow in uncertainty about when and if we will get sick when we can figure out precisely what is wrong through testing and then address just those things. In other words, these biases feed the Flexnerian system in which we live.

They relieve the cognitive dissonance between the inherent uncertainty and complexity of our health and that of our desire to control our health simply. What better way to control things than to let the doctor test us for everything and then to fix – with drugs and procedures mostly – anything that the doctor finds to be "wrong"? That is the very nidus of Flexnerian philosophy and why it has taken such a deep root in the hearts and minds of Americans.

Some real-life examples follow.

Mr. L had a PSA (prostate-specific antigen) blood test to look for prostate cancer. His primary care doctor told him it was not a reliable test, and that even if he found cancer there was no evidence that curing the cancer would extend his life, but he got it anyway. Good thing he did. The test turned out to be abnormal. He dashed to a urologist, who immediately ordered a set of biopsies, one of which showed that he did indeed have prostate cancer. And it was Gleason 7, a high grade. After a series of exhaustive tests, it was ascertained that the cancer was confined to his prostate and had not spread. He asked for the most aggressive treatment. His urologist gave him hormonal therapy and radiation. Within two months his PSA dropped to undetectable levels, and his MRI and PET scans were normal. He became incontinent of urine, leading to more testing by the urologist that turned up nothing. He ended up wearing pads. He also became impotent, but the caring urologist inserted a pump in his penis to enable him to have erections. Now he was cured, and his caring and thorough urologist promised to check a PSA every year for the rest of his life. He was a cancer survivor thanks to his insistence on getting a PSA.

So, what's the problem here?

Mr. L's primary care doctor introduced an uncomfortable cognitive dissonance: that it didn't help to check a PSA because

Mr. L wouldn't live longer or better no matter what the test showed, as recent long-term studies have demonstrated.[3] But that made no sense to the patient. Surely, finding and treating cancer would save his life, and the primary care doctor must be wrong. In fact, thanks to his urologist, Mr. L was able to debunk the primary care doctor's confusing conclusion and pursue what he knew had to be right: checking a PSA would detect a cancer early, leading to a cure and saving his life. Mr. L had many friends whose doctors ordered PSA tests that diagnosed cancer, thus saving their lives too. He could not understand why his primary care doctor would deprive him of this simple test.

Mr. L's decision-making process was cluttered with an array of cognitive biases. Cancers are deadly, so how could a test that detects cancer be bad? How could finding and treating the cancer not be beneficial? For that matter, how could all his friends whose lives were saved by getting a PSA have been wrong when specialist doctors told them that the test and treatment saved their lives? Isn't it better to get the test than to sit around and do nothing as the cancer grows? These biases are often used to justify aggressive interventions in many arenas of health care, from skin cancer screening, to bone density testing, to blood pressure treatment, to stress tests and stents. We assume that if we find a problem and fix it, then we will do better. In fact, about 99 percent of people survive prostate cancer whether or not they receive treatment after 10 years, and 97 percent after 15 years. Getting a PSA does not change the survival rate at all. Had Mr. L never had the PSA checked, there is a 99 percent chance he would have lived a full life not knowing that a harmless cancer inhabited his body, and there is little evidence that his aggressive treatment changed his chance of survival, even if it did impair his quality of life.

We want to believe that through a thorough menu of testing, medicating, and surgically repairing problems that we can fix everything that's wrong with us. Find problems before they harm us. Lower abnormal numbers that the doctor discovers through tests and exams. See specialists. Get things repaired that are broken. Within this system there is no dissonance between what the patient wants and what the doctor is offering. Doctors, too, are victims of the same cognitive biases. Mr. L's urologist wanted to save Mr. L's life, and he convinced himself that through a simple test, followed by a simple procedure, they could do just that.

We are programmed to believe that if something is broken, then we should fix it. It seems very logical, but it is very wrong. And it costs our health system hundreds of billions of dollars a year without improving health or extending longevity; its main purpose is to resolve people's cognitive dissonance and make them feel as though they have control over their health by simply getting a lot of tests. The fact that they know other people whose lives were saved the same way, and the fact that people are living longer now than they did 100 years ago, is proof to them that this approach works. We will only acknowledge the facts and experiences that buttress our own cognitive biases. This is the thinking that fed patent-medicine salesmen back in medicine's dark ages, and it is what feeds Flexnerian doctors in medicine's "golden" age.

When I tell people that health care spending has skyrocketed from $600 billion a year a decade or so ago to $4 trillion now, and that during that time people are not in fact living longer, they tell me I must be wrong. When I tell people that I know many whose lives were ruined by stents and prostate surgery, that I know many more who eschewed such procedures and lived a long and happy life, they scoff.[4] They choose to embrace a narrative, anchored in their biases, that if they are proactive and they embrace all our medical wonders, they can stay healthy. On their side are doctors, media experts, politicians, and health care advocacy groups. So much of our society is embedded in this thinking that it seems normal and right. Any attempt to disavow it introduces strong cognitive dissonance and is usually very quickly dismissed.

Mr. L's son, Joe, was enamored of testing. He was pleased that his cardiologist wanted to get a scan of his carotid arteries. His regular doctor told him that such a scan was unnecessary and questioned why Joe's cardiologist was performing it every year, but one year that answer became crystal clear. The test revealed a blockage in his carotid artery, the very artery that feeds the brain. It wasn't much, but it was enough. His cardiologist told him that if left alone, Joe might suffer a stroke. His doctor said that through a procedure called a carotid endarterectomy (CEA) he could fix the blockage. Joe agreed instantly. "Good thing I got that test," he said. "Had I waited any longer, I could have had a stroke!" So, it was fixed.

Joe did, in fact, have a little stroke – *from the procedure*. He also had a big bleed in his groin where the catheter was inserted, leading to some pain that never went away. But it was worth it. On his next carotid ultrasound, the blockage was gone. A measurable abnormality was found, a precise diagnosis made (cerebrovascular disease with carotid occlusion), and a treatment was instituted that cured him. Who could argue that a simple, harmless carotid test saved Joe from an inevitable stroke that was right around the corner?

Was Joe wrong?

From a scientific standpoint, the test harmed him more than it could ever help him. Turns out that people without stroke symptoms who have their carotid arteries checked get more strokes than those who never get them checked.[5] That's because such tests reveal blockages that would never have harmed people, and the CEA procedure to fix those blockages can actually cause strokes in people such as Joe who never would have had strokes otherwise. In fact, there is no evidence that opening carotid arteries prevents any strokes at all. When we find a blockage and fix it, our cognitive biases tell us that we have prevented a terrible outcome and saved our lives. The very fact that his carotid test now showed his artery to be open was all that Joe and his doctor cared about. He would continue to get that test every year, making both him and his doctor very happy.

A powerful bias that feeds our system is the belief that it's better to be proactive and fix things than to take a chance by not fixing things, even if science shows that the fix is more dangerous than the original problem. People would rather have a bad outcome from doing something than from not doing something.

Let's take the case of afib again. Doctors often exaggerate the benefit of using blood thinners for afib, either by saying that it reduces the risk of stroke by 50 percent or by counting even tiny dots on a CT scan as a stroke. They also minimize the risk of blood thinners. But let's say a patient is confronted by the real risks and benefits of blood thinners. In general, about 6 out of 1,000 people avoid a disabling stroke every year when they take blood thinners, and about 6 out of 1,000 die or bleed in their brains from taking the blood thinners. Damned if you do, damned if you don't. So, how do patients make a decision when it is haunted by so much nuance and is not cut-and-dried?

Some of my patients are very logical. They say, "If a half percent of people are harmed by blood thinners, and a half percent of people are helped, that means that 99 percent of people do just fine whether they take blood thinners or not." Most of those people elect not to take blood thinners unless they have a compelling reason to take them, such as if they get a stroke.

But most of my patients are not so logical, and they focus on the chance of getting a stroke if they don't take the blood thinners. Why? Because of the classic cognitive bias called gambler's fallacy: we'd rather die trying than die not trying. It's our natural proclivity to want to be proactive and do something to avoid a bad outcome even if what we do is just as likely or even more likely to cause a bad outcome.

If you get a stroke because you elected not to take a blood thinner, then you feel horrible. You should have taken that damned medicine. If you get a stroke or die from taking the medicine, well, at least you tried, at least you gave it your best shot. That's how our brains work. That may also be why many patients who are not bothered by cognitive dissonance fall prey to peer pressure. When they don't go on a blood thinner, for instance, a friend, and then a family member, and then another doctor may tell them how foolish they are being. Finally, they succumb and take the pills despite not wanting to. Regardless of their own thought processes, they find it very difficult to surmount the cognitive biases of the people around them, all of whom seem to have an almost religious need to convert them to a Flexnerian way of thinking.

Cognitive dissonance is the fuel that propels doctors and patients into the quagmire of expensive and ineffective care that is now suffocating us, and that has convinced so many doctors and patients to rely on measuring and fixing problems as the only path to good health.

Osler's emphasis on the complexity of the human body and the uncertainty inherent in numbers and measurements are in opposition to our most basic cognitive biases. We want certainty. We want to be able to measure and fix. We want precise diagnoses. We want someone with authority to be able to cure us. We want to believe that the more we probe and treat, the longer and better we will live. No one wants to hear that it's best to leave a prostate cancer or a blocked blood vessel alone. No one wants to hear that high cholesterol may not be that important, that lowering it won't necessarily help us, or that sometimes it's best to have a higher blood pressure, that exercising and eating better is far more effective than fixing all those numbers.

We think we're cured when we can show a demonstrable change, which is why we are all sitting ducks to this approach. Health care and its ramifications vary from person to person, are flooded with uncertainty, and are not related to discrete measurements and numbers. Patients are best served by a doctor who asks them how they are doing and then observes any changes. But we don't want to hear all that.

And this need for certainty drives another potent cognitive bias, our assumption of cause and effect: We measured and fixed stuff, we are doing well, so therefore the measuring and fixing is why we are doing well. Ironically, this bias blinds us to the factors that really contribute to good health. People such as Mr. L and his son Joe, who pursue expensive and aggressive care, ascribe their good health to the doctors who care for them. Contrarily, people who are healthy and who don't do all that stuff – who exercise and eat well, who don't go to doctors often, who refuse to treat high cholesterol or get mammograms – are perceived by people such as Mr. L and son and many others as just being lucky.

Many doctors stoke this belief, likely because they are just as influenced by biases. If, for instance, someone on a blood thinner gets a stroke, the doctor says, "That's just unlucky." If someone who refused to take blood thinners gets a stroke, the doctor will say, "He was stupid not to take one little pill that would have prevented his stroke." This happens all the time. People and doctors both assume that aggressive care paves a path to good health, and the proof of that occurs when people who take that approach have good health. If they don't have good health, well, at least they gave it their best shot. If someone who doesn't follow that approach has good health, well, you know, they are damned lucky, and likely their luck will soon run out. The fact is that sooner or later everyone's luck will run out. That's just the way it is.

CHAPTER FIVE

Most of What We Offer Patients Is No Better Than a Pebble

The first duty of the physician is to educate the masses not to take medicines.

– William Osler[1]

Ms. K came to my office for a regular visit and, as is routine, we reviewed her medicines. I was appalled to learn that her neurologist had put her back on both Aricept and Namenda, pills we had stopped months ago by mutual agreement. Combining the generics of Aricept (donepezil) and Namenda (memantine) into a new nongeneric pill, Namzaric, was a "novel" treatment for dementia and thus could be sold for a hefty price tag.

But my very pleasant and intelligent patient did not have dementia. Ms. K was in her mid-80s and lived alone. Sure, she had a bit of memory loss (who doesn't at her age?), but she was fully functional, independent, and sharp. She could tell you what she ate yesterday and what the president did and said most of the time. Because she thought her mind was slipping – she forgot where she put things and sometimes could not remember people's names, which I told her happens to me every day – she saw a neurologist, who ordered a CT scan of the head, then an MRI, and then put her on a combination of Aricept and Namenda, two drugs used to treat *severe* dementia.

The thing is that Ms. K has a bowel problem, and after starting these drugs she developed diarrhea. That prompted a workup from a gastroenterologist who performed numerous tests, including another CT scan (of the belly this time) and a colonoscopy, before he gave her a few more medicines to stiffen her bowels. No one thought to consider that Aricept causes diarrhea, despite it being listed as among the most common adverse reactions to the drug, along with nausea, insomnia, vomiting, muscle cramps, fatigue, and anorexia (per the FDA website). The neurologist told her that Aricept was "necessary and effective" and that any connection it had to her diarrhea was coincidental. Never mind that when I asked Ms. K to stop the drug, her diarrhea resolved.

I discussed with Ms. K the risks and benefits of Namenda, which is approved for severe dementia only, and likely does not even work for that. In fact, I told her, the combination of these two medicines is no better than either one alone, and even alone both medicines barely do anything, especially for her as she has no dementia. So she stopped them.

That was six months ago, before she followed up with her neurologist.

That's why I was irritated that the neurologist put her on a combination pill of the very same medicines she had just stopped taking, claiming it to be a new and effective treatment for her memory loss. The neurologist told Ms. K that there was very good evidence that both pills worked, that they had been proven to curb memory loss, and that both together were better than either alone, something that she had read about in prestigious journal articles.

"That's just dead wrong. She's quoting the party line and clearly has not looked at the studies," I said to Ms. K, shaking my head. "I told you that these medicines don't work. And the Aricept gave you diarrhea. Why would she put you back on them?"

Ms. K shrugged. "I told her all that," she said of the neurologist. "She said that if you can find something as good as these pills, then be her guest, put me on them."

At that, I put my hand on the rug, grabbed a small pebble that must have fallen off my shoe, and handed it to Ms. K. "This is as good as those drugs," I said. "And without the side effects."

Like most doctors, Ms. K's neurologist relied on Flexnerian thinking to persuade her patient to take the drugs. She diagnosed a disease, a disease that was measurable through a memory test. Never mind Ms. K's reality: she lived alone and took care of herself and knew everything about politics and history. That wasn't enough for that doctor to dispute the test results that proved Ms. K had dementia. Adding insult to injury, she gave Ms. K a set of medicines that in drug-company-sponsored studies improved memory test scores in a handful of people for a brief period of time, thus making those medicines "necessary and beneficial." The neurologist never discussed the side effects, nor did she or the gastroenterologist consider that Aricept could cause Ms. K's diarrhea.[2] They just launched Ms. K into another Flexnerian quest, replete with tests and pills to tackle that issue. That is Flexnerian dogma, and Ms. K was one of its many victims.

Osler had no such illusions about the pitfalls of this approach. He knew that to define a disease by a number completely obscures the nuance and individual variability of disease from person to person, situation to situation. Thinking that a drug used to fix an ill-defined and arbitrarily assigned number can somehow help patients feel and act better is pure folly. Osler would never have diagnosed Ms. K with dementia in the first place. He would have told her, "You have some memory loss, don't worry about it, do more exercise, write stuff down, and focus on staying healthy." He would have looked at the studies done on Aricept and Namenda and realized that they are not compelling and could trigger Ms. K's side effects.

Interventions are said to work because they fix numbers. But if you look at how these drugs affect real outcomes, such as helping memory or avoiding heart attacks, then more commonsense interventions, such as exercising and eating well, usually are more effective at a lower cost and without so many side effects. But common sense doesn't fix numbers. And it doesn't generate profits for the doctors, companies, and other players in our health care industry.

In the case of Aricept, the drug may not improve memory or function, but it does improve the results of a numerical scaled memory test that the pharmaceutical industry helped to create, one that is clinically irrelevant but that is often touted by people such as Ms. K's neurologist as being scientifically valid. It is called the ADAS-Cog (Alzheimer's Disease Assessment Scale–Cognitive subscale), and its relevance to clinical outcome is much disputed.

Osler observed, "The desire to take medicine is perhaps the greatest feature that distinguishes man from animals." "The person who takes medicine must recover twice, once from the disease, and once from the medicine." Osler practiced at a time when medicines were not regulated, when miraculous snake oils and patent medicines flooded the market. But really, what has changed? When the vast majority of medicines are no better than a pebble, and when they are likely to cause side effects equal to or worse than their puny benefit, how are doctors any different than the snake oil salesmen and patent medicine pushers of yore?

Flexner derided patent-medicine doctors and snake oil sales-men no less than Osler did. To Flexner and his crew at Hopkins, only medicines proven effective by science should be prescribed. But what Flexner did not take into consideration is that just because a drug fixes an "abnormal" number, just because a pro-cedure opens arteries and adds more density to bones, it doesn't mean that it is clinically beneficial. To say nothing of how easily drug companies can design studies to fool doctors and patients into believing that their more sophisticated snake oils are really the next wonder drugs touted for their number-fixing properties. But that's what happens when you design a health care system on a model in which finding and fixing measurable things counts as scientifically validated medical care.

Before Aricept, the initial version of this type of drug (acetyl-cholinesterase inhibitors, or ACIs), called tacrine, came out to great acclaim. It was the first "cure" for dementia, according to its drug manufacturer. Early in my career, I gave a talk with a neurologist at our local hospital about the benefits of tacrine, and I learned after just a little investigation that it really didn't work in any meaningful way. I let that point be known in my talk. I was shocked to hear the neurologist skip right over that fact and implore all people with memory loss to start the drug as soon as possible. Any delay in treatment, he said, would lead to a per-manent decline in mental ability. And, he went on, if you take the drug and you stop it, even for a month, you will lose ground and never be able to recover. After the talk, most people in the audience latched on to the neurologist's naively sanguine assur-ances, likely because they so much wanted there to be a drug that would finally cure this horrible disease.

But nothing in the scientific scrutiny of this drug gave him license to make any such claims. In fact, the only place where I heard similar fallacious babbling was from the tacrine pharmaceutical representative, who had visited our office with pens and lunch a few weeks before, and he showed some misleading graphs and charts demonstrating a puny improvement in memory score on one type of test for about a year or less. "And if you stop the drug, even for a bit, then your patient will lose all the memory he gained from the drug and maybe be worse," the drug rep told us.

Could it be that the neurologist heard the same manicured speech from this drug rep, and ate the same catered lunch, and, despite there being nothing in the single drug-company-sponsored study that touted the merits of tacrine, chose to ignore that fact and cling to the company's self-serving propaganda? Probably. He was likely enamored by the graphs and numbers and measurements. He chose to ignore the inconvenient fact that patients and their caregivers noticed no benefit from this drug or the many newer versions that followed.

There are several germane facts that one sees in the studies of drugs such as tacrine, Aricept, Exelon, and other copycat versions of ACIs. First, there is a huge placebo effect when it comes to medicines for memory loss. Thirty percent of patients who take placebo have objective improvement in their memory. When we want to believe something works, often it does.

Second, studies were finagled to demonstrate benefit. Early studies looked at an endpoint called "caregiver score." This is a reasonable way to see if a medicine works. Half the people receive the drug and half the people receive a placebo, and then the blinded doctor (meaning the physician did not know whether the patient had the drug or a placebo) asks a close relative or caregiver if the patient improved after being on the treatment for a while. Thirty percent of patients improve by that criterion on Aricept. That's sounds pretty good, except that 30 percent improve with placebo too.

So, the smart designers of dementia studies found a surrogate endpoint, likely after a lot of trial and error. They invented the ADAS-Cog test and declared that if a patient improves their score by four points on that 70-question test, then they have had a meaningful response to the drug. This criterion worked well for the drug companies, who sponsored subsequent studies. Although 30 percent of pebble-takers did improve their test scores by four points or more, 39 percent of ACI users improved, clearly showing a benefit of this miraculous drug. It no longer mattered that the improvement was not noticed by anyone, such as patients and doctors and caregivers, any more than in those who took placebo. What the doctors cared about was that the drug improved a measured numerical score.

Based on this trick, many doctors dogmatically push these pebble-like drugs and, just like the neurologist taking care of Ms. K, point to the scientific certainty of its benefit. That enables them to sell solutions to a drug-hungry population to the tune of tens of billions of dollars a year.

But there is another shocking fact that the ACI studies demonstrate and that most Flexnerian doctors either don't know about or selectively ignore. The tiny 9 percent difference between placebo and drug found on the 70-question test dissipates very quickly. By 6 months, people taking placebo start to narrow the gap, and by 12 months pebble swallowers do just as well as ACI takers on the test. No randomized study has exceeded 12 months, so it is possible that pebble swallowers surpassed drug users and started doing better. Why else would the companies fail to publish any data after a year?

These facts have not gotten in the way of doctors and patients relying on these drugs as though they are miraculous cures. Recently, I was discussing a patient's condition with his daughter. She explained to me that if Exelon was as ineffective as I suggested, then neurologists would not be prescribing it. After all, a neurologist is much smarter than I am when it comes to matters of the brain. No argument there. However, when I pointed out that her dad was losing weight, a common side effect of Exelon, she chose to ignore that and chocked it up to her mom's bad cooking. She would not take him off the drug, more influenced by her cognitive bias than a disappointing reality.

The placebo effect with these drugs is one reason people think they work. If 30 percent of people see some improvement with placebo, that means that 30 percent of people will have placebo-induced improvement with the drug. To most people, that means the drug is working. This has also led many of my patients' children to notice a sharp decline in mental status the minute I stop one of these drugs. They put mom under a microscope after the drug is stopped and, with their cognitive biases in full force, and their fear of hurting mom reverberating in their head, they can detect a decline when there is none.

On one occasion, a patient's son did not want his mom taken off the drug Namenda, even though I told him it was not likely doing her any good. Namenda is a different type of dementia drug, one that is a bit better than a pebble in people with severe dementia, but no better in people with mild or moderate memory loss. In fact, one study comparing it to placebo and vitamin E found that vitamin E was better, and placebo was equal.[3] The makers of Namenda did not repeat that study or any one like it after that result came out.

For years the patient's son wanted to keep her on Namenda until its cost shot up, at which time he asked me to stop it. I did, and I said I would check back with him in a month.

When a month passed, I sent him an email to check in on his mother. "I'm sorry to tell you," he wrote, "but she is much worse since stopping the Namenda. She is more confused and anxious, and even my sisters said the same thing. I guess we have to start it back again."

It was funny because I did not notice any change in his mom, nor did her caregivers. But her son's observations carried the most weight.

I told her nurse, "It looks like we have to restart the Namenda, same dose."

"Why?" she asked me, perplexed.

"Because the son says she is worse since we stopped it."

The nurse laughed. "What you and the son don't remember," she said, "is that he told me to use up her supply of Namenda before I stop it. She is still taking it. Her supply never ran out."

That's the placebo effect in full force.[4] Even her son had a good chuckle about it.

As for Ms. K, I told her that even though the pebble I picked up was just as good as the drug she was given for her memory loss, I had something better to offer her than a pebble. Something that wouldn't cause her to have diarrhea or be expensive like the new combination pill that her neurologist touted.

"There was a study done recently," I said, "that looked at people with memory loss and dementia. Now, I don't think you have dementia; I hate labeling people that way. But what they found is that something can help treat dementia, prevent dementia, and help memory. And it has no side effects."

She looked at me with great anticipation.

"It turns out that in people who exercise regularly, eat a diet high in fruits and vegetables, sleep well, and practice stress-reduction techniques have minimal progression of their memory loss, and they get better over time. That's what it's all about."[5]

"Well, if it's all that great, why didn't my neurologist tell me about all that?"

That is indeed the question.

As a patient, it's more difficult to distinguish effective medicines from pebbles. Doctors should be able to help you figure that
out; right now doctors are doing just the opposite.

Ms. K understood. "I'll stop the medicine," she said. "But I'm
not telling my neurologist. I don't like it when she gets mad."

As I write, a new medicine has been approved by the FDA
called Leqembi. It is an infusion that, for $25,000 a year (money
that Medicare already stated it was willing to pay), promised
to finally treat dementia. It does reduce the amount of amyloid plaque in the brain, which is a surrogate; we don't know
if amyloid causes dementia, is the result of some other process
that causes dementia, or maybe even protects the brain from the
process causing dementia. It also, like Aricept, improves the test
score by a couple of points in a small number of people for the few
months the very manicured study was carried out by the drug
company. And, although the study excluded anyone who had a
predilection to bleed, it caused a significant number of disabling
and lethal brain bleeds, numbers that will certainly increase
dramatically once it is introduced to the public.[6] Doctors such
as Ms. K's neurologist will likely prescribe it because it meets
many Flexnerian objectives by improving measurable surrogate
markers. And it is likely, too, as drugs such as Exelon and the
combination of Aricept and Namenda become generic, their use
will be marginalized in favor of this new wonder drug at a cost
of tens of billions of dollars for the drug and many billions to care
for all those who bleed in their brains, without any meaningful
improvement in anyone's dementia. Thus is the consequence of
a Flexnerian philosophy of care.

CHAPTER SIX

Turning Pebbles into Boulders: How We Exaggerate the Benefits of What We Do

Medicine is a science of uncertainty and the art of probability.

– William Osler[1]

There is no question that medicines have saved lives – whether they are antibiotics that have prevented deaths on a global scale, blood pressure and diabetes medicines that dramatically reduce strokes and heart attacks and kidney disease, statin cholesterol medicines that (if used appropriately) reduce the incidence of heart disease, and even blood thinners such as Eliquis when people develop clots. But the vast majority of drugs that litter our medical landscape are not as effective as patients are led to believe. Many are used inappropriately, many have more risks than benefits, and many don't work at all when compared with placebo. But given the overall public trust in medicines, these pills have been touted as being necessary and effective, not because they are, but rather by exaggerating their benefit (and reducing their risk) with statistical trickery.

I went to the gym early one morning, and, boy, was it cold. When I woke up, it was two degrees. I trudged into the locker room with a bunch of quiet, freezing men, getting ready to hop on a machine or two. Just then someone came in and announced: "Good news everyone. The temperature just increased 50 percent outside. It's now three degrees!" Everyone laughed, enjoying the man's light-hearted exuberance. If you increase a small number just a little bit, it is a big percentage increase. Go from two degrees to three degrees, and it's a 50 percent increase. So, if you want a meaning-less change to seem significant, just use the percent it increases and not the actual amount it increases, because if he announced, "Good news everyone. The temperature just increased by 1 degree," they would have all thought he was insane.

That percentage – called a relative change – is the prevailing mechanism by which medical statistics are presented to patients, discussed in newspapers, and slapped into medical guidelines. The medical community relies heavily upon relative numbers. In the realm of epidemiology and public health, relative num-bers help define the effect of an intervention or disease on a large population group, but for individual patients, relative numbers serve no useful purpose other than to exaggerate the effect of what is being assessed.

If a drug or procedure generates a negligible benefit that may be little better than a pebble, we can make that pebble seem more like a boulder by using a relative number. When, for instance, doctors talk about atrial fibrillation, they may tell you that using blood thinners reduces your chance of a stroke by 50 percent. That's a relative number. If they use what we call an absolute number, which is the actual reduction in risk from blood thin-ners for you – which in most cases is that 6 out of 1,000 fewer people have strokes – you may be less inclined to believe that taking blood thinners is as vital as your doctor purports it to be.

It's not surprising that most medical studies and pharmaceutical ads present data using relative numbers, which make the results of the study or drug seem much more powerful.

A good example of how relative numbers influence medical thinking and practice is our perception of mammograms.[2] Cancer screening has gravitated to the pedestal of medical necessity, and anyone who dares to question its efficacy is soundly rebuked. Pink ribbons, road races, and a massive promotional campaign remind us that mammograms are crucial to the health and very lives of women. As doctors, we are not expected to ask women if they want mammograms; we simply tell them when it's time to get them.

When most medical societies and doctors talk about the benefit of lifetime mammograms, they'll state that women who get annual mammograms are 20 percent less likely to die of breast cancer than women who never get mammograms. That appears to be a huge benefit of this test, but it is a relative number. All that number tells is that when you compare the two groups, 20 percent more people die of breast cancer in the nonscreened group than the screened group. But 20 percent of what? Certainly, if very few people die, then a 20 percent reduction will be very small. If a lot of people die, then a 20 percent reduction is large. Therefore, we need all that information if we want to know what someone's *actual* benefit is from annual mammography.

This is called the "absolute benefit" of mammograms, and it is the only meaningful way to assess the efficacy and risk of a medical intervention. Out of 1,000 people who get lifetime mammograms, 4 die of breast cancer. Out of 1,000 people who do not get mammograms, 5 die of breast cancer. That is a 20 percent reduction in breast cancer. Reducing one cancer in five people is 20 percent. But in actual numbers, one person out of 1,000 avoids a breast cancer death if they get lifetime mammograms, so 99.9 percent of women don't benefit from mammograms.[3]

We're not trying to dissuade anyone from getting a mammogram. It is up to doctors and patients to discuss the risks and benefits of this and every medical intervention through a clear and unbiased lens. The point is that when we have those discussions, we need to use actual numbers and customize them to a patient's individual circumstances. We have to accept uncertainty and accept that most tests and treatments have tiny risks and tiny benefits that vary from patient to patient. When doctors understand these nuances, we can help our patients decide how to proceed.

When we tell women that being compliant with their mammograms can reduce their chance of dying of breast cancer by 20 percent, we are exaggerating the benefit of that test. But if we tell them that 0.1 percent of low-risk (they don't have a strong family history of cancer or other risk factors) women avoid breast cancer death with lifetime mammograms, they may be less persuaded to get the test. If we then juxtapose that benefit of mammograms against the risk – namely that 40 out of 1,000 people will have a false positive in their lifetime and 3 out of 1,000 will receive unnecessary treatment for a cancer that would not have harmed them if left alone – we will be providing the most accurate information possible to help women make the decision best for them. But that flies in the face of Flexner's first rule of finding problems and then fixing them. Doctors prefer to sell the test, not have patients grapple with the nuance and uncertainty of it.

Virtually every study that is published, every medical breakthrough highlighted by the media, every drug ad on TV is framed in a relative way. When your doctor tells you that you need a test, or procedure, or medicine, it is likely she will state relative numbers to make her case. This is the only way to make small interventions seem much larger and more significant.

An easy way to understand the power and deception of relative numbers is the lottery. Very few people win a lottery, so even the tiniest intervention that increases your chances of winning can show a big relative benefit. Let's say your chance of winning in Alan's state of New York is one out of a million. Let's say, by some quirk or by design, the chance of winning in Andy's state of Maryland is three out of a million. The Maryland Lottery Commission can accurately announce that buying a lottery ticket in Maryland has a three-times higher chance of generating a winner than buying one in New York. The new Maryland Lottery ads state, "Drive down to Maryland and play the lottery here where you will triple your chance of winning!" This way of presenting data is accurate, but deceptive. Yes, you triple your chance of winning, but the *actual* increased chance of winning is only two out of a million.

Such statistical trickery is rife in the health care industry. In fact, the Institute of Medicine estimates that 25 percent of our medical interventions have no or low value, and a trillion dollars of medical spending are wasted on unnecessary interventions, a number large enough to finance universal health care, should we choose to fix this pervasive problem.[4] So, to convince patients to take pills and to undergo tests and procedures, we magnify benefit by using relative numbers.

Take Mr. L, who relayed a discussion he had with his specialist about getting off his medicines. He was not sure they were of value, so he asked. He is 70 and healthy, at least he thought so; being on eight medicines made him question his health.

"I'm not sure I need to be on Lipitor [a statin], especially at such a high dose," he said.

"Why, is something wrong?" his doctor asked. "Your cholesterol is much better."

Mr. L explained that he heard that cholesterol alone is not a risk factor for heart disease, and statins don't necessarily help save lives or decrease heart attacks in healthy people like him.

"That's nonsense," his doctor said. "Statins cut your risk by 20 percent of a heart attack and stroke, and by another 10 percent if we up the dose and push down your LDL below 60. Do you want a heart attack?"

Mr. L did not want a heart attack. He asked about side effects. He said that his legs were weaker since he started the Lipitor.

"Nonsense. Have you been reading the internet? No. Not a single study shows a statistical increase in pain or weakness. If you are weak, don't blame the pills."

Mr. L then asked why he needed to be on three blood pressure medicines.

"Because we want you to avoid a stroke and heart attack. A recent study proved that there is a 40 percent chance of living longer if you lower your pressure a lot. Don't you want to live longer?"

And so it went. Mr. L was of course correct, and so was his doctor. Statins may lower his heart attack risk by 1 out of 1,000, and higher doses may lower it by another 1 out of 10,000, and that could translate to a 20 percent and 10 percent risk reduction, respectively.[5] So, the doctor told Mr. L the truth, just not in a very forthright way. He told it in a Flexnerian way: magnify the benefit, minimize the risk, to always prove that fixing numbers translates into better results. After that visit, Mr. L asked me about his blood pressure.

"I mean, I check my blood pressure and it's all over the map," he said to me. "If my arthritis kicks in, it is high. If I watch Fox News, it's even higher. Sometimes after I'm sitting in the sun it's really low. So, which one is accurate, the high numbers or the low ones? Sometimes I don't even know if the blood pressure cuff I have is all that accurate, even though it was pretty highly rated on Amazon."

"Don't get too focused on the numbers and don't check it so much," I told him. "It's just going to drive you crazy. We don't know what the perfect number is; it varies from person to person, from moment to moment. We have some basic parameters, like most of the time it should be under 150, and we don't want it ever under 110, but otherwise, it's going to bounce around."

People don't like uncertainty. They usually appreciate doctors who tell them exactly what their numbers need to be and what has to be done to get those numbers in the correct range. Luckily, Mr. L was one of those rare patients who could see through the relative-number haze, who knew that all these medicines were making him feel bad, and who disputed the benefits being sold to him. He stopped most of his medicines and did just fine.

It's fun to watch the omnipresent pharmaceutical commercials dazzle us with impressive relative numbers, and then we to go back to the studies and see how inconsequential the benefits of these "necessary and lifesaving" drugs actually are. In Osler's ideal world, doctors would be trained to see through such trickery and would revel in tearing apart these false messages. Doctors, according to Osler, must dig into the roots of medical information, not simply believe what they are told. In school, they would be taught how to read medical studies and to interpret them accurately and in ways that are applicable to their patients. In the Flexnerian world in which we live, doctors more willingly accept a protocol that suggests that an intervention that "fixes" some definable endpoint would inherently be beneficial. They don't do the hard work of figuring out the truth behind the ad.

When the AMA derided drug ads because it was too difficult for doctors to fight against all their misinformation, they were acknowledging that today's doctors are taught in a Flexnerian framework in which they are unable to understand the deceptive nature of relative numbers. Sadly, little of this is taught in medical school, and little is discussed by the doctors and professors who train our young doctors. And thus relative numbers rule the roost.

CHAPTER SEVEN

Numerical Epidemics

The problems of disease are more complicated and difficult than any others with which the trained mind has to grapple; the conditions in any given case may be unlike those in any other ... [T]he physics of a man's circulation are the physics of the waterworks of the town in which he lives, but once out of gear, you cannot apply the same rules for the repair of the one as of the other.

– William Osler[1]

A few months ago, I went to sleep thinking it was just an ordinary night. But when I woke up the next morning, 30 million people had a diagnosis of hypertension who had not had it the night before. We had a blood pressure epidemic on our hands. The newspapers were full of front-page stories alerting Americans to this new threat. The most erudite and well-respected physicians implored us all to get checked and treated immediately lest we suffer heart attacks, strokes – even death.

Welcome to the world of numerical epidemics. Once we base our definition of disease on numerical abnormalities, we can change the numbers in a way that expands the number of those who have the disease. This has been occurring in dramatic fashion the past 20 years, especially since Medicare (by congressional decree) relinquished the task of defining normal numbers to specialty medical societies. Hence the American College of Cardiology can change the definition of an abnormal cholesterol reading or abnormal blood pressure reading such that more people will be labeled with a diagnosed disease related to these numbers. Likewise, the American Society of Nephrology can broaden the definition of what constitutes abnormal kidney function and expand the scope of those now diagnosed with kidney disease. The list goes on and on, from diabetes to dementia to skin cancer; the criteria for being declared sick are rapidly being broadened, instigating epidemics of diseases across the medical horizon.

These fabricated crises affect well more than half the population and drive a measure-diagnose-treat crusade to eradicate sickness by prescribing medicines, ordering tests, seeing specialists, and undergoing procedures, all in an effort to normalize errant numbers. We are squandering trillions of dollars, often to the detriment of our patients, merely to push a number across some arbitrary line of what we call "normal."

But are we helping anyone?

Without a doubt, treating high blood pressure and high sugars in a measured and patient-centric way has saved hundreds of thousands of lives. Helping high-risk people with osteoporosis can similarly improve the lives of people we treat intelligently. But when our zeal to fix all numbers transcends the science, when all patients are viewed similarly regardless of their individual risks, when numbers eclipse the meaningful health of those we are treating, and when what constitutes a "normal" value is constantly altered to make more people appear sick, we have all the makings of a Flexnerian epidemic.

When Flexner and his colleagues insisted on reconstructing health care upon a bedrock of science, they assumed that if you can test someone and determine what is physiologically aberrant in his or her body, you can address that abnormality and perhaps fix it. Science to the architects of the Flexner report is not fickle or subjective, it is measurable and absolute. But they ignored the malleability of scientific "facts." Studies can be designed to reach foregone conclusions. Cognitive biases can distort our views of what is medically relevant. Benefits of certain interventions to fix abnormalities can be exaggerated and risks minimized. And the very term "abnormal" is hardly objective because it has to be defined by someone.

Certain groups – whether the American College of Cardiology or the Centers for Disease Control and Prevention (CDC) – can influence our definition of normal, especially when assessments are based on medical studies that these groups handpick to use as the barometer of normal. These studies are only as reliable as those who design them, but their influence carries great weight.

Mr. S reads the *Washington Post* regularly, and in 2018 he came to see me about the front-page headline regarding new blood pressure standards. A systolic reading of 140 used to be a normal pressure, but now it was deemed to be 120. This bold declaration, which created 30 million new hypertensives overnight, emanated from the SPRINT study, which concluded that aggressive treatment of blood pressure in older people results in a 25 percent decrease in stroke and heart attack, and a 40 percent cut in death. When SPRINT defined what a normal blood pressure was, a hypertension crisis gripped the nation.[2]

Mr. S graphed his and his mom's blood pressures over time. At ages 68 and 92, both fit in the category of old as defined by SPRINT, but the study did not look at people as old as his mom. He showed me the graphs. "Most of the time, we're way above

120," he said. "Mom especially. Her blood pressures seem to be all over the map. We need more medicines, doc. I'm going to see my heart doctor in a couple of weeks, but I'm afraid that if we don't get the numbers down now we could get a stroke any time."

As an engineer, Mr. S placed great value in the significance of numbers. That's why he created spreadsheets and graphs whereby he could demonstrate the fluctuations and averages of his and mom's numbers. It was crucial information, he said.

The danger of basing a new normal on a single study – and then proclaiming from that study that we have a numerical epidemic that requires aggressive and immediate treatment, as so many doctors and media outlets did – is rife with flaws. The primacy of numerical measurements in diagnosis glosses over salient differences between people, some of whom might require different normal numerical values than others. It also fails to recognize the harms of treatment and the way that "fixing" one number can affect the body more broadly.

SPRINT looked at a few thousand highly screened people, all of whom had severe heart disease, which was not the case with Mr. or Mrs. S. It found that by adding an extra medicine to those with blood pressures over 140 systolic, and getting that pressure below 120, there was substantial improvement in outcome. But what does a 25 percent *relative* reduction in heart attack and a 40 percent *relative* reduction in death actually mean? How many people actually benefited from aggressive blood pressure lowering in this very select group?

It turns out, not many: 1 out of 1,000 people treated aggressively avoided a heart attack or stroke, and 2 out of 1,000 lived longer by pushing pressures below 120 systolic. But we don't know how much longer they lived. Not only does the study fail to reveal that fact, it also doesn't tell us if people live longer because of lower pressure or from some other benefit the add-on medicines might confer in regard to their underlying severe heart disease.

Also, though SPRINT claimed to measure adverse outcomes of aggressive treatment, it did not adequately assess the more subjective effects of low blood pressure that I see every day in my office: dizziness, fatigue, falls, increased confusion, among others. Mrs. S was a perfect example. Her blood pressure fluctuates widely, as is true of many her age, and whenever her heart doctor pushed her pressure too low – usually at the behest of her son – she stayed in bed all day and was very confused. The numbers looked great, but Mrs. S didn't. Also, lowering the blood pressure aggressively triggers other problematic side effects, some of which were seen in SPRINT but largely ignored by those who touted the study's miraculous findings. There was no mention of the 5 out of 1,000 people in the treatment group who developed severe kidney disease over the brief trial period, and the 10 out of 1,000 who were hospitalized for dangerously low blood pressure.

Mrs. S's kidney function declined with the addition of her new blood pressure medicine. Already she had been given a diagnosis of chronic kidney disease, stage 3, something with which 90 percent of my elderly patients had been labeled ever since the definition of kidney disease changed. None of these people ever get sick or need dialysis; the diagnosis is merely an inconsequential numerical blip that was now defined as an illness.[3] But now Mrs. S believed that she had a disease. Mr. S brought her to a kidney doctor, who performed pages of labs regularly and an occasional X-ray. Until now, her kidney function had stabilized, but suddenly with the new pressure medicine it bumped up. "We should stop the medicine," I told her son. "Her pressure is too low, and her labs look worse. She feels terrible."

"Mom's kidney doctor begs to differ," he said. "She wants mom's pressures as low as possible, and she is closely monitoring many of mom's kidney tests to be sure we're on the right track."

Performing tests is one thing. Interpreting the outcome is another. Again, through an Oslerian lens, we simply cannot declare that there is a "normal" blood pressure below which everyone should fall. Everyone is unique, everyone has their own "normal" number, and it is up to a discerning doctor who understands his or her patient well to interpret the blood pressure reading in a way that makes sense for that particular patient. But Mrs. S's doctor had one goal in mind: *normalize the number.*

Unfortunately for Mrs. S, soon after her kidney doctor insisted she be put on another pressure pill, she promptly fell down and broke her wrist. "Purely a coincidence," her son later told me. "She tripped."

Many studies have demonstrated the danger of aggressively lowering blood pressure, some of which, such as a large Department of Veterans Affairs study, showed worsening renal function and a higher death rate in people aggressively treated who had underlying kidney disease, a fact that escaped the notice of those who declared the immediacy of our new hypertension epidemic. In fact, a study published after SPRINT received little attention, but it showed an increase in deaths among people treated aggressively when they did not have severe heart disease, which was the case with Mrs. S and son.[4]

Dr. Osler frequently taught that a doctor cannot simply treat a number; he must treat the patient. Mrs. S feels better with higher blood pressure. Maybe her body is pushing her pressure up to get blood through her many narrow arteries, and by lowering the pressure too much she is putting herself and her organs in danger. Also, her blood pressure is not the same from minute to minute, so how can we possibly gauge what her pressure really is and what it should be? Her son, and her specialty doctors, didn't care about all of that nuance. They read the guidelines, and they vowed to fix her. After all, this was an epidemic.

Another measurement that has reached epidemic proportions is cholesterol. All of my patients want their cholesterol measured, and most want it fixed. Cholesterol is a surrogate marker for heart disease. Everyone assumes that if your cholesterol is high, then you could have a heart attack. If you drive the number down through pills, then your risk of having a heart attack disappears.

Is cholesterol really a surrogate for heart disease, and is its significance the same for every person? The answers are no and no.[5] I have patients with tremendously high total cholesterol levels, 400-plus, in fact, enough to give a doctor a heart attack. And yet they don't have any heart disease. For several of them I have ordered a calcium score, which tells us how much plaque is caked on their blood vessels, and they have scores at or near zero. Just to let you know, anything under 100 is normal, between 100 and 400 is marginal, over 400 indicates that you have enough plaque to cause a heart attack.[6] How in the world can they have such high cholesterol and have no plaque? The answer is fairly simple. Cholesterol needs inflammation to stick to blood vessels. You can have a lot of cholesterol and no inflammation, and you won't have plaque. You can have very little cholesterol and lots of inflammation and get plaque. I have patients with normal cholesterol who are riddled with plaque and who have had heart attacks. In fact, just as many people who present to the hospital with a heart attack have normal cholesterol as have high cholesterol.

Some people are very inflammatory – people who smoke, eat poorly, don't exercise, are obese, have a family history of heart disease, have diabetes – and the goal is to treat the cause of inflammation, not to measure and "fix" the cholesterol surrogate marker. We have elevated the cholesterol measurement into something far more important than it is. Why? One reason is that you can't measure inflammation accurately, but knowing your patient and understanding the causes of inflammation can clue you in. Still, today's doctors like discrete measurements they can fix. ✗

The definition of what constitutes "normal" cholesterol, by the way, keeps dropping lower and lower. Consequently, the number of people inflicted by the cholesterol epidemic is rising. Some cardiology groups say it affects half the population. Half of people over 70 are on cholesterol medicines and get their cholesterol checked regularly, despite no evidence that lowering cholesterol works in that age group. Many of my very old patients adhere to strict low-fat diets, sometimes losing weight and feeling miserable in the process. They or their children believe this to be necessary, despite what I may say. So, if cholesterol is not very important, why are we so determined to measure and fix it?

Our obsession with cholesterol began in the 1950s when a scientist named Ancel Keys published the landmark Seven Countries Study in which he studied seven countries and found a strong link between cholesterol and heart disease. This landed him on the cover of *Time* magazine and made cholesterol the latest medical celebrity. But there was a catch. Keys actually studied 22 countries, and he eliminated the 15 that did not demonstrate the cholesterol/heart disease link he sought to demonstrate. France was one such country in which higher cholesterol consumption led to lower rates of heart disease, something Keys labeled the French Paradox. But if we dig up the parts of his study that he didn't publish, there were more paradoxes than countries that fit his model!

A decade later, Harvard researcher Mark Hegsted published another landmark study in the *New England Journal of Medicine* proving that fat and cholesterol were the main culprits in inducing heart disease. Hegsted went on to script our nation's dietary guidelines, which stressed a low-fat diet. It also turns out that Hegsted and his coauthors were each paid $50,000 by the sugar lobby to finagle the study results in a way that made fat look bad and sugar look good.[7] Ironically, the move toward a low-fat diet (which is still in vogue today) led to increased consumption of sugar and white flour, two of the most potent triggers of inflammation. Hence, a low-fat diet, even if it lowers cholesterol, could increase body inflammation through altered dietary habits, and consequently increase plaque and heart attacks, because inflammation causes cholesterol to be stickier. This explains the French Paradox and the rise in heart disease in this country following the new guidelines.

Mr. S graphed his and his mom's cholesterol over time and insisted they be checked at least every year. My attempts to explain that all studies conducted on people his mom's age showed no benefit of lowering cholesterol, and no risk of high cholesterol, fell on deaf ears. "That's not what mom's heart doctor said," Mr. S noted. "He wants the LDL cholesterol under 80, and right now it's not there. We may have to increase mom's Lipitor."

Mr. S was on a drug called Zetia because his cholesterol was not low enough from taking his high-dose statin. Zetia is illustrative of the flaws inherent to using a numerical measurement to define disease. Zetia does a great job of lowering cholesterol in general, but no study demonstrates that it reduces death or heart attacks.[8]

What causes heart disease is not the cholesterol that we can measure in our blood, but the cholesterol that sticks to our heart arteries and creates plaque. If you have enough plaque – even if you have no blockages in the heart and thus a normal heart stress test – you can rupture that plaque and trigger a stroke or heart attack. Because drugs such as Zetia don't lower inflammation and only make a number look good, they don't help prevent heart attacks or have any other meaningful outcome.

Interestingly, statins, such as the Lipitor Mr. S takes, can help reduce heart disease in people with plaque. These strongly anti-inflammatory drugs work well on heart and brain arteries and can reduce disease there. They don't work on everyone, though, and they have a lot of side effects – especially in the elderly. But they do help younger people with heart disease regardless of the cholesterol measurement. People with low or high cholesterol equally benefit from statins if they are at risk for heart disease. It's not about the number, as Mr. S and Flexner contend. It's about the health risks of each individual person.

Cholesterol is a nifty way for people to believe that they have control over their health. Measure a number, fix a number. But, Osler told us long ago that a person's health is not that simple. Mrs. S certainly does not benefit from lowering her cholesterol, and in fact the treatment puts her at high risk of injury and discomfort. Mr. S could easily mitigate his inflammation by eating better and exercising, but he chooses to ignore those difficult remedies and to graph his cholesterol numbers, falsely assuming that if he can keep that number down through medicines then he will be healthier. It is a simplistic way for people to fool themselves. Number-fixing is a tonic that fits well into our cognitive biases and makes us feel proactive, while generating large profits for drug makers and doctors, even if it is doing little to reduce our risk of becoming ill.

Nothing has stoked the public's awareness of numerical epidemics more than diabetes.[9] Mr. S incessantly checks his and mom's sugars; both are well graphed and associated with the time of the day and to what they ate. They see endocrinologists, who check copious labs several times a year and make sure to normalize everything that drifts too high, including blood sugar and its most prolific surrogate marker, the hemoglobin A1c. "Drop the sugar as low as possible and avert diabetes." Mr. S tells me this all the time, extolling the wonderful job they are doing with him and mom with keeping that sugar curve flat.

But just how bad is the diabetes epidemic?

As numerical diagnoses go, it is among the worst. It is also among the most telling about how epidemics are created and how divergent they are from a person's, and a society's, real health. In 1958, 1.6 million Americans had diabetes. By 2019, that number rocketed to 29.1 million. Some of that increase certainly was from poor dietary habits. The very diets advocated by doctors and cholesterol gurus – low-fat, high-sugar – have dragged down the health of Americans ever since Ancel Key's landmark cholesterol study. We still eat to lower our cholesterol, and in the process increase our body's inflammation and trigger diabetes. But the epidemic also has more nefarious roots, and treating diabetes aggressively can, as with our other epidemics, hurt us more than help us, despite what our doctors and cognitive biases might tell us.

As we saw with the hypertension epidemic, if we change the definition of what a normal measurement is, then we can increase the amount of people who have the disease, thus instigating an epidemic. That is exactly what happened in the realm of diabetes. In 1998, the American Diabetes Association (ADA) lowered what is considered normal sugar from 140 mg/dl to 126 mg/dl, thus doubling the number of people who had diabetes. A 1998 article by Steven Woolf and Stephen F. Rothemich revealed the justification for this shift.[10] It was based on ONE study, whose conclusions diverged from virtually every other study that sought to find a numerical value of sugar that was too high. Woolf and Rothemich show that there is little benefit in treating anyone for diabetes unless their sugars are above 200, and studies also demonstrate a real risk of overtreating diabetes and pushing sugar too low. In fact, several landmark studies demonstrate conclusively that aggressive control of type 2 diabetes (the form of diabetes that inflicts most older people) causes more death, heart attacks, and disability than more measured treatment. None of this registered when the ADA constructed its new guidelines; there was a diabetes epidemic, and we needed to use every means possible to get people's sugars as low as possible, as Mr. S often reminded me.

In today's atmosphere of numerical hyperdrive, millions of people with perfectly normal sugars now believe that they have diabetes. They check their sugars obsessively, falsely believing that by graphing and perhaps lowering those numbers they will live longer and healthier. They see diabetes doctors and check their A1c several times a year, and then check other labs and see other doctors who can help them reduce the chance of having a diabetic complication. Doctors keep pushing the numbers lower, despite a complete lack of evidence that this will help their patients. It feels good to have low numbers, something it's easy to achieve with our many new medicines. It appeals to our cognitive biases, it is so simple, and it gives us control over our health.

But it is deceptive.

As with cholesterol, the sugar and A1c are just numbers, more fickle and more variable than our epidemic-focused medical community will acknowledge. What causes the complications of diabetes is inflammation, and with diet and exercise we can reduce this pernicious dagger much better than we can with drugs. In fact, many diabetes medications lower blood sugar but don't reduce the meaningful outcomes of death, heart disease, or kidney disease. That's because they don't address inflammation. We may feel good with low numbers, but we are not healthier. In fact, many diabetes medicines – and lowering sugars too aggressively – make us less healthy, as countless studies have shown, especially in elderly people.

Even more frightening than the deception tied to our diabetes epidemic is an epidemic that we have fabricated primarily to sell more drugs, and one that has entered the hearts and minds of many people, including Mr. S, who himself is beset by it: prediabetes. Now, anyone who has a sugar over 99 is labeled as having this new disease. My patients who get labs have an asterisk near their sugars when they are 100 or higher, causing many to panic and a few to insist on medicines. With prediabetes, we have created scores of people who are now believed to be sick, an epidemic to end all epidemics. In fact, with diabetes and prediabetes, 85 million Americans are now labeled as being ill with this disease, almost half of all adults.

There are many prediseases that are now defined by numbers, identified by doctors, and often treated or closely monitored, despite little to no evidence that they will become dangerous any time in the future. Pre-osteoporosis is labeled as "osteopenia," predementia is called "mild cognitive impairment," pre-skin cancer carries the label of "actinic keratosis." The list goes on and on. In a recent article, Dr. Kenneth Lam called prediabetes a "risk factor twice removed" because, rather than being a disease, it is a potential risk factor for diabetes, which itself is a risk factor for true illnesses. And even as a risk factor twice removed, it rarely predicts who will get sick.

According to an article in *Science*, ADA doctor Richard Kahn invented prediabetes because "he needed a pitch to persuade complacent doctors and the public to take seriously a slight elevation of blood sugar." Despite a complete lack of evidence that people with prediabetes are at risk of being sick, or even at risk of becoming diabetic, both the ADA and the CDC "declared war against prediabetes," instigating a buffet of tests and treatments in an effort to squelch this newly defined epidemic. Says John Ioannidis about prediabetes, "You have a combination of two forces. One is to expand the definition of disease and to get more people classified as being sick or in need of treatment. And second, direct endorsement of specific interventions that [doctors and organizations] have direct conflicts of interest with. It's really very worrisome."[11]

According to the *Science* article, the ADA has strong ties to the pharmaceutical industry. It's no coincidence that its advocacy of finding and treating everyone with prediabetes and diabetes has led to a bonanza for the makers of diabetes drugs. The ADA receives between $18 and $27 million every year from drug companies, and 7 out of 14 ADA experts who recommended prediabetes treatment received between $41,000 and $6.8 million from companies that had a vested interest in prescribing more drugs. Such conflicts of interest are common in health care, but what is more concerning is how quickly doctors and patients got on the prediabetes train. Drug use for newly defined diabetes and prediabetes has escalated exponentially. New drugs are coming out regularly that lower the surrogate marker of A1c, but have no proven value to the people taking them. But yet, clinical guidelines and specialist doctors continue to push for lower and lower sugars and more testing, even though such behavior has been demonstrated to be more harmful than helpful. All of this is because of the soothing myth of believing that if we fix the number, we help the person.

I berated Mr. S that the aggressive number-lowering he advocated for his mom was making her more prone to falls, but he had an answer for that: "No problem, doc, I get her bone-density tests every two years, and now we have her on Prolia, so she has nothing to worry about on that score." He showed me graphs documenting her improved bone density. Yes, low bone density – osteoporosis – is yet another numerical epidemic barraging our Flexnerian medical landscape, and as with diabetes, there is a precondition – osteopenia – that has made this epidemic even worse.

Several years ago, I was in New York City giving a talk on health care when I picked up the *New York Times* and found a front-page article highlighting the osteoporosis epidemic and the need for doctors to take it more seriously. Several bone-density experts from major academic centers stated that millions of people were going to break bones because we were not testing and treating enough for bone loss. We have drugs to fix abnormal bone density, and the fact we weren't using them was derelict.

Bone density can be measured through a machine. If the number is lower than some arbitrary cutoff whose value was determined less by scientific scrutiny than by industry, then a person has a diagnosis of osteoporosis. If it's not quite that low, but still lower than "normal," then the person has a diagnosis of pre-osteoporosis, or osteopenia. Once people are labeled with such diseases, then a plethora of treatments are available, and with those we can improve bone strength and stop fractures.

"Wait a minute," said an older gentleman sitting in the front row of one of my talks. I thought he was asleep until he popped up. "Measuring bone density is a tiny part of the mechanism of how a bone breaks. What about flexibility of the bone, the bone matrix, the padding over the bone? Why are we just measuring density? You can have good density and still snap a bone." Of course, he was quite right. I later learned that he was a 92-year-old retired engineer and was much more astute than the experts who had frightened the world with this new epidemic.

We measure bone density because that's an easily calculable number. Flexnerians love numbers, and when we can measure a number, tie a diagnosis to that number, and then fix the number, we believe we have accomplished our goal as doctors. But, as the man said, many other factors contribute to fractures, none of which is captured in a bone-density test. These include the strength of the bone matrix, the fragility of bone, the flexibility of bone, the fat pads and muscle strength around bones, torque, and other physical factors of a rod that would lead it to bend rather than break. Doctors, though, are less concerned about those other details, which include fall risk, muscle strength, inflammation, and even weight. They are focused on bone-density measurements alone, and they can even plug those measurements into a drug-company-programmed calculator and determine a FRAX score, which provides your precise risk of breaking your bones in the next few years. Many people like Mr. S appreciate such certainty and precision, and they also crave a measurement that they can fix. That's why he put his mom on a drug called Prolia, which increases bone density and, in his mind, will lower her chance of breaking a bone.

Drugs for bone density have been well studied, and many similar to Prolia, called bisphosphonates, have been prescribed to the tune of tens of billions of dollars annually by doctors who marvel at their ability to not only improve bone density, but also to reduce fracture risk. Studies – conducted by the makers of the drugs – have shown an approximately 20 percent reduction in hip fracture over five years, and a 50 percent reduction in spine fracture. Those are the *relative* numbers typically quoted by bone density experts, bone specialists, the media, and even Mr. S. But how much do these drugs actually help? Is there a downside to their use?

Out of 1,000 people who take such drugs for five years, two hip fractures are prevented in moderate-risk people, and 10 hip fractures are prevented in high-risk people. Spine fracture reduction is more impressive, at 40 out of 1,000, but there is a caveat. Just as blood thinners reduce the risk of primarily silent strokes, so do bisphosphonates reduce spine fractures found on X-rays but that exhibit no symptoms. In fact, the vast majority of reduction in spine fractures are meaningless. In addition, studies for these drugs highly screen all participants, impairing their ability to produce generalizable results.[12]

First and foremost, if you don't want a fracture, don't fall. Also, exercise regularly, lower your inflammation through a good diet, and stay flexible. These drugs may be helpful for those at high risk for a couple of years, but for low-risk people a pebble is just about as good. But there is still another problem with these drugs – their ability to prevent fractures wanes over time. After about five years, patients on these drugs start building fragile and easily broken bones, even if they are very dense. You see, the mechanism of action of these medicines is to block the body's ability to break down bone, something that we naturally do to keep our bones healthy. Thus we are accumulating unstable, old, and low-quality bone over time. Sure, this builds up density, but it builds it up with bone that is ripe to crack in half.

In 2019, Merck faced a multibillion-dollar lawsuit for deceiving patients about the long-term dangers of Fosamax, a bisphosphonate. That is because all of their published studies stopped at five years, but their unpublished data clearly showed that the drug stops working in three years and increases fracture risk after five years. Out of 1,000 people who use these drugs longer than five years, 10 people will develop spontaneous fractures where their bone just snaps as they are walking. Thus, prolonged use of the drug actually increases the risk of fracture rather than helping, even as the magical and deceptive surrogate measurement of bone density improves. Sadly, fixing the bone-density epidemic may be causing an epidemic of fractures.

Mr. S was very proud of his mom's FRAX score, which had declined from 20 percent to 8 percent, thanks to the use of Prolia and paying attention to her bone health. "See, doc," he said, "we fixed her." But because of his and her doctors' aggressive care in helping her through all her many numerical disorders, she was hardly fixed. Her low sugars, drops in blood pressure, and statins made her more tired, unsteady, and confused. She lost weight and stopped participating in activities. She also continued to fall and complained constantly of dizziness. As her numbers improved, she declined, until finally she fell and broke her hip. In the hospital she deteriorated and, a week after the fracture, died. "Well, doc, at least we gave mom the best shot possible," her son said to me. "It was just bad luck and her age that did her in."

But it was hardly just bad luck. Even with her improved FRAX score and her stellar numbers, Mrs. S was a victim of our Flexnerian system and the false message it sells us. We fixed her numbers and destroyed her health. We did not view her as a human being, but rather as a collection of measurements that were amenable to treatment.

Manufactured numerical epidemics have a common thread: they use measurements to make a lot of people believe they are sick, and then offer quick fixes to help people think they are better. They exaggerate the danger of the numerical aberration and the benefit of the cure, and they assess success purely through a numerical lens, discarding the nuance and complexity of one's health that cannot be reduced to simple measurements. In the process, these epidemics have enriched many members of our health care network, have escalated the cost of care, and have falsely reassured tens of millions of people that drugs can repair a damaged body by measuring and fixing a simple number. Although this approach appeals to our cognitive biases, and is anchored in the bedrock of Flexnerian science, it is both dangerous and deceptive. Fixing numbers often causes more harm than good, and rarely does it address the real determinants of health. When we can take a pill rather than working on our diet, quitting smoking, or exercising, and if we can prove the benefit of that pill by showing how well it lowers a number, we are putting ourselves into a deleterious haze. Yes, there are epidemics, but they are not numerical. They are Flexnerian.

CHAPTER EIGHT

The Pitfalls of Screening for Diseases You *Might* Have

We did much for the patient and as little as possible to the patient.
– Bernard Lown[1]

Bernard Lown was a cardiologist and humanitarian working to both advance the science of health care and curb its excesses. His book *The Lost Art of Healing* shows how compassion and a strong doctor–patient bond are the most important ingredients in healing. He founded the Lown Institute and ultimately inspired the Right Care Alliance, which brought together doctors and others interested in improving health care under an umbrella of science, compassion, and dignity. It is there where Alan and Andy met, and in many ways Dr. Lown and his organization inspired this book. When we discuss health screening, we see the impact of Dr. Lown's gaze, as shown in the above epigraph, on how we should evaluate certain "truths" pushed on patients that often have more to do with profits and illusion than compassion and scientific reality.[2]

Patients often ask me to do whatever tests are necessary to make sure they don't have cancer or any other really bad diseases. It's called screening: look for diseases before patients exhibit symptoms, then fix the problems before they can rear their ugly head. Many of my patients believe that they have had their lives saved this way, always by a caring and thorough doctor who, thank God, performed that "necessary and lifesaving" screening test *just in the nick of time.*[3]

Most blood tests we order are screening tests. We send off a survey of chemical measurements, not because patients have any particular symptoms, but because it's their yearly visit. As thorough Flexnerian doctors, this is what we do. We acquire data. In fact, the entire physical exam – whether it's listening to your heart or your neck, feeling for lumps, or sticking our fingers up your rectum – is characterized as screening when you present without any particular symptoms.

Screening has a very Flexnerian ring to it. It epitomizes the allure of the test-diagnose-fix approach to health care, and the American public has bought into this philosophy hook, line, and sinker. Screening can pick up some disease and perhaps even prevent people from dying of illness (especially by finding a high blood pressure or high sugar level, or picking up a curable cancer), but with that benefit comes many serious pitfalls. When your likelihood of having a disease is low, then testing for that disease in the absence of symptoms is tremendously inaccurate. But that doesn't deter us from spending billions of dollars and assuring millions of people that they do or don't have certain diseases, just so we can erase some uncertainty and make them feel safe.

We have come to accept, for instance, the necessity and value of annual mammograms for women of a certain age, typically 40 to 75. Most doctors say simply, "It's time for your annual mammogram," and most patients accept the validity of that declaration, and doctors accurately cite a 20 percent reduction in breast cancer death over a lifetime among women who have annual mammograms compared with those who don't.

But, as we discussed in chapter 6, that 20 percent reduction is a poor representation of actual benefit. It sounds impressive, but the actual benefit is much smaller, as is seen in a KFF Health News video made with the help of Andy and his colleague Erik Rifkin.[4]

When Andy and Erik showed the Kaiser video to several insurance companies – and even to some patient advocacy groups – mostly to demonstrate the necessity of providing patients with accurate information before they can make a good decision, a look of horror came upon the faces of those watching the video. "Well, your point makes sense, but we can't possibly show anyone a video that questions the validity of breast cancer screening. It won't fly, we will be attacked," one insurance company executive told us. Even when Medicare tried to reduce the frequency of breast screening to every other year, based on solid scientific data, they were assailed by pro-women advocates, such as US senator Barbara Mikulski (D-MD), by lobbying groups such as the American Radiology Society that touted the 20 percent life-saving power of the lucrative test, and by many patient advocacy groups. Suffice it to say, recommendations for annual mammograms have not changed and never will.

But there are downsides of mammography, and it is illustrative of the pitfalls that haunt many of our screening tests, most of which are typically less beneficial and more harmful than statistics they promote.[5] Many of the patients whose lives were "saved" by mammograms actually were harmed by having their cancers discovered. How can this be? Approximately 20 percent of breast cancers are indolent, a number that increases with age.

This means that they just stay there and mind their own business, being contained by the body's immune system, and growing so slowly that they will never spread or kill the host. Some even regress and disappear. So, in a large number of older women who think their lives were saved, the discovery of a harmless breast cancer through mammography leads to surgery, radiation, and/or chemotherapy that is unnecessary and potentially harmful. This is especially true because the prevalence of cancer increases with age, so the more we look, the more of these harmless cancers we'll find. Of course, because we don't know which cancers are indolent, and because we are unwilling to watch the cancers to see if they progress or regress, virtually everyone diagnosed is subjected to aggressive "lifesaving" treatment.

This week I had a patient tell me that even a short delay before treating her tiny breast cancer found on a mammogram could be lethal; the surgery and radiation treatment were scheduled immediately. "Thank God we don't have socialized medicine, or I'd be dead," she told me. For decades a localized breast cancer called "carcinoma in situ" was treated with all the guns at our disposal. Now we know that it need not have been treated at all. We thus exposed hundreds of thousands of women to dangerous interventions, and labeled all of them as breast cancer survivors, a label they will carry the rest of their lives. This is a crucial ramification of Flexnerian screening dogma that many people do not perceive. Finding cancers early doesn't mean we are saving your life. In many cases, it may cause you unnecessary physical and emotional harm.

Mammograms, like all screening tests, are burdened by a high rate of false positives. When you test a large number of people who don't have symptoms, many of the abnormal measurements you discover are not abnormal at all; they are just a variant of normal. According to Jeanne Lenzer's *The Danger within Us*, about

9 out of 10 abnormal mammograms in low-risk women are false positives, an astonishing statistic about which most ordering doctors are unaware.[6] To Flexnerian doctors, an abnormality is an abnormality; scientific measurements are not to be questioned. It is estimated that with lifetime screening, about half of women will have at least one false positive, inciting fear, further testing, and even biopsies, which themselves can give more false positive alarms and prompt more fear and testing and, God forbid, uncertainty. Yes, screening leads to much more uncertainty than we realize, because hearing that you may have cancer but not being sure is about as bad as it gets on the uncertainty scale. Some women have multiple false positives, and their annual mammogram is one of the most frightening ventures of their lives. And mammograms can miss cancers, too; someone with signs of cancer can be falsely reassured with a normal mammogram. Either way, there is no certainty to this test.

This is not to say that mammograms should be avoided, only that they are not as scientifically valid and unquestioningly necessary as most Flexnerian doctors dogmatically purport them to be. Given that there are approximately 167 million women in the United States, and that lifetime mammograms save 1 out of 1,000 people who get them, that's a lot of lives saved across the population. It's just that for each individual woman grappling with whether to get the test, the benefit is small, and there is some risk, so the decision must be individualized. There is no right or wrong answer, no one right path the woman must pursue. It's up to a good doctor to explain the risks and benefits as they apply to the woman sitting in front of her, and then let the patient decide.

In the world of cancer screening, there are three basic categories: turtles, rabbits, and birds. Birds are cancers that, even if we catch them early, are already too far gone; cancers such as ovarian and pancreatic are so aggressive that screening for them will not save a single life. Rabbits are cancers that, like breast cancer, have a predilection to cause harm and may be more easily eradicated if found and treated early. All cancer screening should be directed against rabbits, which include things such as breast and colon and maybe some lung cancers. As with breast cancer screening, we'll see with lung cancer screening that even screening for rabbits provides limited benefit and substantial potential harm. Perhaps the most onerous flaw of rabbit screening is that Flexnerian doctors assure their patients that the test is scientifically valid and is an accurate gauge of underlying disease. That is Flexnerian logic; science is absolute, what the test shows must be right.

Turtles are those cancers that progress so slowly, if at all, that finding and treating them early derives no benefit. These cancers just hang around minding their own business right up until a patient dies; if they are going to kill us, usually finding them early doesn't prevent that unfortunate result, and treating them does not help people live longer. But, with screening, we can find turtles, tell a patient he or she has cancer, and then fix that cancer, touting the lifesaving feats that our precise testing can offer. When we find and fix a turtle, we have done nothing to help our patient; in fact, we often expose him to unnecessary harm. But people don't want to hear that. They are convinced that their lives were saved by the very thorough and caring doctor who ordered the test and removed the cancer. They are now cancer survivors, labeled with a lethal disease by a medical system that thrives when we can convince more people that they are sick.

Prostate cancer is the poster child of a turtle, something we discussed and cited in chapter 4, but it is worth mentioning again in this context. About a quarter or more of men who die have prostate cancer sitting harmlessly in their bodies, having probably been there for years or decades, not bothering them at all.

Millions of men have these turtles; if we test all of them, we'll find them. It is estimated that about 99 percent of prostate cancers do not kill a person even 10 years after discovery, and treatment of prostate cancer does not change the prognosis. The same amount die whether treated or not, and the vast majority of people with prostate cancer do just fine without any intervention.

So, why even look for it?

It turns out that turtle hunting is a big business. Urologists in particular make a lot of money by finding and fixing prostate cancers. Not to mention that patients beset by cognitive biases believe that it's always better to find and remove any cancer than to leave it alone.

Therein lies an unfortunate reality of screening. In a medical society built on the premise that if we measure and fix things, then we will be healthier and live longer, people have a hard time grasping the flaws of our current screening processes. As with all tests and screening, a blood test to detect prostate cancer (prostate-specific antigen, or PSA) gives us a precise number that opens up a window to a horrible ailment that may be silently lurking in our bodies. Such scientific precision makes us think that one test can save our lives, and so it brings us down a very long and dangerous road about which we are totally blinded.

Mr. D is an elderly but active man, a spy in his former life, whose doctor ordered a PSA as part of a thorough exam and laboratory screen. It was high, and a biopsy showed cancer. He had hormonal treatment and radiation. His doctors said that they would monitor his treatment's progress by following the PSA level; they could not assess treatment efficacy by asking if any of his symptoms resolved because he had no symptoms. Nevertheless, the patient and his wife were thrilled that he would be cured. In the world of *fix the number, not the patient*, the treatment was a great success. His PSA dropped from 90 to below 1 in a matter of months. There was only one catch. Since starting his treatment, Mr. D was exhausted. He couldn't walk because of leg weakness, and he could barely breathe. When I first met him after his treatment sent him to a nursing home, his wife still extolled the treatment that eradicated his prostate cancer, and she questioned my advice to stop it.

"Will we monitor the PSA if you stop the treatment?" she asked me.

"There's no reason for that," I tried to explain. "It's likely to go up, but we don't care. We're not going to treat the number. You see what the treatment did to him."

"Then how will we know if the cancer is spreading?"

"We won't," I told her. "But that's okay. The cancer isn't the problem. The treatment is. If he starts feeling poorly, then we can talk about what to do."

Mr. D may have improved once we stopped the treatment, but the damage was done. He remained wheelchair-bound in the nursing home for the rest of his life. We never did check his PSA again. He had no cardinal signs of metastatic prostate cancer, no weight loss, no bone pain, no urinary issues. He was just weak and remained that way until he died in his sleep one night.

Medicare alone pays about $1.2 billion over three years for ineffective prostate cancer treatment. That's small fries compared with many unnecessary medical interventions, but it does help prop up the salaries of urologists, whose society endorses such treatment. What makes prostate cancer similar to other Flexnerian screening tests is that the cost is incurred by measuring and fixing a number in a healthy patient without symptoms, potentially triggering harm and even more downstream cost.

In college, I remember my friend's father was diagnosed with prostate cancer. A medical nihilist, he decided to treat the disease with vitamins and alternative treatments, much to the chagrin of his doctors. Twenty years later, he was still alive and well. He never did check his PSA again. I thought my friend's dad was being reckless to eschew proven therapies for a deadly cancer. That my friend's father survived, well, I figured that was a lucky fluke. But it turns out that he could have just as easily wiped his hand with cow manure every four days and done a dance in the moonlight around an oak tree, and there was a 99 percent chance of his prostate cancer not killing him. It wasn't the vitamins. It was the fact that his cancer never should have been looked for in the first place, and it certainly demanded no treatment.

Mrs. E was almost 90 and in fairly good health. As part of her check-up, she showed me a small nodule on her leg. She wanted to know if it was dangerous. I told her not to worry about it. Her friends disagreed. She went to a local dermatologist, who biopsied it and found a squamous cell cancer, which she had removed through what is called a Mohs procedure.

"What you so callously dismissed turned out to be cancer," she told me indignantly. "Thank God the skin doctor recognized it and took it off. I'd probably be dead had I let it sit there too much longer."

The surgery, which costs Medicare $15,000 to $25,000, removed the cancer no better than an $80 scalpel would have done, and it left its claws on my patient's very fragile 90-year-old skin. The wound never healed. It bled and then became infected, enlarging as it spread down her leg. She went to a wound clinic almost every week for many months, took antibiotics, and lived with pain and some degree of disability. A year later, the wound finally resolved, tens of thousands of dollars later, to the detriment of my patient's health, all for a cancer that if left alone would have just harmlessly remained there.

In fact, especially among the elderly, squamous and basal cell cancers neither kill nor maim the vast majority of people.

Removing them is a different story. About 20 percent of elderly people who have skin cancers removed suffer the complications we just mentioned.[7] They think their lives were saved, but instead their Flexnerian providers broke the most basic law of health care: inflicting harm beneath a veil of deception.

In 2018, I attended a talk at the Lown Conference – "a non-partisan think-tank advocating bold ideas for a just and caring system for health," according to their website, and it is a group that speaks the language of William Osler – and heard a dermatologist speak about an "epidemic of skin cancers" being tossed upon the American public with the test-diagnose-treat mantra. He said that one dermatologist in his practice billed for 214 cryotherapy surgeries (freeze-gun treatments of harmless precancers) at a cost to Medicare of $8,700, while another billed for 20,000 cryotherapy treatments in the same year at a cost to Medicare of $227,000. Same patient population, likely same outcome, but one doctor is a thoughtful Oslerian who provides measured patient-centered care, whereas the other practices with a Flexnerian knife and removes anything that is deemed to be abnormal. Likely the more aggressive doctor told his patients that he was saving their lives, and the patients were happy for such thorough service; with the cancer gone, so was their fear and uncertainty. And the aggressive doctor was awarded for his Flexnerian beneficence by hefty insurance payments.

As with diabetes, osteoporosis, high cholesterol, and hypertension, skin cancer is now considered to be an "epidemic." How is it an epidemic? Because by finding so many harmless cancers and precancers that in the past more doctors would have left alone, dermatologists have caused a dramatic increase in skin cancer diagnosis. In other words, dermatologists created the crisis and are benefiting from it, with a tremendous boost in their incomes during that time.

The skin cancer epidemic started in the 1980s when the American Academy of Dermatology hired an advertising firm to improve the status of dermatologists. Their suggestion was to transform the role of dermatologists from the doctors you go to for a pimple or a rash to skin cancer experts. They suggested that dermatologists conduct free skin cancer screenings to identify and treat all those cancers that had been neglected, thereby igniting public fear that skin cancer was both pervasive and potentially deadly.

The lingering effect of that advertising blitz is with us still today.[8]

Skin cancer detection and removal is a multibillion-dollar industry that has enriched many and helped few. The few studies done to assess the efficacy of skin cancer screening show no benefit in terms of lives saved. We label many millions of people as having cancer, but because the vast preponderance of those cancers are dormant, we don't prevent death. According to the US Preventive Services Task Force 2014 statement, "The current evidence is insufficient to assess the balance of benefits and harms of visual skin examination by a clinician to screen for skin cancer in adults."

And yet, a large number of my patients see dermatologists, and the majority of them get frozen, cut, diagnosed, and treated. They become cancer survivors who get surveillance checks, usually twice a year. Dermatologists don't have to discuss much with their patients or think too much about what to do; it's all algorithmic. In 10 minutes, they charge Medicare as much money as doctors who spend far more time treating complex chronic illnesses and conversing with their patients about difficult issues that inflict them. Flexnerian medical care pays well!

Precancers, like prediabetes, are even more suspect in terms of their potential harm. Studies indicate that few of them ever progress to cancer, most spontaneously regress, and the cancers they do evolve into are typically harmless. A multibillion-dollar industry has blossomed by frightening patients into believing that they have a disease – precancer, called "actinic keratosis," or AK – that if treated regularly by cryotherapy or excision will avert a potential malignant catastrophe. Many of my patients adhere to that myth, and dermatologists gladly stoke it. The aforementioned dermatologist said at the Lown Conference: "AKs are the low-hanging fruit, easily frozen by those dermatologists who look on the practice of medicine as a business, not as a calling. Their greed harms and scares patients as it enriches con men in white coats. What they do is not patient care, but patient-assault with a cryo-gun."

What about melanomas, the most egregious and deadly of skin cancers? Unlike squamous and basal cell cancers, and their precancerous AKs, melanomas do kill, so wouldn't an early detection program reduce the chance of dying from that? Because of enhanced screening, the incidence of melanoma has increased threefold since 1975, but the death rate remains the same.[9] In other words, we are finding and treating a lot of the indolent melanomas, but the lethal cancers continue to kill at the same rate as they always did. Finding a melanoma early will not necessarily affect whether it will kill you. Like many aggressive cancers, the most lethal melanomas have already spread once they are detected, and all the others that we find are more like turtles. Our surveillance and slicing help no one.

I should add that the sunscreen industry has also benefited from our skin cancer "epidemic," even though there is not a bit of evidence that the use of sunscreen prevents any skin cancer deaths. In fact, by denying us vitamin D, sunscreen may well be causing more harm than good. And now, of course, we have a vitamin D deficiency epidemic. It never seems to end.

The proliferation of testing and screening has led to a huge jump in cancer diagnosis across the board. Many of my patients believe that they have had their lives saved by finding a mass on a chest X-ray that turned out to be lung cancer. The X-ray was done for other reasons, typically requested by a surgeon before an operation in a patient without symptoms, and a shadow appears. The patient then gets the mass biopsied and, if found to have cancer, a surgery and other treatments (radiation, chemo) to eradicate it.

But as with most screening, lung cancer screening is haunted by a plethora of pitfalls.[10] Lung cancers can regress; 20 percent of them are either stable or disappear. Those found on chest X-rays will kill a person or remain dormant regardless of when they are found. And chest X-rays are beset by so many false positives that it is more likely an abnormal X-ray will harm a person than help them. That is why most organizations, such as the US Preventive Services Task Force, give chest X-rays a grade of F as a screening tool: they don't save any lives, and they kill and hurt more people than they help. ✗

Lately, the radiology pundits have introduced a newer and better way to screen for lung cancers in smokers and ex-smokers: low-radiation CT scans. Medicare is willing to pay tens of billions of dollars a year for this test; if only they would pay even a fraction of that cost to help people stop smoking! We wrote a review article about this test in the *American Family Physician* (*AFP*) journal, and it is instructive to look at this test as a barometer of what screening tests accomplish, both good and bad.[11]

The test's supporters, including the American Radiology Society, cite data to show that after five years of annual CT scans, the death rate from lung cancer in those who are scanned is 20 percent lower than in those who are not scanned. This is based on a few recent studies, starting with the National Lung Screening Trial (NLST) in 2011, the first study to demonstrate any benefit from screening for lung cancer. Previous studies demonstrated no benefit of screening, and even if those studies are pooled together with NLST, there is no benefit. Still, NLST suddenly made lung cancer screening a viable test that many pundits believed should be widely disseminated, and subsequent studies verified the NLST results.

The 20 percent (*relative benefit*) drop in lung cancer death touted by NLST translates to an *actual benefit* of 3 people averting lung cancer death out of 1,000 people screened over five years, meaning that 99.7 percent of high-risk people who are tested do not derive any benefit. Is there harm? Yes. About a quarter of people without cancer who receive screening CT scans are told they have an abnormality that may be cancer. Of those, many need PET scans, biopsies, and even surgeries to prove they don't have cancer, and some of those tests and procedures lead to harm and even death. Also, because 20 percent of lung cancers are dormant, we are finding and treating a lot of people for cancers that screening discovers but that are harmless. Not only that, radiologists discover other abnormalities when they perform a screening lung CT (such as kidney nodules!) that drive patients down yet another road of uncertainty and potential harm.

After we published our article in *AFP* discussing the risks and benefits of lung cancer screening, we were greeted by letters accusing us of potentially killing tens of thousands of people by introducing nuance about this "necessary and lifesaving" screening test. The American Academy of Family Physicians, and many other reputable groups and doctors, do not endorse lung cancer screening for two reasons. First, the jury is still out as to its effectiveness. Medicare is conducting a review of all screening performed in the community, and many of us believe that this will be more revealing than the very staged and restricted trials conducted under ideal conditions that showed variable results and at best very small benefit. Second, we still must grapple with the high false-positive rate that leads to stress, overtreatment, and harm.

Flexnerian screening advocates do not accept such uncertainty. To them, lung cancer screening makes perfect sense. It finds abnormalities early before they cause symptoms. It labels people with disease and allows those diseases to be addressed and treated. It saves lives. No one in the screening community is willing to acknowledge the small number of lives saved in the most sanguine of these studies, preferring to magnify the benefit by using a deceptive relative number.

I recently saw a patient who got a chest X-ray in an urgent-care center when he went there for a runny nose and dry cough. The care center owned the X-ray machine and thus was anxious to use it as much as possible, even though typically a slight cough in the setting of a cold would not trigger a doctor to order an X-ray. As it turned out, the X-ray was abnormal, and a subsequent CT scan showed a mass that may well be cancer. The patient never smoked, was not short of breath, and his cough resolved. He was tossed into the lap of a lung doctor, who demanded that he get a biopsy immediately or he would die. My poor patient, who doubted that he was sick, did not want to pursue that course, but was scared by the doctor's dogmatic absolutism. We talked, and he agreed to wait. Many years later, he is alive and well, and refuses to ever get another X-ray.

Tests performed on people without symptoms are inaccurate and lead to false-positive results. Some save lives, but they can kill or maim others who don't have illness. Screening, when done sensibly and after a meaningful and thoughtful conversation between doctor and patient, can have utility. But the screening epidemic that has overrun our country has not helped most people live longer or better. It has led to a lot more cancer diagnoses, a lot more fear and unnecessary treatment, a lot more doctor visits and tests, but not to a lot of lives saved.

Osler was correct in imploring doctors to accept and embrace uncertainty if they truly want to help their patients. Few doctors follow that advice. They interpret tests through the lens of absolutism. Screening tests are just another example of pretending that we can stop disease just by measuring and fixing every abnormality that may lay hidden beneath (or on) the skin of an apparently healthy person. Don't talk to patients, don't weigh risks and benefits, rather, just test for everything all the time. That's screening. Flexnerians use deceptive numbers to prove that it works, but reality tells us another story, and the cost of these efforts is astronomical. Blind screening is Flexnerian at its core.

CHAPTER NINE

When Science Becomes Dogma

The greater the ignorance the greater the dogmatism.

– William Osler[1]

When I entered my residency, there was an attending doctor who was, we were warned, "a bit of a nut." He had a zealous belief that stomach ulcers were caused by bacteria. Most legitimate scientists wouldn't listen to him because the cause of such ulcers had been established and need not be questioned. It was remarkable that this physician remained in academics. But, as with most freethinkers, Barry Marshall had the last laugh. A jovial and light-hearted man, he talked all about *Helicobacter pylori*, a bacterium he believed triggered ulcers.

This was medical heresy. The drug companies that sponsored most research and the scientists who believed in a predetermined dogma regarding the cause of ulcers scoffed at him. They knew what caused ulcers. It was an overproduction of acid, and the only treatments were drugs that blocked stomach acid. Undeterred, Marshall conducted experiments, finally swallowing a bunch of *H. pylori* bacteria. Turns out that Marshall was right. He gave himself an ulcer.

I met Marshall early in my residency. He was a pleasant self-effacing attending doctor, who, I could tell, was not going to let the orthodoxy of his profession thwart his crusade. No one gave him much credence at that time, and they found him to be a misguided doctor, but he did not care. Three years later, when I left the residency, he was on the cover of *Virginia Magazine*. Smartly, he patented the breath test for *H. pylori* and became a multimillionaire. Soon after that, he won the Nobel Prize in Medicine. Barry Marshall refused to be shackled by a Flexnerian dogma, which preached unbending adherence to one right answer. Because of his willingness to confront the system, we are all better off. As is he.

Critical thinking and questioning of established dogma have no place in the Flexnerian worldview. There is always one right answer, preordained by science. And it applies to everyone. Marshall was a heretic, until his discovery was sanctified by the American Gastrointestinal Society after several studies showed it to be true. Pharmaceutical companies concocted drugs for the disorder, and an entire industry grew around it. Now, *H. pylori* is dogma, and no one dares to question it. I often wonder what Marshall thinks about all of that.

Dogmatic one-right-answer thinking is exceedingly difficult to dislodge when it takes root.

Mrs. C found that out when she witnessed a temper tantrum by her husband's lung doctor. Her husband had pulmonary fibrosis – scarring of the lungs – which has an unknown cause and no good treatment. Typically, fibrosis leads to progressive shortness of breath. He was doing all right, but the lung doctor put him on a new drug called Esbriet, which apparently helps slow the condition. He had been on the drug for more than a year and was no better or worse. But he was appalled by the drug's price, so he asked me what to do.

I found a single article that touted the drug's benefit. Apparently, the study was conducted for less than a year, and financed by InterMune, the drug company that created the drug and which Roche purchased for $8.3 billion. The study focused on improvement in lung measurements (a surrogate endpoint) and not symptoms, employing relative values to demonstrate that people on the drug experienced a 50 percent reduction in lung capacity decline. There was no change in how people felt; they were just as short of breath on this drug as on placebo. People on the drug died less, but the reduction was small, and it was unclear to whom it may apply. Esbriet costs $80,000 a year. Its sales are about $1.5 billion a year for a very uncommon disease. A literature search reveals a great deal of controversy as to whether it works in any meaningful way, with most of the positive press generated by Roche.

I found an article about the drug that showed no improvement by any measure after a year of use, and I showed it to my patient. "Likely this drug is not doing anything for you," I said, "but talk to your lung doctor and show him this article and see what he says."

Big mistake.

I knew there was trouble when my office received a message that the lung doctor called and demanded to talk with me. "How dare he tell my patient to stop this drug," he yelled at my receptionist. "I am the expert. He has no right to put in his two cents!"

It turns out that Mr. and Mrs. C visited the lung doctor, and Mrs. C said, "My husband's primary care doctor told us that my husband can stop the drug, it doesn't work." After that, according to Mrs. C, fireworks started to fly.

Had I been confronted by Mrs. C's skepticism, I would have explained to her what the research shows, and then listened to her concerns, not the least of which was the drug's steep cost. There is nuance in every treatment, and it's up to us to understand that and to listen to our patients. There is never one right answer. There is never singular dogma.

Sadly, many of my patients fall prey to medical dogmatism, believing that their doctor's aggressive posturing is caring and thorough. Optimistic about the benefits of treatment, not to mention fueled by their own cognitive biases, they leap right into the Flexnerian soup, slurping up tests, procedures, and drugs they are told are necessary and lifesaving. Some of these "necessary and lifesaving" interventions are not even appropriate for them, given their other health conditions and concerns, and most patients are never told the pros and cons of going that route. It's always the same dogmatic response: "Do it and I will save your life. If you don't do it, you may well die."

The allure of hyperbole is not new to our medical *Zeitgeist*. Doctors have always wanted to be the heroes, that's in our DNA. Back in the day of the snake oil salesmen and the butcher surgeons, doctors proclaimed that what they were peddling was necessary and lifesaving. Ironically, although the prime purpose of Flexner's scientific revolution was to purge the medical field of charlatans who promised patients the moon, a vast amount of our nation's health care budget is being spent on medical interventions that are proclaimed to be necessary and lifesaving but are as effective as snake oils from the darkest times of our medical culture.

Mr. G was a relatively healthy man. He has a lot of risk factors for heart disease, including obesity, diabetes, and high blood pressure. He ate poorly and did not exercise. He had been a smoker until recently, and likely was still sneaking a few. We were treating him with an aspirin a day and a low-dose statin, Lipitor. His diabetes and blood pressure were well controlled, but his numbers were not crazy low. They were reasonable and they varied based on the time of day and what he had eaten. As for exercising and altering his diet, well, that was much too difficult, but he said he would keep trying. Besides, he said, "I hardly eat anything, really."

His wife worried about her husband and talked to a friend, who scared Mrs. G.

"Your husband may be a time bomb like I was," this caring and concerned friend said to Mrs. G. "Don't wait for your regular doctor to act only after he has a heart attack. Act now!"

And so, Mrs. G brought him to an army of specialists. He was put on insulin and had a few dangerous drops in blood sugars. "Unless we get his A1c below 6.5, he will become very sick," his new endocrinologist told him. He saw a kidney doctor and was diagnosed with stage 3 kidney disease (the same "disease" that afflicts 90 percent of my patients now based on shifting definitions of "normal") and put on a handful of vitamins and supplements. Both these doctors ordered pages of tests every few months, most of which did not lead to any treatment, but which he was told were medically necessary. He saw a cardiologist, who ordered an annual stress test, echocardiogram, and Holter monitor (a 24-hour heart monitor), *just to make sure.*

"Things can change fast," said the cardiologist. "It's necessary to do these tests every year so we pick up problems before they occur." On one occasion he had a catheterization that led to hospitalization. He bled from it and had a small stroke, but thankfully, he recovered. He saw other doctors, had skin screening and some moles removed ("Just in the nick of time," Mrs. G told me), had a PSA and needed a biopsy that was normal ("But we'll have to check this closely, get a prostate MRI, keep a close eye on it," his urologist told him), and now spent most of his free time checking his sugars (which, by a miracle of technology, he could do four times a day and map on his iPhone), going to doctors, checking and graphing his blood pressure and oxygen levels, and worrying about his health.

This was all done in the name of medical dogma. None of these necessary interventions were discussed with him. All, he was told, were necessary. Did he need to check sugars four times a day? Did he really need to be on insulin, which only made him eat more and gain weight? Was there science behind any of this, or were his doctors just doing it all because they had been programmed to fix numbers?

What about the annual stress tests? We have discussed the biology of heart attacks and blood vessels. When a person is very inflammatory, or just unlucky from a bad family history, his blood vessels become cluttered with plaque. At any time, some of that plaque can rupture. When that happens and the body tries to fix the rupture, a blood vessel becomes closed off and he gets a heart attack. If it's a small vessel, he may never know it happened. If it's large, he may become very ill or die. When we do a stress test, all we can see is whether there is a diminution of blood flow of greater than about 70 percent in one or more heart artery. So, people such as Mr. G could have his entire heart vasculature riddled with plaque, but none of it blocks off flow and thus he has a normal stress test and is told he is fine. In fact, it is estimated that about 85 percent of people who present with a heart attack would have had a normal stress test the previous day. Stress tests do not measure plaque, only blockages, and because fixing blockages does not prevent heart attacks or plaque rupture, even that is an exercise in futility.[2]

Cardiologists perform hundreds of billions of dollars of stress tests and echocardiograms every year. Not because of any scientific validity, not because of any utility to the patient, but because these tests have been inscribed into the bible of Flexnerian dogma. Study after study showing no value to these tests has not cut back their use. Doctors tell patients it is necessary to find and fix block-ages, and patients eat that up; it appeals to their most basic cognitive biases, especially because so many of them know of a friend or family member whose life was "saved" by such testing.

"We are living longer than before," many of my patients tell me. "So, clearly all this technology and medicine and procedures are saving lives and helping us cheat death."

Again, cognitive dissonance. We are living longer, so therefore stents and aggressive medical treatment must be the reason. It is an assumption many people make.

It is true that from the 1920s until the early 2000s, the lifespan of Americans increased, but it has slid backward the past 20 years. This is true of death from heart disease too. But even though we spend tens of billions of dollars finding blockages and opening people's arteries, the rate of heart disease death has not decreased because of this. In fact, most of the improvement in heart-related deaths occurred before we were conducting billions of dollars of stress tests, echocardiograms, and cardiac revascularization. We as a medical society have improved in our ability to rapidly diagnose and treat heart attacks, slow the progression of heart failure, and use pacemakers and defibrillators to treat dangerous heart rhythms. Once we started finding and fixing heart block-ages, the death rate from heart disease stabilized, but it no longer improved.

In many Blue Zones – areas of the world where people live the longest – there are no stents. No statins. No aggressive monitoring and treatment of abnormal numbers. Rather, there is a good diet (not a low-fat diet, but a good diet with some fat), exercise, lack of smoking, and lifelong socialization.[3]

Why are we living longer? One reason is better management of chronic diseases. We can control blood pressure and diabetes now, whereas before we could not. However, controlling those conditions does not mean aggressively treating them: moderate control does the trick. Aggressive control often makes people worse and has not led to improved longevity. We also can help people with plaque-cluttered arteries with statins and can treat some cancers better than before. But there are much more important reasons we are living longer, and they have nothing to do with aggressive medical care.

First is the ability to prevent and treat infections. In the past, we were terrible at this, and infections were the typical cause of death of most young people, and even a lot of the elderly. That is what happens when you drink water in which someone else has defecated. Now, we are much wiser.

Second is a reduction in infant and maternal mortality. This was a common occurrence back in the day, and now it's very rare. Both children and mothers died young, and so they skewed the average life expectancy. Think about it this way. Let's say way back when, in a small community, a lot of children died young or at birth. So, in a given year, 20 children died before age 2, and 20 adults died at age 80. The average life expectancy of the community is 40. Now let's say that no kids are dying, and that 20 adults are still dying at 80. Now, the average life expectancy of the community is 80. Just by reducing infant mortality we have increased life expectancy from 40 to 80. That certainly makes it seem as though our wonderful medical technology has helped us to live longer, but that is not the case. Throw in infection control, immunization, and treatment of chronic illness, and that pretty much tells you why we are living longer.

It's not from stress tests and stents.

In addition to his annual stress tests, Mr. G is being exposed to aggressive treatment for his cholesterol, diabetes, and blood pressure, which may cause fatigue, weakness, and confusion, all symptoms that Mr. G has experienced since he began his *lifesaving* interventions. Ironically, those drug-induced symptoms are exactly what is now preventing him from exercising, the very intervention that would help him the most. In fact, after being put on insulin to obtain a "perfect" sugar, Mr. G started gaining weight, even as his sugar dropped to dangerously low levels. And the low-fat diet that was prescribed for Mr. G is not effective in preventing plaque and plaque rupture.

All of the medical interventions sold to Mr. G as being necessary and lifesaving are in fact myths, now having become medical dogma despite scientific evidence to the contrary. Yes, Mr. G would benefit from a statin because statins stabilize and reduce plaque, thus cutting heart attack risk. But he was already on a statin before his head-first dive into a Flexnerian sea of doctor-prescribed dogma even started, so he was being maximally treated. The only things lacking in Mr. G's treatment were exercise and a good (low-processed carbohydrate and high-fruit/vegetable/fiber) diet, something not discussed by number-obsessed doctors.

Science is the bulwark of a good health care system. It is science that has led to a near elimination of infant and maternal mortality, curbed infectious disease, and helped us to sensibly manage many chronic diseases. These are the reasons we are living longer. But now science has been co-opted by those who wear it as a mask to justify billions of dollars of interventions that help no one other than the health care delivery system.

I feel sorry for Mr. and Mrs. G. It's easy to see how they fell prey to the Flexnerian deception. The fault lies not with them or with the drug and device companies who profit from dogma. The fault lies with the doctors who peddle it deceptively. We should be smarter than that. An Oslerian doctor would be. An Oslerian doctor would have a better understanding of medical science, and about how to best use that science to take care of her patients.

And the fault lies with insurance companies, including Medicare, that don't have the guts to pay doctors more to take care of patients than to push useless and dangerous snake oil on them. Until the payment and medical education systems are changed, doctors will act no differently than the snake oil salesmen of old; science and caring – the best ingredients of a good doctor – easily evaporate in a cloud of well-compensated dogma.

CHAPTER TEN

There's an App for That!

The practitioner too often gets into a habit of mind which resents the thought that opinion, not full knowledge, must be his stay and prop.

– William Osler[1]

One day I was on vacation with my family, and I feared it would rain. Opening the weather app on my phone, I saw a picture of sunshine. The sun would be out all day.

"Looks like it will be a good day after all," I said.

"But it's raining," said my son, as he looked outside and saw dark clouds with pouring rain.

I nodded and smiled. "You must be wrong. Look at the app. Sunny. All day."

It is easy to manipulate numbers so that "facts" proclaimed by technology diverge sharply from reality. Whoever designed the weather app on my phone inputted certain data to generate an "accurate" forecast. Somehow, it just didn't work. To most of us who live in a world of common sense, if our weather app says it's sunny and we look outside to see rain, we'll believe our view through the window.

Sadly, medical science is not as easy for most of us to decipher. The multiple apps and protocols and calculators designed to help doctors determine the best course of treatment are not more reliable than my phone's weather app, and far too often these "scientifically impeccable" tools show sunshine when it's raining. Unfortunately, Flexnerian doctors are not trained to look out the window. They rely on numbers and calculations, even if such information is contrary to the best interest of their patients, something they would know if they took the Oslerian approach of actually talking with patients and being guided by their unique circumstances.

An app is only as good as the inputted information used to derive its calculations. Put in limited or dubious data, and what the app spits out will be inaccurate. Most doctors have no idea what data are used to create the protocols and calculators upon which they rely as verified gospel. For instance, if a doctor uses a calculator to determine whether a statin will help her elderly patient prevent a heart attack, she will believe the calculator's assessment even if the studies upon which the calculator bases its conclusions are all conducted on young people with existing heart disease. If the patient complains of leg pain from the statins, the doctor's calculator may state that such pain is very rare, even though in this particular patient it happens to really exist.

In fact, if the doctor listened to the patient and kept up with medical science instead of relying on numbers generated by a flawed calculator, she would know that the statins most likely triggered the patient's pain, and that statins in someone her patient's age have no demonstrable benefit at all.

At a recent conference I attended, a speaker proclaimed that as doctors "we must manage by facts and not feelings." Facts, of course, are numbers and data. Feelings are what a patient tells us; the subjective stuff that we can't measure. This speaker – perhaps inadvertently – repudiated the very essence of Osler's philosophy in favor of an impersonal, numbers-driven approach to patient care, the very core of what Flexner has stamped upon our medical system.

At the same conference, another doctor quoted Einstein (but it is likely someone else said this): "Not everything that counts can be counted and not everything that can be counted counts."

A quick story.

We have talked about atrial fibrillation (afib) and the risks and benefits of using blood thinners (anticoagulants, such as Coumadin or Eliquis) to prevent strokes; there are small risks and small benefits of these drugs, and they vary based on the particular health, age, and characteristics of the patient. At the very same conference, one of the speakers pulled out a calculator and showed how a simple tool can enable a doctor to determine the precise risk of stroke in someone with afib, and how much that risk will be mitigated with a blood thinner. Now all nuance evaporates in the absolutism of an app.

It takes a good Oslerian to ascertain who may or may not benefit from these medicines because there is so much variability to their use. But doctors now have calculators that spit out the precise risk of stroke if a patient does not take a blood thinner, the assumption being that stroke risk will be fully remediated if they just take the pill. The calculator does not determine risks of the drug – such as bleeding in the brain – nor does it take into account factors that may escalate those risks. But it has become the mainstay for doctors to scientifically and precisely tell a patient why the blood thinner is necessary and lifesaving. Sadly, like the weather app, what is spit out from the calculator often diverges sharply from reality. The app is constructed by using selective studies, by looking at strokes that are not clinically relevant, by focusing on people not likely to bleed or likely to benefit, by eliminating the elderly (to whom the majority of blood thinners are prescribed), and by minimizing risk. Some patients clearly would be more harmed than helped by blood thinners, but the calculator says otherwise. Relying on a weather app without looking out the window is bad science and bad medicine.

In her excellent book, *Weapons of Math Destruction*, author and mathematician Cathy O'Neil discusses the dangers of inputting flawed data into an algorithm and hoping that the calculated result will be accurate.[2] Although she does not study any health care data, her observations are germane to what is occurring in the medical field today: inaccurate science is trumping patient-centered care, as doctors increasingly rely on apps, calculators, clinical practice guidelines, and protocols rather than on the fine art of individualizing treatment to each patient based on a knowledge of that patient and the most relevant and verifiable medical science. "Models are, by their very nature, simplifications. No model can include all of the real world's complexity or the nuance of human communication. Inevitably, some important information gets left out," says O'Neil.

Osler, or even Einstein, could not have said it better.

Mathematical models are weighed down by inevitable error caused by selective data input. In medicine, the designers of such models select which studies to include in their calculators (a blood pressure app may use SPRINT study data but ignore other studies that contradict SPRINT), which endpoints those studies will look at (all strokes rather than disabling strokes), and how to measure the outcome (50 percent vs. 6 out of 1,000). "A model's blind spots reflect the judgments and priorities of its creators," O'Neil says.

Because input is invariably distorted, and because protocols and calculators are not transparent (those who use them do not understand how they work or who programmed them or even what was inputted into them), these scientific tools have become dangerous; they are viewed as absolute and dogmatic, and carry more weight than reality itself.

The afib calculators are a perfect example of illogic. Given the tiny benefit of blood thinners in preventing stroke, a caring and thinking doctor would never in her right mind tell a patient that he is going to get a stroke if he does not take them. How in God's name is that patient-centric or accurate? The calculator does not accurately distinguish an older patient who falls from a younger patient with multiple risk factors for stroke, does not determine the risk of bleeds in someone who has bled before, does not even acknowledge that most blood thinner studies exclude elderly patients and many others, such as people who have bled or who have poor balance or who have had any reaction to blood thinners in the past.[3] Rather, it bases its results on flawed and selective studies while generalizing its results to everyone.

On top of that, the calculator looks at all strokes, and does not distinguish between clinically apparent strokes (ones of which we are aware) and those that are a mere blip on a CT scan. When a doctor's calculator spits out that her patient has a 27 percent risk of having a stroke in the next three years if he does not take a blood thinner, what kind of stroke is she talking about? The calculator does not tell us. Nor does it tell us other ways to mitigate stroke risk. Is a healthy man who exercises and eats well and whose parents lived into their 90s at the same risk as an obese smoker? What about someone who had a stroke already while on the blood thinner? Apps like this provide limited conclusions, have limited generalizability, and tend to exaggerate benefit and minimize risk.

And yet, the calculator has become a dogmatic god in the determination of treatment for afib, an unassailable tool that provides patients with a precise way to determine if they should take a certain medicine. In fact, it almost invariably demands that the patient take the drug. It doesn't get more Flexnerian than that!

Osler stressed the uniqueness and complexity of each patient, and the danger when quick fixes are applied. Medical apps such as the afib calculator do not allow for such thoughtful and individualized care. They are blind to nuance, patient variability, patient choice, and real outcomes. What is needed is a discussion between doctor and patient, not a calculated result that leads to a robotic response by a doctor who barely cares about the patient sitting in front of her. Such a doctor does not look out the window and see rain clouds; she stares at her calculator and sees only sun.

O'Neil says, "To create a model, then, we make choices about what's important enough to include, simplifying the world into a toy version that can be easily understood and from which we can infer important facts and actions." And she says that these models "tend to favor efficiency. By their very nature, they feed on data that can be measured and counted."[4]

That is why we are throwing so many people on so many medicines that have a tiny actual benefit and telling them that they will die if they don't take the pills. That is why we are putting so many people through so many tests that are "absolutely necessary lest they die," and why we have convinced the public that medical interventions are lifesaving and necessary, when in fact they likely are not. Protocols and algorithms are deceptive, and they almost always favor doing more, likely a ramification of the selective data inputted by those who seek a preordained output.

Models are most dangerous when they are expanded to large scale, when they become national protocols or the accepted status quo.[5] In the context of afib, if a protocol causes one person to die of bleeding, that is bad enough. But if we put millions of vulnerable patients on blood thinners, despite the risk of bleeding, we have created a catastrophe.

We saw this poignantly with COVID-19. Virtually every projection about COVID-19's course, every bit of "proof" that drove our policymakers and doctors to declare what must be done to curb its spread, every declaration of what was scientifically valid and what was not, was calculated by a model. Epidemiologists input selective information into models; some ("masks save x number of lives per 1,000 people who use them") were pure speculation and have no scientific basis, others were far too generic and thus misleading. What these models spit out was perceived through the eyes of the press and our medical leaders as being scientifically derived and unassailable, when in truth it was just as inaccurate and misleading as a bad weather app. The reality of COVID-19 was far from what the models were telling us, but we as a society did not look out the window, we just kept looking at the app, even as it was proven to be wrong over and over again. The result was devastating.

Medical protocols and calculators often become national standards, to which all doctors must adhere, in the form of "quality indicators." In this new medical era of "quality and value," much of physician pay is based on our adherence to protocols to prove we are following quality guidelines. We are expected to have all people with afib on anticoagulants. We are expected to put all people with thin bones (osteoporosis) on medicines to strengthen their bones. We are supposed to put all people with a calculator-derived "high" risk of having a heart attack in the next 10 years on statins. We are expected to push all people's blood pressure below a 120 systolic reading because the model tells us their chance of stroke will be reduced. The lists go on and on. Patient nuance, variability, and preference are not part of these dogmatic protocols. Doctors who speak with their patients, who treat their patients as individuals rather than as points of data, who are cognizant of side effects of interventions, who give their patients choices, are likely to be penalized by insurance companies that demand "quality" care, by lawyers who view protocols as standard of care, and by patients who believe that such doctors are not thorough.

Hence, it is better to overtreat, overtest, and not talk with our patients about the pros and cons of interventions if there is a protocol or calculator that has already told us what to do.

Poor Osler. He would have had a stroke if he saw all this transpiring, even if he were put on a blood thinner.

Models harbor another flaw that makes them dangerous: measuring their success based on a few good results. O'Neil uses the example of stop and frisk as a way to show this. In New York, Mayor Michael Bloomberg sanctioned a policy whereby people who looked suspicious to the police (Black, poor, dressed a certain way, living in certain neighborhoods, hanging out with certain people) could be stopped by police and frisked even if they had not exhibited any suspicious behavior. Says O'Neil, stop and frisk "is built on a simple and destructive calculation. If police stop one thousand people in certain neighborhoods, they'll uncover, on average, one significant suspect and lots of smaller ones ... Even if the hit ratio is minuscule, if you give yourself enough chances you'll reach your target ... If stopping six times as many people led to six times the number of arrests, the inconveniences and harassment suffered by thousands and thousands of innocent people was justified."[6]

In other words, if we put thousands of people on blood thinners or statins or bone-density medicines or high-dose blood pressure medicines, and if one or two of those people avoid a bad outcome, then we have succeeded, according to biased goals. As with stop and frisk, which uses relative numbers to claim success (we found six times as many criminals using this method than we would have found otherwise), the absolute number of people helped is puny, and the amount of people harmed and forced to endure interventions of dubious benefit is huge. But we'll proclaim success if just a few people benefit.

To determine the validity of an algorithm, its designers typically choose an outcome measure that is easily calculated and easy to obtain, even if clinically irrelevant. Often it is a surrogate outcome, such as lowering cholesterol, preventing all strokes or all spine fractures, or lowering A1c. When surrogate outcomes become the measure of success of an algorithm or calculator or protocol, the result is that doctors and patients are deceived into thinking the intervention works much better than it actually does. And, of course, most medical models don't look at the negative ramifications incurred by the aggressive intervention.

Tellingly, we use a model to choose the very medical students who likely would comply with models. Based on Flexner's medical education model created in 1911, to which we still adhere today, medical students are picked based largely on their ability to memorize and regurgitate obscene amounts of scientific information. We're not talking about relevant medical science comprehension and problem-solving skills, we're talking about scientific facts in physics, chemistry, biology, and organic chemistry that all can be looked up and need not be memorized.

One of the most significant factors in medical school admissions is the MCAT (Medical College Admissions Test), a model-created exam that purports to be able to measure scientific competency through a marathon-length standardized test, again focusing on memorizing huge quantities of information and spitting it back in a one-right-answer multiple-choice format. There is no nuance on the MCAT. No answers that can be right or wrong based on circumstance. It is yes or it is no. People who think too deeply or see many possible right answers fare poorly on the MCAT. People who see the world as black and white, right and wrong, do well. So, students are chosen in a way that discourages critical thinking, discourages assessing answers based on variable situations, and encourages blindly following what they are told and repeating it back in the exact format that is expected of them. In other words, medical students are chosen by a model to make them more amenable to believing models. It's brilliant.

The MCAT is a big moneymaker for the testing companies and thus is hard to dismantle. But there is a more profound reason that medical schools rely on this one test: it provides schools with a single discrete data point – a test score – that is sold as being objective and a good way of comparing students with each other. The fact that it is not predictive of medical acumen is not important; that is too soft and unmeasurable an endpoint. Rather, the MCAT has been validated in a self-serving way that makes it look sound: students who do well on the MCAT are also likely to do well on other standardized tests throughout medical school and beyond.[7] Utilizing scores on a standardized test to validate performance on another standardized test is self-selecting for people good at taking multiple-choice tests. Hence, we pick students who are good one-right-answer multiple-choice thinkers, the very type of doctors who are apt to rely on Flexnerian calculators and protocols.

All model-based apps can be validated in that way. An afib calculator is always right if our endpoint is all strokes and if we don't consider bleeds and bad outcomes in our equation. Once the model veers from clinical significance, once we assess it based on meaningless criteria, it will always succeed.

And now another story about afib told in the context of our oft-touted afib calculator. MM has afib and is on a blood thinner. Her cardiologist told her that she would get a stroke if she stopped it. His calculator documented a risk of stroke that was very high unless she took the "necessary and lifesaving" blood-thinning pills. At least three times, MM developed a major bleed, sending her to the hospital, and after each episode the cardiologist called me begging me to put her back on her blood thinner.

"She could get a stroke any day," he said to me. "Her calculated risk is higher than 18 percent."

One day I visited her apartment, and she was bleeding again, badly. I told her we would try to keep her out of the hospital, but that she had to go off her blood thinner and never go back on it. Even though I explained that the risk of a disabling stroke was low, she insisted that I call her cardiologist right then and there because he had scared her so much about getting an imminent stroke as soon as she stopped the medicine. This is a gross simplification of my conversation, but it's accurate.

"She is bleeding again," I said to her cardiologist. "We have to stop this medicine, it's not worth it."

"Her risk of stoke is well over 20 percent if we stop it," he said to me. "We just can't do that."

"She has a higher chance of bleeding," I shot back.

"No," he said. "According to the calculator, her bleeding risk is not significant, less than 1 percent."

"Actually," I said. "It's 100 percent, because she's bleeding right now."

"No," he said. "I don't know where you got that number, my calculator says otherwise."

"But she's bleeding even as we speak!" I insisted.

"I don't think so," he said. "Her risk of bleeding is low. I'm worried about a stroke."

There it was. The app told him that his patient would not bleed, so the fact that she was bleeding did not alter his one-right-answer Flexnerian approach to care. This is the current status of medicine today in the United States. Science has been severed from reality. The efficacy of medical interventions is exaggerated and impersonalized through the use of flawed generic weapons of math destruction; the patient has lost her place to the protocol and has been replaced by a number.

Seven years later, MM has not had a stroke and has not bled while off the blood thinner. MM was shocked by her doctor's myopic thinking process in the face of a crystal-clear clinical reality. She shouldn't have been. In this day and age of Flexnerian medicine, that type of thinking is standard operating procedure.

CHAPTER ELEVEN

Whatever Happened to Common Sense?

Common sense in matters medical is rare, and is usually in inverse ratio to the degree of education.

– William Osler[1]

One day during the COVID-19 pandemic, I found a group of men in a park conscientiously standing six feet apart outside and wearing masks. And then each of them pulled out a pack of cigarettes and started smoking. They would slide down the mask just long enough to suck on their cigarette and blow out the smoke. It was quite a scene!

Being the brazen person I am, I approached them.

"Why are you wearing masks outside?" I asked. "And not getting near each other?"

"Just trying to be safe, man," one of them said to me.

I said nothing, just staring at the man's cigarette. He looked at me, then at the cigarette, then at me, and then laughed. "Yeah, I get it," he said. "Doesn't make much sense, does it?"

No it didn't, and he understood that. Unfortunately, for today's Flexnerian-trained doctors, where numbers trump reality far too often, and where calculators and protocols are trusted more than the patient sitting in front of us, common sense has become a lost art and one that doctors don't realize they have lost.

Mr. L had a cough. It was dry and hacking and had been there for months. We dismissed the common and most worrisome culprits. He was on no medicines that could cause cough. He had no other associated symptoms and had no wheezing or sputum. He remained active and was not short of breath. In fact, the cough was not terrible, it was just annoying and would not go away. He was also a lifelong nonsmoker who was in great shape otherwise. Just a bit of diabetes and high blood pressure.

There is always a question about whether to get an X-ray. I mean, what's the big deal? It's just an X-ray. Not much radiation, very little cost. But the real issue is the lack of accuracy of this test. In someone with a low probability of having cancer or infection, X-rays often show findings that prove to be false positives. If those show up – like a nodule or shadow or something like that – we need to do CT scans and sometimes even biopsies before we can prove that there is not a problem. Studies show that even in people with a high probability of having cancer (i.e., smokers), people who get X-rays are more likely to die and be injured by the results of inaccurate testing than will be helped by the test.[2] In someone such as Mr. L, with no worrisome symptoms, a normal exam, and no risk factors for a bad disease, such as cancer, even ordering a simple X-ray deserves some pause. And by the way, X-rays notoriously miss stuff too; people with cancer and infections can often have normal X-rays. So, these are not great tests.

I relay this snippet of information about X-rays because, at least in the Oslerian world, every intervention we toss at our patients has consequences, good and bad, and those need to be contemplated and discussed before we just order a bunch of stuff. We must use common sense, a knowledge of our individual patient, a grasp on the most robust science available that applies to the situation, and a big dose of critical thinking before flooding our patients with tests, medicines, and procedures; that is Oslerian medical care. So, even something as simple as an X-ray needs to be assessed through this lens.

In the Flexnerian world, an X-ray is another data point that helps an impersonal physician-scientist make a decision about treatment. Forget its flaws; you put enough data together, and then you will have the right answer.

One of the most evident deficiencies of Flexner's scientific method, and something I encounter every day in the medical community, is a commonsense gap between a reality staring us in the face and an alternative reality composed of numbers and protocols and models. In a patient without lung symptoms or signs of disease who has an abnormal X-ray, do we believe what we are hearing and seeing with the patient, or do we believe the X-ray? Similarly, in a patient with signs and symptoms of, let's say, pneumonia who has a normal X-ray, do we believe the X-ray and not treat the person, or do we trust what the patient is showing and telling us?

The case of Mr. L illustrates the ramifications that occur when common sense collapses. After a good discussion of risk and benefit, we ordered the X-ray and it was, thankfully, normal. I advised him that the two main causes of a chronic cough are silent postnasal drip and silent acid reflux. Because his symptoms occurred primarily when he lay down at night, and because he often ate dinner late, acid reflux made the most sense. So, we started him on a reflux medicine and behavior modification for a few months to test our theory. I didn't need tests and consultations. My conclusion resulted from talking to Mr. L and using some basic common sense mixed with scientific knowledge about reflux-induced coughing. I told Mr. L I would see him back in two months to ascertain the result of our intervention.

For Mr. L, those were a long two months. Soon after seeing me, he had a routine visit to his cardiologist to follow up on a heart murmur he had for 20 years. He went annually and often received an echocardiogram, for reasons that make no medical sense, but he wanted it anyway. His cardiologist asked about symptoms, and he mentioned the cough.

"Well, maybe it's something else," the cardiologist said. "Let's get a stress test for you."

A stress test? What in the realm of common sense could a stress test possibly reveal that would lead a patient to cough? Even a blocked artery doesn't trigger coughing.

The stress test was mildly abnormal – as so often it is.

"You have to have a heart catheter to see if you have any blockages," the cardiologist told him.

Mr. L had no symptoms to indicate blockages, and even if he had a clogged artery or two, he was already on a statin because of his diabetes. So, he was receiving maximal treatment for any heart blockage. Had they found a blockage in the catheterization, it should not have changed treatment because opening up a blocked artery in someone without symptoms and who is already on a statin is more dangerous than leaving the artery blocked.

He went for the catheter. There was a complication; one of his arteries in his groin bled profusely; the cardiologist thought that was because Mr. L was taking fish oil. Regardless, he had to stay overnight in the hospital. Mr. L was lucky; 1 percent of people who are catheterized get strokes, so it could have been worse. But the hospital itself is potentially dangerous – it's a leading cause of death from medical errors, infections, and overtreatment – and now Mr. L was tossed into another dangerous situation unnecessarily.

Mr. L survived his hospital stay and his groin bleed improved. Unfortunately, his dive in an ocean depleted of common sense did not end there.

"We found a 70 percent blockage in one of your arteries," the cardiologist told him the next morning. "We're going to have to put in a stent."

He was shipped to a nearby teaching hospital where doctors put a stent in a branch of his barely blocked right coronary artery, not a high-risk blockage, and of course, given he was on statins, opening up any blockage would confer no benefit. He left the hospital on very high-dose statins, two antiplatelet agents, and Eliquis. Eliquis? Yes, he had gone into atrial fibrillation (afib) after the stent for a few minutes, and they did not want him to have a stroke.

The risk of his having a major bleed with his current regimen of blood thinners (Eliquis, Plavix, and aspirin) is 7 percent in the first year.[3] The benefit of Eliquis in a man who had a few hours of afib is, well, about the same as a man who had no afib. Most afib after a stent placement resolves on its own, but now his cardiologists told him he would be taking Eliquis for life. He had immediate consequences of his high-dose statin: his legs ached badly, and he was weak. But, when I saw him, he was not upset about all that.

"Thank God for my cough," he told me. "If I didn't have the cough, they wouldn't have discovered the blockage, and they said I could have died of a heart attack at any time. Sometimes fate has a good outcome. There is only one problem."

"What?" I asked him.

"I still have the cough."

I have two cartoons I show my patients. One depicts a doctor looking at a patient who is sitting on an exam table with an arrow through his head. The doctor says, "I think you may be suffering from an arrow in the head, but I want to run a bunch of tests just to make sure."

The second shows a doctor staring at his computer. Behind him is the patient sitting on the exam table with his wife. The man is bleeding everywhere, has arrows in him, a hatchet in him, and looks almost dead. The doctor, who makes no eye contact with the patient, says with alarm: "I am really worried about your cholesterol. We will have to address this immediately."

Although perhaps a bit exaggerated, these cartoons effectively illuminate the commonsense gap that has crippled US health care under a Flexnerian umbrella. Because Flexnerian doctors are more focused on data and testing than on their patients, numbers always trump common sense. Osler was all about the patient. Look at the patient, talk to the patient, understand the patient. Only use medicines and tests if absolutely necessary, because both are burdened by pitfalls that can be injurious, and both can be inappropriate to the individual patient sitting in front of you. Tests are often inaccurate and lead us down very dangerous roads when done inappropriately. Medicines are harmful much of the time with little to no benefit. And yet, often without much thought, doctors flood patients with both, using their brains much less than a robotic measure-and-fix mentality.

Some doctors cry the tears of "defensive medicine" to justify why they test and medicate patients in a way not commensurate with their medical condition: they are trying to avoid a lawsuit. This has some validity. As someone who has recently been sued for not ordering a chest X-ray on a patient without symptoms who subsequently developed lung cancer, and who has had this case linger for almost two years before squandering large chunks of my time and sanity during a two-week trial, I get it. Our system rewards overtesting and overtreating in many ways. We are paid more. Patients think we are more thorough.

And we deflect being targeted by lawyers should an outcome go south.

That is the consequence of breathing in Flexnerian fumes from the moment we enter medical school, from spreading the myth of a test-diagnose-treat philosophy to ourselves and our patients so zealously that it becomes the gauge by which we are judged. In other words, our complete repudiation of Oslerian common sense has created an atmosphere where we are now forced to rely on tests and numbers or else we can be paid less, dinged on quality indicators, and sued. It is self-defeating, to say the least.

Common sense lapses are everywhere across the Flexnerian landscape.

I witness doctors ordering cholesterol levels on people every year, even though patients are already on cholesterol medicines and would not benefit from being on any more, or they aren't on cholesterol medicines and refuse to take them, or they are not at high risk of disease and the cholesterol level is irrelevant to their particular situation.

I see doctors ordering bone density scans every two years on women who explicitly say that they would not take medicine for osteoporosis even if it were discovered.

I watch doctors order annual stress tests and echocardiograms and carotid ultrasounds (on their own machines, of course, which is very lucrative), even though their patients already are on maximal medicine for any problems that may be uncovered and even though they are having no symptoms.

I see urologists ordering PSA blood tests even as they tell the patient, "It's not a very good test."

I see doctors treating patients in the emergency department for high blood pressure with strong medicines, even though they showed up there with bruised bones and never had high blood pressure before. Does it take a medical degree to understand that blood pressure goes up when people are in pain? Why would a doctor in an emergency department who does not know the patient feel compelled to treat a transient elevation in blood pressure that common sense tells us is caused by pain and science tells us is the wrong thing to do? Why is their only lens that of number-fixing when even the data tell us that it is best to leave the pressures alone?[4] Because, in a system where numbers trump patients, doctors lack common sense.

Take the case of Ms. D. She was having diarrhea. She was on two medicines that cause diarrhea. But rather than address that, her gastroenterologist ordered copious tests on her blood and bowel movements, performed a colonoscopy, and started restricting her diet. She then lost weight. That made her diarrhea seem more serious. She had two CT scans, and then an upper endoscopy.

When she saw me, I stopped the two medicines. One was Aricept, the pebble-like memory medicine we have already discussed. The other was Metformin, a very good diabetes medicine that, unfortunately, can cause diarrhea.

"How are we going to treat mom's diabetes now?" her daughter asked me.

"Well," I said with a smile. "We may not have to. She lost so much weight, she may have cured it herself."

How is that not simple common sense? Certainly her daughter understood it immediately, and she had no medical degree.

The deprivation of common sense often has tragic consequences. A few years ago, I took as a patient a 35-year-old mother with likely irritable bowel syndrome (IBS), who, before I met her, underwent about six surgeries, saw too many doctors, and became addicted to narcotics from these interventions. She ultimately died from an overdose of her medicines, leaving behind a husband and 11-year-old son – and a raft of medical bills. Any doctor who came to know this unfortunate soul, as I did, would have learned how much stress she was under, how little she tolerated pain, and how many of her symptoms were easily explained or caused by the "fixes" tossed at her. She was lulled onto a train of tests/procedures/medicines to delve into and repair her abdominal pain, was assured that this test or that surgery would fix it, was given drugs to get her past all of her surgeries, and fell deeper and deeper into a pit of no return.

All along, no one addressed her anxiety and low pain threshold, no one reassured her or told her that interventions could make it all worse, no one helped her through what was ultimately not a medically repairable condition. Doctors failed her by convincing themselves and her that if they could just test her enough and fix what they found wrong, then she would be cured. In the end, that process made her more ill and, finally, killed her.

In the mind of Osler, every test we order needs to make sense to the patient sitting in front of us. We must understand what we are looking for, how we would treat anything we might find, what the negative consequences of the test may be, and what the consequence of not getting the test might be.[5] This same rule applies to medical procedures and medications; there are pros and cons to every intervention. Every patient and situation is different. Common sense is crucial to any decision we doctors make; our thinking must involve taking into account the obvious.

For instance, why on earth would we get a routine electrocardiogram for a patient without any symptoms of shortness of breath and who runs marathons, when we know just from talking to the patient that his heart is fine? Why would we check cholesterol on a 90-year-old patient in whom there is no correlation between cholesterol and disease and in whom cholesterol-lowering medicines don't even help, and may well hurt?

If we do an MRI on the backs and knees of people over 70, people who have no pain in those areas, about 85 percent of them will have abnormalities. These include bulging and slipped discs, compression fractures, severe arthritis, and cartilage tears, among others.[6] So, when an elderly patient presents to the office with back and knee pain, what will we gain by doing an MRI? Common sense tells us that it is a worthless test if done without a very specific purpose, which might be ascertained by a history and exam. If people have abnormalities on the test, likely they were there before the pain even started and have nothing to do with the pain. And yet, rather than grasp that bit of common sense and explain it to patients, doctors just order the test much of the time, often leading them down the road of treating a problem that may make the pain worse or trigger something else. These tests cost a fortune, often lead to unnecessary interventions and surgeries, and do not improve the outcome. Where is the common sense in ordering them? Again, by Flexnerian logic, tests provide information, they are necessary, even if common sense may tell us otherwise.

In fact, in older people, virtually any test we order might show an abnormality, so we have to order tests with great care. Even elders who are doing just fine likely have heart valve issues, blocked arteries everywhere, arthritis that does not hurt, nodules and cysts on kidneys and livers, bone compression fractures, osteoporosis, high cholesterol, anemia, thyroid issues, and a lot of skin cancers. None are helped by interventions when patients lack symptoms referable to them. Yet we will look for them even when not indicated, and we will fix what's broken even if it's not improving our patient's health or well-being. Much of the cost and harm inflicted by our health care system is caused by doctors ordering tests that lack all common sense.

Our bodies are riddled with problems we often compensate for or fix ourselves, or sometimes these "problems" (such as high blood pressure in very old people) are our body's attempt to avoid disease (by pushing blood past blocked arteries, for instance, in the case of high blood pressure). And yet, through our Flexnerian glasses, we feel compelled to find and "fix" every problem we encounter, even if common sense and a thorough knowledge of our patient and of science should tell us otherwise.

That is why, thanks to our excessive CT scanning, we have uncovered so many previously unrecognized kidney cancers. In fact, the rate of kidney cancer has quadrupled recently from scans done for other reasons, and yet the death rate from kidney cancer has not improved at all.[7] The same is true for blocked arteries. If we perform carotid ultrasounds on patients without symptoms, we are likely to find blockages as people age. But what does that mean if they are doing well? I have patients where both of their carotid arteries are blocked 100 percent. How is that possible? Because the body is good at bypassing and thus fixing its own blockages. But if we do a test and find a blocked artery, we will feel compelled to fix it ourselves, and the patient will think we have saved their lives. We have done no such thing. We have given the body a new problem – the stent and medicines – for a patient who was doing just fine on his own.

Common sense works the other way too. Sometimes a test shows nothing, but the patient is sick. Sometimes, too, a study will tell us not to intervene, but the patient's presentation tells us otherwise.

Take the case of Mr. F and Mrs. L. Mr. F is a runner who injured his right knee. The injury was more of an irritation at first, and the exam was not revealing. He had no pain with movement of his ligaments or twisting his cartilage, there was no swelling, and he seemed to have good strength. In fact, he could still walk and run well, but it hurt just enough to annoy him, and over the course of weeks and then months, it simply did not go away. After a long discussion, we obtained an MRI, and it showed a small cartilage tear.

"Studies show," I told him, "that the surgical repair of those tears is no better than just waiting. One study compared a group of people who had their cartilage fixed by a scope called an arthroscopy to another group who had pretend repair with an arthroscopy, and both groups did the same after six months. I would suggest we order physical therapy, give you some pain medicine, and let time heal it."

Six months after that, the knee was still hurting; in fact, it was getting worse, and he was less able to engage in his usual activities. But he clung to the study I quoted and would not think about getting an arthroscopy. As with all studies, the generic subjects in the study do not match the patient sitting in front of us. Mr. F was not getting better, and it made sense now to try to fix his cartilage tear. This is true in people with back pain, in people with persistent chest pain, and in people getting weaker and losing weight; sometimes tests, procedures, and medicines can be helpful even if studies claim that they are not. As Osler says, the patient will tell us that.

Mrs. L had a different problem. She had severe abdominal pain and was losing weight. She came to me and various specialists; we ordered labs, scans, and two colonoscopies. "I don't know what you have," I told her, "but it's not cancer." And yet, everything about her presentation smelled of cancer, even if the tests told me otherwise. A year later, when her bowel blocked, a surgeon opened her up and found cancer everywhere. The tests missed it. Sometimes even cancer can be sneaky; it can evade our tests. People can have normal labs, normal scans, and yet the patient is screaming out to us that she has cancer. We ignore her pleas, and instead focus on the test results. And often they lead us astray by being too normal.

Common sense should guide us in the right direction, not the tests we perform. In fact, our tests should only be done to confirm our basic medical instincts or to challenge and supplement our observations. If the tests don't match the patient, we always should follow Osler's prime directive: The patient will tell you the diagnosis. Listen to the patient.

One of my colleagues suggested that we should introduce a course on common sense in medical school. "More to the point," I responded, "We need courses in common sense starting in first grade."

I believe that our entire medical education must be infused with a patient-centric approach rooted in common sense, as William Osler had been doing at Johns Hopkins more than 100 years ago. And that form of thinking, of learning, must continue even after we get out of school.

We need to always ask how interventions can help or hurt our patients, how we can use medical facts and technology in a constructive and commonsense way, and why each patient is unique and thus our interventions must be customized to their particular clinical realities. Common sense begins and ends with the patient. Abnormal numbers, tests, and exam findings mean nothing when viewed apart from the patient. We as doctors need to know how to be judicious, how to explain to our patients when an intervention makes no sense or when it does, and how to ignore abnormalities when our patient is living in peace with them. Our mantra should be what we are taught from day one of medical school: first do no harm. Unfortunately, in our Flexnerian world, that bit of commonsense advice has drifted far from how doctors are treating their patients every day: measuring, diagnosing, and fixing is our dogmatic mission, common sense be damned.

CHAPTER TWELVE

The Drug Epidemic
(It's Not What You Think)

The young physician starts life with twenty drugs for each disease, and
the old physician ends life with one drug for twenty diseases.

– William Osler[1]

Ms. L would not get better, despite the vigilant and devoted
attempts of her two daughters. She was old, as she was quick to tell
you, and had some dementia. She had lots of aches and pains, and
a ton of chronic illnesses: a past heart attack, two stents, osteoporosis, urinary incontinence, high blood pressure, thyroid disease, gastroesophageal reflux disease, arthritis, and poor vision. She had a
poor appetite and was often dozing; a psychiatrist told her daughters that she was depressed. She was being treated for all of these
with more than 20 medicines and supplements. She saw an army
of specialists. Each doctor told the daughters that every medicine
was "necessary and lifesaving." She continued to get tests. At 87
she recently had a colonoscopy, a CT scan of her abdomen, and
a cardiac echocardiogram. She was losing weight. She had belly
pain and diarrhea. Her daughters tried to push her to eat, they

hovered over her, they visited every day, they brought her from doctor to doctor, test to test, and flooded her body with every new medicine and supplement that they or her doctors or their friends could think of. Nothing worked. Ms. L was dying.

After much discussion, Ms. L's daughters agreed to put their mom in hospice; they realized that there was nothing more they could do. I was taken aback early in her hospice course, when we agreed to remove virtually all of her medicines, that one of her daughters asked us to still check her cholesterol levels to make sure that "it wouldn't go too high off the Lipitor," to check blood pressure a few times a day, and to maybe get a bone density measure while she was off Fosamax. We did not do any of those things.

As the weeks and then months passed, Ms. L's daughters continued to visit, but they no longer nagged her to eat or dragged her to doctors. Rather, they sat with her, they talked, and they laughed. And then something amazing happened, something that those of us who practice Oslerian medicine see every day. She got better. She started to eat, she gained weight, her diarrhea resolved, her aching muscles improved. Soon she was walking and was much more animated and mentally sharper.

After about six months, hospice dismissed her. That is when one of Ms. L's daughters said to me something I will never forget: "Now that mom is off hospice, should we check all her labs to see where she is and then start her back on her medicines?"

The benefits of most drugs are vanishingly small, despite medical claims to the contrary. The risks are large because they are cumulative. At least half of Ms. L's drugs increased the risk of falls, of tiredness, of weakness, of worse memory. Many of them caused muscle pain, low blood pressure, depression, appetite suppression, and diarrhea. Ms. L's terminal condition for which she was put on hospice was in effect instigated by pills prescribed in an effort to make her numbers look good and to "fix" her. She was the victim of Flexnerian doctors who touted exaggerated statistics and calculators to buttress their "fix everything" mantra with a religious zeal. Her devoted daughters were also victims, transformed from loving caretakers into the unwitting instruments of their mother's decline.

Many studies have demonstrated the devastating effects of polypharmacy, especially in the elderly. Polypharmacy is simply the consumption of multiple medicines and supplements, typically more than five or six drugs. In the past it was often difficult to convince people to take a drug, and the number of drugs available to take were small, but now the average elder is on almost 10 drugs. This epidemic – and it's a real one – has led to serious health concerns that are the direct effect of Flexnerian thinking.

The issue of polypharmacy was tackled by the Lown Institute's 2019 report on "medication overload."[2] The Lown Institute is a medical think tank in Boston whose primary purpose is to evaluate overtreatment and medical disparity. We are members of Lown's Right Care Alliance. We collectively direct its primary care council, and we in fact met each other and developed ideas for this book at one of its conferences. According to the Lown report, "The epidemic of medication overload is bound to get worse, given the rapid aging of the population and the trend of increasing medication use. Over the next ten years, there will be at least 4.6 million hospitalizations of older Americans and fifteen times as many outpatient visits for side effects from medications. Yet the enormity of the problem is invisible to the vast majority of families and patients, most policymakers, and even many health care professionals."

But what if someone such as Ms. L is on 20 drugs and all of them are *absolutely essential* to her survival according to her doctors? If we stop her Eliquis, she will get a stroke. Stop her Lipitor, she will have a heart attack. Stop her Norvasc and her blood pressure will soar too high and she may die. Stop her Fosamax and her bones will break. That's what Ms. L's daughters thought, because that is what their mom's specialist doctors told them. The alluring trap of a Flexnerian approach is that we can "fix" our patients one number and one organ at a time by dispensing medicines promoted as necessary, lifesaving, and harmless. Studies tell us that once people start taking more than five drugs, then the already tiny benefit of each drug diminishes, and the side effects accumulate. But that did not figure into the numerical calculations made by Ms. L's specialists, each of whom only cared about one of her numbers, one of her organs, not the totality of her as a human being.

Drug company studies exclude people who are older, who have multiple chronic conditions, and who are on too many medicines. Drug companies know: they don't want real patients to cloud their manicured results, and so they invite only ideal patients into their carefully designed studies so that they can "prove" the benefits of what they are peddling. Their results are published in esteemed journals and touted in newspapers and ads as being scientifically valid. No one seeks to look behind the curtain to see how much or whom they help, or what happens when they are tossed into the gut of someone on other drugs or who has other problems.

No wonder we are all taking so many medicines and believe the myth that we are healthier – maybe even alive – thanks to these pills of scientific wonder. After all, look at our numbers; they are so much better, and so we must be so much better too.

According to the Lown report, medication overload will cause the premature deaths of 150,000 older Americans in the next decade and reduce the quality of life for many millions of people, at a cost of $62 billion to our medical system. On a given day, 750 older people are hospitalized from serious side effects of their medicines, and in the past decade 35 million people sought treatment for (and 2 million of them were hospitalized for) adverse medication reactions. More than 40 percent of older adults take 5 or more prescription medicines and 20 percent take 10 or more prescribed drugs. There has been a 300 percent increase in polypharmacy in the past 20 years, which coincides with the increased medical specialization of our society.

The Lown group ascribes this epidemic of polypharmacy to multiple factors. First, in our nation we have developed a culture of prescribing. This is, of course, a consequence of Flexnerian thinking by both doctors and patients. "Advertisements linking prescription medications to happiness and health, the increased medicalization of normal human aging, the hurried pace of medical care, and the desire of both health care professionals and patients to 'do something' have fostered a shared expectation that there is a 'pill for every ill,'" says the Lown report.

The report points to information and knowledge gaps as the second cause of medication overload: "Clinicians and patients lack critical information and skills they need to appraise the evidence and make informed decisions regarding medications." We have shown how data are manipulated to make drugs seem far more beneficial and far less harmful than they actually are.

Finally, the Lown report explores the fragmentation of care as one of the causes: "There is a pervasive lack of communication between a patient's various providers. Often, more prescriptions are written to treat what appears to be a new condition, when in reality prescribers are treating a side effect of another drug. This 'prescribing cascade' can lead to a cycle of debilitation and even death." Much of this is related to our specialized society, where there is a doctor for every organ, and each of those doctors wants to find and fix everything in his or her organ of interest without having any concern for the person as a whole.

In effect, the Lown report describes exactly what happened to Ms. L and to very many other people in our deeply flawed system.

Interestingly, though usually extolling the virtues of medical treatments, Flexnerians often find some drugs to skewer; it happens every few years. As with the medicines they promote as being absolutely good, the ones they demonize are absolutely bad. There is no nuance, no patient-directed assessment of these medicines. In classic multiple-choice thinking, either a medicine is all bad or it's all good. There can only be one right answer.

Two demonized drugs come to mind: opioids and proton pump inhibitors (PPIs). Pharmaceutical companies pushed narcotics upon doctors and patients through deception and subterfuge, and now they are paying for that perfidy. Prescription narcotics have caused a great deal of misery among many, including death and addiction. But such drugs also have a useful role. Many patients, including some who are old and riddled by arthritis, benefit from low doses. Such drugs can be the difference between a life of independence and mobility and one of dependence and misery. It is rare that elderly people get addicted to these drugs, and often opioids are the safest choice to help with pain.

But, because of our all-or-nothing thinking, it has become increasingly difficult for patients to have access to these medicines without feeling as though they are addicts, or for primary care doctors to even prescribe them. Once a drug hits the Flexnerian bad list, there is little that can be done to revive it.

PPIs, such as Prilosec and Nexium, were also massively overprescribed when they came out, both because of a deceptive advertising campaign from drug companies and because they seemed to help the very common problems of acid reflux and gastritis – and peptic ulcer disease – that afflict so many. Despite the fact that many people take these drugs who likely don't need them, and that there are side effects and drug interactions associated with their prolonged use, overall their harm is minimal, and there are certainly people who benefit greatly from them.[3]

But then, after several studies linked these drugs to heart disease, kidney disease, and even dementia, the public clamor for their exorcism prompted many in the medical community to demonize them. The studies were observational and thus could not prove cause and effect. One study, for example, found that more people who had heart disease used PPIs than people without heart disease.[4] But that does not mean that PPIs cause heart disease. People with heart disease tend to smoke more, eat worse, have chest pain, use drugs that cause stomach irritation, and thus are more likely to have acid reflux and gain some benefit from PPIs. Thus, there is no cause and effect between these drugs and heart disease, only an association. One may say that heart disease causes people to take these drugs, not the other way around.

Still, the media expunged that nuance and declared that PPIs cause heart disease. All of the sudden, people who benefited from these drugs stopped taking them. It is not a question of a drug being all bad or all good; it is one of degree and utility. That subtlety is lost in the Flexnerian mindset that stresses one-right-answer thinking. Once the drug was declared to be bad, the medical community pounced on it. After all, it looks good in the public eye if overprescribers assail a few drugs here and there. That makes it seem that they are being conscientious stewards of medication use.

Supplements and over-the-counter remedies, also overused, are another target of doctor-prescribers who equate them to glorified placebos. Recently one of my patients asked his neurologist

162 | A Return to Healing

if he could try medical cannabis for Parkinson's. The neurologist nearly had a seizure, telling the patient that it was akin to witchcraft to use treatments that have no verifiable efficacy. The neurologist then prescribed that same patient Exelon for his "dementia," somehow feeling comfortable using a drug that has been shown not to work, while rejecting a treatment about which the jury is still out.

Most supplements and alternative treatments are barely regulated and not well studied.[5] However, some have been beneficial to my patients because they either work or have a placebo effect. As with all drugs, supplements need to be assessed as best we can through whatever information we can gather. It is unlikely they will ever be well studied because pharmaceutical companies monopolize all drug research in this country, and the last thing they want to do is show the benefit of a supplement. The makers of Namenda (for memory) tried that a long time ago by comparing their drug with vitamin E, and when people on vitamin E did better than those on Namenda, the study was buried and will never be repeated. Although prescription drugs do have more science through which to evaluate them, much of the research is not valid and is deceptive.

In the end, pills of all sorts must be viewed with skepticism. We escaped the era of patent-medicine salesmen and snake oil doctors, but in many ways we are right back in the same conundrum. All medicines, whether drugs or supplements, should be looked at objectively. Very few have significant benefits, some can cause harm, and the accumulation of too many of them is typically dangerous. Each patient is unique, and so too must be our treatment of them. Pills are never the entire answer; they are just as often the problem as the solution.

CHAPTER THIRTEEN

Flexner and the Care of the Elderly

Frankly to confess ignorance is often wiser than to beat about the bush with a hypothetical diagnosis.

– William Osler[1]

An elderly patient named Ms. R called our office somewhat upset: "I just looked at my labs, the labs that the doctor said were normal, and everything looks off. It says I have stage 3 kidney disease, that I have an abnormal MCV (whatever that is, but I bet it's important), that my sugar is too high, and that I have high cholesterol. How can that be normal? It seems to me that I'm falling apart."

From a Flexnerian standpoint she was indeed falling apart. All the numbers that our doctors use to gauge someone's health naturally change as people age. In fact, most of them become quite abnormal because the "normal" range of numbers is typically determined by studies conducted with younger people. In what medical guru Nortin Hader describes as the "medicalization of aging," we ascribe diagnoses, perform tests, and prescribe treatments for changes (both numerical and clinical) that are normal and common as people age.[2] Instead of enabling and facilitating a person's healthy aging process, instead of helping them to be more functional and happier as they age, we simply make them feel sicker. We label them with diseases, such as Ms. R's phantom kidney condition, and then send them to specialists and flood them with medicines. The average older person is on a mountain of medicines and supplements, virtually none of which has been proven to be helpful at their age, and virtually all of which have deleterious side effects that can be life-altering. The average older person is also exposed to seemingly endless tests and procedures to investigate "abnormalities" that likely are normal for them, interventions that cause far more harm and angst than benefit.

Several salient facts about numbers should give us a great deal of pause when we pursue Flexner's logic in diagnosing, testing, and treating elderly people. For one thing, we don't know what normal numbers are in the elderly. Some studies give us insight, but virtually every study is conducted on young healthy people. What is the ideal blood pressure in a 90-year-old? What about sugar, kidney function levels, blood counts? What if someone feels better with a higher pressure or sugar, and what if "fixing" those numbers makes them feel worse?

We also know that numbers vary widely from person to person, and even within the same person. An elderly person might have a very low blood pressure while eating breakfast, and then have a "dangerously high" pressure after falling and breaking a rib. Never mind that the low pressure may have caused the fall; when the patient enters the emergency department, her blood pressure is so high that they want to treat it immediately, thus exacerbating her problems. Numbers fluctuate more in the elderly, and when we act rashly to fix something, we often trigger a cascade of woe. Geriatrics is the act of slow care, of contemplative care, of minimizing medical assaults on the body and accommodating change.[3] It is palliative, focusing more on a person's concerns, symptoms, and functions than erratic and ill-defined numerical abnormalities largely defined in the young. In fact, palliative care in the elderly typically translates to a longer life and a better life, the very antithesis of the Flexnerian ethos of aggressive number-based care.[4]

As our bodies age and break down, we are very good at repairing ourselves. Thus, we may have several blocked blood vessels that we already bypassed, and we are keeping our blood pressure higher to get through some of the others. Our back may be riddled with arthritis, but we find ways of accommodating. We can always find abnormal measurements in older people. In fact, certain numbers, such as body mass index (BMI) and cholesterol, actually increase in healthy elders and decline in sick older people, so they are hardly a predictor of illness. The question we always have to ask is, What do they mean, and should we even care?

Think about Bernie Sanders's heart attack. Do stents work for acute blockages in elders like they do in younger people? Some studies suggest not, and virtually all studies are conducted in the young.[5] We have already discussed how most studies of statins and of blood thinners are conducted in people under 70, whereas most prescriptions for these drugs are written for people over 70. The few studies of these drugs done with the elderly demonstrate less efficacy and far more side effects. Pharmaceutical companies understand what they are doing when they study the young and market to the old, but Flexnerian-oriented doctors don't, and thus they focus on number normalization and not on patient care that is age-appropriate.

Dementia tells us a bit about the Flexnerian approach to medical care for the elderly. We have medicalized dementia and made it seem so scientific that we can divide it into discrete and precise diagnoses – Pick's disease, frontal-temporal dementia, Lewy body dementia, Alzheimer's – and we have various drugs and drug combinations to fix it all. A patient's husband recently approached me, after I took his wife off Aricept because of lack of efficacy and side effects, and handed me an article that "proved" that dementia drugs work because they fix cognition. The lead investigator stated, "Our results provide strong support for current recommendations to treat people with Alzheimer's disease with cholinesterase inhibitors."[6] When I looked at the article, out of a memory test score of 0 to 30, these drugs on average improved the test score by 0.18! In fact, in the study just as many people suffered a progression of their dementia as placebo. To make it worse, the study controlled for no other variables, and we know that people who tend to take these drugs are also more likely to exercise, eat correctly, socialize, and have the social supports that improve outcome in dementia. Hence, this study twisted data and mangled facts to "prove" something that was false, claiming that we can fix discretely defined forms of dementia with medicines that somehow improve memory testing. That doctors believe such findings blindly without using the arts of common sense and critical thinking – without realizing that a tiny bump in memory test scores for a brief period of time does not translate into meaningful clinical success – says a great deal about how their Flexnerian brains are programmed. They want to be able to fix the unfixable, and numerical success allows them to claim victory on that score.

We spend $5 billion a year on dementia medicines, a price tag likely to escalate since the FDA approved Leqembi, which, using Flexner's language, improves definable abnormalities – amyloid plaque in the brain, which is a surrogate marker, with a tiny bump on the memory score – but does not help people with dementia in any meaningful way. And it leads to brain bleeds. But because we are so focused on medicalizing aging, in labeling dementia as a physiological condition defined by memory tests and plaque deposition, we can peddle drugs to treat these definable numbers – many of which are abnormal in people without dementia – and claim success, something that appeals to doctors and likely will lead to tens of billions of dollars of sales and tens of billions of dollars of hospital bills to deal with the medicine's pernicious side effects, but no improvement in anyone's life or cognition.

We spend billions more to diagnose causes of dementia, all sorts of labs and scans that doctors repeat over and over again, even though a good history and physical exam would negate the benefit of virtually all those tests; only 6 out of 1,000 tests for dementia show a reversible cause, and most of those are done at the primary care doctor's office.[7] Entire industries and professions revolve around diagnosing and treating dementia by viewing it through the Flexnerian lens.

And yet, it is all an illusion. Many people simply become forgetful when they age. Others do develop dementing illness. But all this measurement, all this precision, all this specialization, all these drugs have not helped anyone to get better. In fact, if anything, they impede the acceptance and normalization of aging and turn it into irrelevant measurements and false hope.

In 1965, when President Lyndon Johnson launched Medicare, there was no diagnosis of dementia on the books. No Alzheimer's. No Pick's disease. No Lewy body dementia. It's not that these diseases are brand new, it's just that society did not feel the need back then to medicalize something that was common and untreatable by doctors. When people became more forgetful as they aged – it was part of aging. That's just what happened. Lots of stuff happens. I mean, we can devise medical diagnoses and treatments for wrinkles, for hair loss, for being tired and

lol

sleeping poorly, for peeing too much, for constipation, for joint pain, for shaky hands. Guess what? We have. We literally have diagnoses for every symptom that affects us as we age. We label every symptom as being a manifestation of a disease, a new diagnosis; we have tests for each one, specialists, drugs, and procedures. Everything that happens to us as we age, everything we used to think was normal and expected, is just one more notch in our long list of illnesses with which we must now contend. Yes, we have medicalized aging. And now, everyone thinks that he or she is sick because that is the very ethos, the business model, of our Flexnerian medical society: to make you ill and promise you a cure, to measure you and then fix those measurements we deem to be aberrant.

There are treatments for dementia that work. Exercise, good diet, and stress reduction have been shown to prevent memory loss and slow progression of dementia. Acceptance of memory loss by caregivers, love and compassion even when people get confused, and socialization all help the patient with memory loss and their loved ones. But in our quest to define memory loss numerically and then treat it with drugs, we rarely tread down that road. Our medical system does not pay for adult day care, for home health aides, for exercise programs, for caregiver education and help. No, it pays for drugs and tests, and ascribes a diagnosis to every aspect of our mental decline. This is why Flexnerian medical care does not facilitate aging. It causes accelerated anxiety, polypharmacy, and excessive specialization. It will not acknowledge an acceptance of aging that is compassionate and effective.

What might Dr. Osler have said to someone who presents to his office with memory loss?

"You are right, Ms. B, you are getting more forgetful, it's very common at your age so don't stress about it. There is no cure for it, and no tests that will help us beyond what we have already done; knowing a score on a memory test like your friend told you about is not going to make anything better or change what we can do. But there are things you can do to help. Write everything down. Get help from your son with things that are hard for you to do. Take some long walks. Start writing a journal; write down the story of your life for your grandkids. Try something new, something like drawing; there's a great class at the senior center. And get rid of all that bread and pasta you are eating. There's a better way to eat to really make you feel better, and I'll tell you about it. And you can still have your apple pie! Don't worry, Ms. B; worry is the worst thing you can do. This happens to a lot of people. But, along with your son and your friends and family, I promise we will get you through this."

No new labels of illness. No tests. No drugs. Just compassion and a lot of common sense.

And it's not like the Osler who just spoke with Ms. B did not know his science. He knew it quite well. He understood that labels do not help us take care of our patients, that in fact most diagnoses are too broad to be of value because each individual patient manifests his or her memory loss quite differently and thus doesn't fall into one precise category, that tests don't guide better treatment, that the drugs don't work, that exercise/diet/ stress reduction/socialization/mental exercise are the most effective means of helping curb memory loss and dementia, and that reassurance and compassion are the best treatments of all. He knew his science well. He just didn't flaunt it. He cared about his patient, and he showed that.

Let's meet Mr. P, who, sadly, did not benefit from the Oslerian script. His doctor worried about his numbers; he had some decline in his kidney numbers and was followed closely by his kidney doctor for many years. That doctor was keeping a close eye on him and was very thorough; lab tests every two months, an ultrasound twice a year. "He told me to eat less protein," Mr. P said, but he was not sure which foods contain protein, so he stopped eating fish. Every visit the nephrologist sat with Mr. P and his daughter and told him that he was getting close to needing dialysis. They put a specialized IV line in his chest. They brought him to dialysis classes. And then, they decided it was time.

The problem is that Mr. P, who was in his mid-80s, was not at all ill. He walked five miles a day and enjoyed time with his girlfriend. He had an active social life in an over-50 community; he loved it there. With dialysis, his daughter uprooted him from all that and moved him 30 miles away, to an assisted-living facility with a dialysis unit attached to it. He never saw his girlfriend again.

Because of the strain on his body caused by dialysis, and by moving away from the life he loved, Mr. P deteriorated rapidly. He became more withdrawn and morose; he joked and laughed when I first met him, but that trait evaporated, as did his energy. Each day after dialysis, he fell asleep, and the next day he was weak and tired. He stopped his daily walks. He ate less and lost weight. He was seen by more specialists, told he was depressed, given medicine for that, more blood pressure medicine, medicine for his bone density, told to use a walker; it seemed to never end. One day he went for a simple procedure – the placement of a shunt in his arm to make dialysis easier – and he died. In a sense, kidney disease did kill him, but not because of the disease itself.

When I had first met Mr. P, I looked over his numbers, the ones that everyone was so worried about, the ones that pushed him into dialysis. "I'm telling you, a lot of my patients have worse numbers than you and are worse off than you, but I tell them they are just fine," I said to him. "Why the hell are they putting you through all of this?"

He just shrugged and said, "Well, that's what my doctor says I have to do."

If we were to test and examine older people thoroughly, we would find sickness everywhere.[8] Even with elders without any symptoms, MRIs make them look like they are on death's door. If we look at carotid or heart blood vessels, we will find blockages. All my elderly patients have fluctuations in blood pressure and a ton of abnormal labs. Most have bacteria in their urine. Most have cysts or masses on many of their organs. A good number of men have prostate cancer that's just sitting there. Almost everyone has at least one skin cancer somewhere on their body. They have cataracts, even though they may be seeing just fine. They all have some heart irregularities. Should we treat all of these? Should we monitor them with more tests and specialist visits? You test them for one thing, you end up finding 10 more problems.

If we look at the elderly thoroughly through a Flexnerian lens, there will be no end to tests, diagnoses, and treatments we feel compelled to offer. That is exactly what is happening in our society, and it feeds the medical system hundreds of billions of dollars a year. Not only does this dance tear the guts out of my healthy elderly patients who now believe they are beset by copious illnesses that need surveillance and treatment, but it's also tearing Medicare to shreds by financing a destructive and expensive health care philosophy geared to fixing numbers and not to taking care of patients.

Half of the elderly are on statins, and there's no evidence they work. There is evidence of increase in the risk of falls and aches. Elderly people are being aggressively treated for blood pressure, which makes them dizzy and forgetful and tired and prone to falls. We have so many elderly people on novel blood thinners, such as Eliquis, which barely work in people this age, but can cause lethal bleeds, especially if they are prone to falling. The list goes on and on. What is even worse, when an older person develops a side effect from a medicine, far too often she is shipped to a doctor who labels that side effect as another disease and instigates even more testing and treatment. This prescribing cascade triggers polypharmacy, which may be the most toxic and deadly disease from which far too many elders suffer. We as a medical society are simply unwilling to allow our elders to age gracefully and be free of stress. Instead we carve them up into diseases and they become our most vulnerable – and profitable – victims of Flexner's legacy.

It's always instructive to take a step back and realize that in the areas of the world where people live the longest – where there are no doctors filling up people's charts with diagnoses and deluging them with tests, procedures, specialist visits, and medicines – elders age well. They remain active, they eat healthy diets, and their every complaint is not viewed as a license to test-diagnose-fix. These are the Blue Zones – Ikaria in Greece, Okinawa, and Costa Rica.

All elders have some symptoms. They hurt, they have urinary difficulties, their balance worsens, they are tired and more forgetful, and, yes, they have wrinkles. But these are not amenable to medical cures. To aggressively lower blood pressure, sugar levels, and cholesterol; to carefully follow kidney function and to perform sophisticated tests and procedures on people who urinate too much; to think we can lick memory loss if we hit it with enough tests and drugs; to fix abnormalities in the knee that have been there for 20 years; to measure and "fix" bone density while not preventing falls – in all this we are not helping them stay alive longer or to live better lives. We are doing just the opposite. We are adding to their anxiety, their misery, and their disability. We are making them sick.

Thank goodness Medicare enabled our elders to get care when they need it, something to which they had limited access before 1965. Now, though, it encourages and pays for a quest to fix aging itself, to identify every problem and to finance expensive treatment for them even without proof of efficacy. Many of Medicare's quality guidelines were scripted by specialist societies that have a vested interest in making as many people as sick as possible. So, now Medicare is sinking under its own Flexnerian weight. At its inception in 1965, there was no dementia. Now dementia is a rampant illness, broken down into multiple, more specific diagnoses, instigating unnecessary tests and specialist visits, and pushing handfuls of medicines into trusting seniors. The outcome of dementia is no better now than it was in 1965. People aren't living longer or better. They are feeling sicker. And Medicare is going bankrupt in the process.

When we impose Flexner's medical strategy on the elderly, the results are disastrous. Measuring and testing everything, labeling people's normal aging processes as diseases, using treatments that have never been shown to work in an older population of people, relying on generic protocols and calculators instead of listening to and responding to the patient individually; these are barbaric techniques.

Virtually no studies include the elderly, and for good reason; the pharmaceutical companies that design and sponsor the studies know that their drugs won't work. They know that their devices and surgical treatments don't work either. They know that fixing numbers and repairing broken body parts do no good. So, no one studies the elderly. They don't have to; Flexnerian doctors will test and treat older people even without any proven benefit of their pursuit. And hopeful and frightened patients are willing participants in that charade. There is no compassion and common sense in much of what we do in our care of the elderly. Only cost.

CHAPTER FOURTEEN

Shared Decision-Making in a Flexnerian World

There are only two sorts of doctors: Those who practice with their brains, and those who practice with their tongues.

– William Osler[1]

A nurse and I were looking through the medicine list of a new patient admitted to our nursing home. The man was on five pages of the usual array of medicines: blood thinners, aspirin, statins, bone density medicine, two blood pressure medicines, two dementia medicines, an antidepressant, two medicines for his prostate, six vitamins/supplements (D, fish oil, probiotics, multivitamin, eye vitamin, turmeric), and several more. The nurse just shook her head.

"Doesn't anyone know that these medicines don't work?," she said.

"Tell me about it," I said. "But I'm not his doctor. He's just here to recover from his hip fracture."

She laughed. "Well you don't have to be a brain surgeon to figure out why he got a hip fracture. Who can walk with all this poison flying through his blood? I guess the Fosamax didn't work this one time to stop him from breaking his hip. Another promise broken I guess."

She was pleasantly cynical.

Then she told me a story. Her father was in a hospital in Florida and was quite sick. He had dementia and was living with help at home. When she arrived, she saw that the hospital doctors had started him on several new medicines. She demanded to talk to them.

"I want my dad off this garbage Aricept and Namenda; they don't work and they'll make him sicker. And I don't want these depression medicines."

The doctor pushed back. "He needs these," he told her.

"Well, I don't think so," she said. "And I want them stopped."

"No," he told her. "He needs them."

"I'm his power of attorney," she snapped. "What gives you the authority to say what he needs?"

"Because I'm his doctor. I know what he needs."

Very often that's all a Flexnerian doctor can offer in defense of treating people in a way that is antithetical to their health and wishes. They play the doctor card. They may refer to clinical guidelines, calculators, and quality indicators to buttress their unassailable position, but typically they simply flex their doctor muscle and say, "I am the doctor, so I know what's best." Their Flexnerian guts adhere to the inherent value attained by measuring a lot of stuff and then fixing the things that are broken. That's Flexner's prime directive. That's how they have been educated and trained. That's all they know. So, doctors believe their calculators, not their patients and not even what their eyes may show them. They rarely involve their patient in the course of his or her own care or even acknowledge what the patient has to say; they rarely dwell on the larger consequences of how their prescribed interventions will affect their patient or even if the patient wants to pursue that approach. Osler's philosophy of compassionate, intelligent, patient-centric care is absent in today's medical landscape.

The irony is that shared decision-making and patient-centric care are catchwords incessantly tossed around by doctors, insurance companies, and the media. The medical establishment claims to want patients to be active participants in their own care. And then they reward doctors who do just the opposite. Cardiologists don't get paid nearly as well if their patient, after an honest discussion, decides not to have regular stress tests or get that stent. This is true across many specialties. And virtually every doctor is graded by how many of his or her patients have perfect numbers, or get certain vaccinations, or are up to date with that mammogram or colonoscopy. Talking with our patient be damned; it's best we just tell the patient what to do!

That's the double-speak built into the terms *patient-centered care* and *shared decision-making*; we want our patients to make the decisions that WE (based on dogma) know are best for them. We don't want them to make the wrong decision; in fact, we are not allowed to let them make a wrong decision, or else we will suffer! It doesn't matter if someone has had too many false-positive mammograms and wants to stop. It doesn't matter if statins cause falls and leg pain and are not likely to be very effective. It doesn't matter if a patient feels worse when her blood pressure is lowered too much. It doesn't matter if patients just don't want to do all this stuff. To doctors, any patient who drifts from the prescribed norm is risking his or her life, and risking the doctor's quality score, and thus must be redirected. Shared decision-making in the Flexnerian universe only works if the patient makes the "right" decision. Their only shared contribution to that discussion is when they say, "Yes, thank you, doctor, I will do that."

Let's talk about atrial fibrillation (afib) again and the case of Ms. R.

I met Ms. R several years ago, and when I asked her if she was taking a blood thinner for her afib, her smile faded and she yelled at me. "No, I'm not, and you're just going to have to deal with that."

Then she told me her story.

On two separate occasions in the past 10 years, her primary care doctor sent her to a cardiologist to deal with her afib, which was not even bothering her.

"The first time he wanted to put me on Coumadin," she said. "He told me that I had to get my blood checked every month and that I had to watch everything I eat. Forget that, I told him. I'm not doing that. And you know what he did? He kicked me out of his practice. He told me that if I didn't do what he thought was right, if I was going to get a stroke because I was being stupid, then he no longer would care for me. Then he walked out of the room."

I had heard similar stories too many times, I told her. She continued.

"Last year I saw a new cardiologist who my friend told me was reasonable, and that doctor insisted that I go on a medicine called Eliquis. He said it's a much better medicine than Coumadin, and I didn't even have to worry about what I ate or check blood levels; I just take it and not worry. I told him that I saw an ad on TV by a lawyer group that said that anyone on Eliquis who bled or had a relative who died of bleeding should contact them immediately. I told him that it scared me. He said I shouldn't be listening to those moronic ads on TV by a bunch of lawyers. So I asked him, "Why should I listen to you?" He said because he was an expert in afib and he knew my best interest. I told him I didn't want to take that medicine. He pulled out a calculator and said, you are stage 4, or something like that, and you will almost certainly get a stroke if you don't take this medicine. I said I don't care, I'll take that small chance of having a stroke rather than take a medicine that will make me bleed to death. So you know what he said? He said he was firing me as a patient since I refused to do what was right. So, that's two who kicked me out. Are you going to be the third?"

That is shared decision-making in the era of Flexner. And no, I was not the third, I still take care of her, and no, she has not had a stroke almost a decade later.

The doctor's calculator did not know my patient. It was fed with data that had nothing to do with her. She is prone to bleeding; she had been transfused before because of a stomach bleed, and she bruises all too easily. She was also admittedly clumsy and trips a lot. And she was afraid to take anything that could make her bleed. She called it a phobia and wouldn't budge from her stance, a stance that the calculator's "one right answer" approach refused to acknowledge. No subjects like my patient were entered in the data used to create the cardiologist's calculator.

Most patients blindly trust what doctors say. Ms. R's doctor probably has fired very few of his patients. The others have made the "right" decisions.

Can shared decision-making exist in a society that is overly specialized, that financially encourages procedures and does not allow enough time for doctor–patient discourse, and when doctors are trained and rewarded to do more and talk less? Can shared decision-making exist when doctors are taught and tested in a multiple-choice format that claims there is always one right answer that is the same regardless of who the patient is?

Can shared decision-making exist upon the road that Abraham Flexner paved with absolutism, dogma, and one-right-answer thinking?

A similar example occurred to a colleague, Erik Rifkin. At almost 80, Erik is a medical nihilist. He is not a doctor but has a great deal of common sense when it comes to medical decisions.

His book *The Illusion of Certainty*,[2] co-written with Edward Bou-wer, changed my medical life by showing me why everything that my medical education claimed to be gospel really wasn't. In other words, it verified my own observations and beliefs. Erik does not see doctors (other than socially), does not take supplements or medicines, and eschews all screening and blood tests. He eats well, is vibrant and active, and walks all the time. He still jumps off boats and snorkels and climbs many flights of steps regularly. One day he called me and told me he wasn't right. He was feeling awful and had some chest pain that he thought was indigestion. Except, Erik does not get indigestion, and Erik minimizes everything, so it was pretty clear that if he called me he was dealing with something likely very serious. I sent him to the hospital.

He was having a heart attack. This is where our medical system is at its best; we do a great job taking care of critically ill people. In the past people died or became impaired by the type of heart attack Erik was experiencing; now, lives are saved and people walk out unscathed. It's pretty amazing. Erik had two stents placed in his blocked arteries. As much as we talk about the lack of benefits that stents have when performed in people with stable heart disease, they are effective in situations like this. A heart attack occurs when plaque ruptures and, in its attempt to fix the rupture, the body creates a clot that blocks the artery and stops all blood flow. If a doctor then puts a stent through that blockage, blood flow is restored and the heart is saved. That is what happened to Erik, and he could not have been more thankful.

Unfortunately, things deteriorated quickly after that, and it prompted Erik and I to write a story about it in *JAMA Internal Medicine* to assess shared decision-making in the hospital.[3]

Erik was told he may need another stent, that his situation was not stable, that he had to be on blood thinners. Every time a new group of doctors came to him, they wanted to do more: "All these proclamations were tossed at me with little discussion of my prognosis, the uncertainty of the potential benefit, potential harms, why such interventions were needed or treatment alternatives." He demanded that the doctors explain the risks and benefits of everything. Eventually, likely frustrated by his incessant need to be involved in the decision-making process, Erik said that the doctors stopped pushing him. They did not want to discuss these issues. Either he agreed to the procedures, or they would not offer them.

Erik was on two antiplatelet agents. Blood thinners of sorts, Plavix and aspirin are standard of care to prevent stents from closing. As to how long he had to stay on them, the doctors each had a different answer. But then Erik developed a brief episode of afib and was told he had to start taking Coumadin on top of his two other blood thinners, or else he would get a stroke. When Erik asked what the chance was of having a stroke if he did not take Coumadin, the attending physician declared that it was 4 percent. Erik knew well that the benefit was far lower than she was quoting, and the fact that his afib persisted for just a few minutes made the issue moot in his mind. But he played along.

"So, you are telling me that there is a 96 percent chance that I won't have a stroke if I forgo the Coumadin?" he asked. "Those sound like good odds to me. I'll take my chances without it."

The attending doctor was not pleased. She questioned Erik and again insisted that he take the medicine. When he asked what the downsides of taking Coumadin were, she minimized any risk. When he persevered, she stormed out of his room. Later, she sent a medical resident back to talk to him; the resident said that the doctor was very worried that he would have a stroke and hoped that he would reconsider his decision. Erik had a nice talk with the resident about the value of shared decision-making.

By the way, the risk of serious bleeding and death from taking Coumadin on top of Plavix and aspirin is about 6 percent in a year, something hardly negligible. Either the attending cardiologist did not know that or chose not to share it. Either way, Erik was being told that he had to take a drug. He was given deceptive information and told that essentially he had no choice in the matter.

When he left the hospital, Erik was very weak and short of breath. He could not get up his steps and slept a lot. He was worried about his heart. We talked, and I saw him. His blood pressure was dangerously low. His high-dose statin was likely tearing apart his muscles. And he was a nervous wreck, something very uncharacteristic of him. The medical system had beaten down its greatest foe. So we went through the literature, and together decided to stop his two blood pressure medicines and to cut back his statin to a low dose. Within a few weeks he felt great and was back to his usual cynical and pleasant self. He met with a cardiology friend of mine, who told him not to worry. "The doctors will keep making you feel sick," the cardiologist said. "You're not. You're fine. Go on with your life. Put all of this behind you."

That was the last doctor Erik saw, four years ago.

The inability to incorporate shared decision-making into a Flexnerian world is antithetical to good patient care, but it flows naturally from Flexner's absolutist creed.[4] This is especially true today when there are protocols to tell doctors and patients what to do; patient-centered critical thinking evaporated a long time ago. Everything now is mechanized. There is nothing new on the horizon to make us think that our number-focused one-right-answer system is going away any time soon.

Shared decision-making and patient-centered care lay at the very heart of Osler's medical philosophy. We still talk about it, but through our Flexnerian lenses we are incapable of practicing it.

Our medical-industrial complex has grown so large, and so invested in the status quo, that it bucks any attempt to move in a reasonable direction. But all change starts and ends with the patient, and if we are going to progress as a medical society, that must always be our focus.

PART TWO

The Cogs of the Flexnerian Medical-Industrial Complex

CHAPTER FIFTEEN

The Foundations of Our Health Care Infrastructure

If Abraham Flexner were alive today, what would he be attacking? Surely he would ... be appalled at commercialism in medicine. He would insist on evidence-based decision making and probably his pleas for integrating the humanities and medical science would resonate with many.

– Flexner biographer Michael Nivens[1]

In 2011, a group of medical scholars commemorated the 100-year anniversary of Flexner's report with a series of articles. One that struck me in its even-handedness was that by Yale physician Thomas Duffy.[2] After extolling the report's role in providing a fledgling US health care system with a firm organizational and scientific foundation, Duffy spoke of its many flaws. As author Michael Nivens states in this chapter's epigraph, Flexner himself may not have envisioned that his report would morph into our current system. Flexner did critique the evolving health care system under the American Medical Association (AMA) hegemony during much of his life.

Duffy writes that "the oversights of Flexner and his associates need not have occurred if these leaders had recognized the primary role of physicians as beneficent healers," and that under the Flexnerian system "doctors had become neutered technicians with patients in the service of science rather than science in the service of patients." Duffy concludes, "There was a maldevelopment in the structure of medical education in America in the aftermath of the Flexner Report. The profession's infatuation with the hyper-rational world of German medicine created an excellence in science that was not balanced by a comparable excellence in clinical caring. Flexner's corpus was all nerves without the lifeblood of caring." I couldn't have said it better myself.

Flexner's primary goal of constructing a top-down, one-size-fits-all, basic-science-rooted health care system has largely succeeded. Many in our society – from specialized doctors to hospital and insurance company CEOs to drug and device companies – have been enriched by a system that has hijacked compassionate, rational, patient-centric care. And so we find ourselves in a web of organizational and normative snares as we attempt to dismantle Flexner's structural edifice. It is a daunting, if not impossible, task. Still, if we want to embrace health care as a right for every American, if we believe that all should receive effective and compassionate care, and if we want to use our amazing health care technology in the service of patients rather than to generate profit for a few, then we must try.

That requires us to understand the roots of the health care system Flexner's report constructed.

There's no doubt that Flexner's remodeling of medical education is his most enduring legacy. Flexner stressed classroom work, laboratory research, and a squadron of nonpracticing scientists as teachers and mentors. Not only did clinical medicine take a back seat to the memorization and regurgitation of facts, but students had no exposure to patients or clinically oriented teachers until late in their training. From the outset, medical schools immerse their students in the study of rigid scientific rules with one right answer. They rely on full-time, nonpracticing, scientist-doctors for teaching and put students in the lab rather than in patient-driven community practices. Only later do they plunge students into the care of real patients, typically instructed by doctors immersed in Flexner's prime number-fixing directive.[3]

Many in Flexner's day protested such a system. According to Osler biographer Michael Bliss, Osler "could not see how the heads of department could be cut off from active practice" without losing touch with medical science as it applies to real patients. Sending a letter to Johns Hopkins after his school adapted Flexner's changes, Osler "began by condemning Flexner's 'very feeble grasp of the clinical situation at the Johns Hopkins Hospital' and offering a spirited defense against untrue statements about 'the very men who have done so much, or more, than any others to build up the reputation of the school and to advance the best interests of the profession.'"[4]

Osler wasn't the only one who hoped to move medical education in a more clinical direction. Many progressive leaders of the day rebuked Flexner's report and its implications. According to Flexner biographer Michael Nevins, "Harvard's Francis Peabody complained that Flexner's approach weakened 'the soul of the clinic' and pleaded for a more patient-oriented, less academic place to reach medical students and for 'more of the spirit that gives life.'"

Ironically, as time progressed, Flexner himself challenged the strict science focus of medical education that evolved over the decades. Two of his biographers, including Michael Nevins, who is quite critical of his accomplishments, agree on this point. Nevins states that Flexner strongly supported a background in humanities and in humanism among medical students, not the science orgy that premeds must imbibe today. Another Flexner biographer, Thomas Bonner, states that Flexner's educational style emphasized learning by doing, not memorizing and regurgitating.[5] Unfortunately, the educational system his report initiated promoted just the opposite.

Another fatal flaw of Flexner's system – one that prevented his intent from becoming his legacy – is its reliance on private-industry funding and top-down protocol-based control of all facets of the health care industry by large medical conglomerates.

Flexner worked for the Rockefeller Foundation for more than a decade after his report and used that organization's financial tentacles – among others – to pay for the reforms medical schools implemented to stay compliant with the new regulatory framework. Flexner is said to have channeled in excess of half a billion dollars from the Rockefeller Foundation and other philanthropic organizations to institutions he championed, a move that forever distorted the system of medical education in the United States. "Whether their motives were shrewd business instincts, or noblesse oblige," says Nevins, "the influence of these industrialists and financiers was profound, some would say pernicious."[6]

Many other contemporaries eschewed the undue power and hegemony exerted by industry over health care. Flexner's use of corporate funding irritated former colleagues and mentors from Hopkins, who quickly saw that the power base of health care had shifted away from them and into the hands of large foundations. Scientists initially supportive of Flexner's reforms, such as "Bacteriologist Hans Zinsser, regretted the growing power of foundations over educational decisions of universities, noting that too many conditions were attached to each grant, and that there was danger that control was passing to a 'self-perpetuating body of gentlemen," writes Nevins.

Osler had no taste for the dependency of doctors and medical schools on industry or on top-down rules. Early on, he boycotted an AMA meeting, fearing the group's intrusion into medical care and institutions. Later he warned that pharmaceutical companies were exerting too large an influence on medical education, hospitals, and doctors. "Far too large a section of the treatment of disease is today controlled by the big manufacturing pharmacists, who have enslaved us in a plausible pseudoscience," Osler said. "The remedy is obvious: give our students a first-hand acquaintance with disease and give them a thorough practical knowledge of the great drugs, and we will send out independent, clear-headed, cautious practitioners who will do their own thinking and be no longer at the mercy of a meretricious literature which has sapped our independence."[7]

Today, a similar influence is exerted by pharmaceutical companies who supply the research grants that pay for the full-time faculty and medical school operations, thereby controlling virtually all medical research. Our proliferation of medicines, tests, and procedures is a direct result of this embrace of corporate money.

In addition to corporate control of education and health care, Flexner's reforms expanded the power of medical organizations, such as the AMA, upon whose report and ideas Flexner's were based. Since 1911, the AMA has certified and micromanaged medical schools, controlled the certification and practice of doctors, and determined how doctors are paid. Ultimately, it grew strong enough to influence and shape the direction of Medicare (which it initially opposed) and the entire medical reimbursement network.

Today the AMA is but one of many organizations that define appropriate standards of care for doctors, control who gets paid for what, inform the press and public what is "necessary and lifesaving," and lobby Congress and statehouses to assure that health care expenditure remains high and narrowly focused on their own constituents. Some very respected groups – such as the Centers for Disease Control and Prevention, Food and Drug Administration, American Cancer Society, American Diabetes Association, and Alzheimer's Association, among others – receive the bulk of their funding from industry and thus are likely to push drugs and interventions that benefit their sponsors. Other large groups – such as the American College of Cardiology (ACC) and American College of Radiology (ACR) – extensively lobby Congress and insurance carriers to pay steep prices for tests and treatments that financially benefit their doctor-members, while disseminating information to the media and public to buttress their claim that what they do is necessary and lifesaving.

In Flexner's day, most doctors were oriented to primary care. In fact, internal medicine and family medicine were considered specialties at that time. Internal medicine and family medicine doctors, all of whom train for three to four years after medical school, now are the pillars of primary care, which essentially implies that they care for the entire patient. But especially since the advent of Medicare in 1965, and concomitant with the expanding influence of medical societies and the growth of medical procedures, our health care system has become dominated by specialists, further perpetuating the test-diagnose-treat philosophy with which we live. Flexner did not advocate specialization, but his system encouraged its growth and proliferation.

Because groups such as the AMA, ACC, and ACR exert such a tight grip on how doctors are evaluated and paid, they have assured that procedural-based specialists earn more than the cognitive, patient-oriented doctors Osler believed to be the bulwark of an effective and compassionate health care system. Doctor-technicians who slide a stent in an artery are reimbursed far more for that single procedure than physicians who must grapple with, for example, an elderly person living in poor conditions who has multiple chronic illnesses and frequent flares of serious sickness.

Osler, among others, did not perceive specialization as advantageous to the profession. He believed that sick humans were beset by a wide range of problems that could not be isolated piece by piece. A good doctor is one who understands and treats the entire person, not a single organ or slice of the person. "The family doctor, the private in our great army, the essential factor in the battle, should be carefully nurtured by the schools and carefully guarded by the public," Osler said.

Alas, ours is a medical society controlled by organizations with money, dictated by self-serving, all-powerful medical societies, and favoring the specialization of care by doctors who are told to follow a script and adhere to the mantra of test-diagnose-treat. The gentle, thoughtful, and wise generalist who knows her patient well and who is skeptical of promises and miraculous cures has faded away amid the tide of the medical-industrial complex that Flexner unleashed.

CHAPTER SIXTEEN

The Financial Ramifications of Our Medical-Industrial Complex

The natural man has only two primal passions, to get and beget.
— William Osler[1]

The system in the United States is hardly the wonder that its medical proponents claim it to be. The United States ranks 26th in the world in life expectancy, 37th in the world in overall health care outcomes, and yet we spend twice as much per capita than do other leading nations.[2] How is this possible? The answer is embedded in the growth of a philosophy that places so much emphasis on drugs and procedures that it has sprouted a multi-trillion-dollar cash cow that cares less about outcome and more about feeding itself.

Part of the problem lies in the growing separation of wealth in our nation. More than 20 million Americans still do not have health insurance, and being uninsured increases the risk of dying by as much as 40 percent. It is estimated that more than 45,000 deaths occur every year because of a lack of health insurance, according to a 2009 study conducted by researchers at Harvard Medical

School.[3] Even more are likely dying because of high-deductible plans, which have proliferated recently. High-deductible plans are much cheaper because the patient is required to pay a large portion of their initial health care costs, often as high as $7,000.

It is certainly the case that a great deal of testing and treatment that insurance enables is both unhelpful and dangerous. But testing based on symptoms, certain screening tests, and many treatments do help, especially in cases of chronic illness, infectious disease, and catastrophic care. High-deductible plans dissuade many patients from seeking health care for conditions that can sometimes be serious, leading to delays in care, increased costs, higher complication rates, and even death. In fact, a 2020 study published in the *International Journal of Environmental Research and Public Health* confirms that uninsured and underinsured individuals delay care for emergencies, leading to higher mortality rates.[4] How many died in the COVID-19 epidemic who were either uninsured or underinsured will probably never be known, but it is likely more people died from avoiding care during COVID-19 than from the disease itself. How many are dying every day from other treatable ailments?

But even health insurance is not a buttress against our profit-driven health care system. The concept of medical bankruptcy does not exist in most of the world. A recent Harvard University study shows that medical expenses are the leading cause of bankruptcy in the United States, resulting in 62 percent of all personal bankruptcies, with 80 percent of the medical bankruptcies occurring among insured patients.[5] Working-class families often lose their homes and other assets to care for themselves and their families. A patient of mine recently had to sell her house to pay medical bills, and ended up temporarily in a homeless shelter. But that's what we have in our country today, largely thanks to our Flexnerian legacy. We spend so much on meaningless dives into health care that even insurance often doesn't cover the escalating expenses of genuine illness.

The problem is, as more people share in the health care bonanza, the more expensive it becomes, and the more it feeds itself. Adding to our woes is that we do not have a primary-care-based and patient-centric system in place. We have clinics, private offices, hospitals and their controlled community practices, urgent-care centers, and pharmacies delivering fragmented patient care with no comprehensive approach or equitable access to care. We have almost totally neglected the concept of integrated health and preventive medicine, as embraced by Osler, in favor of a system based on both acute care and splintered specialty care. More than 90 million Americans have at least one chronic illness, and 70 percent of us die slowly from genuine chronic diseases, such as hypertension, diabetes, cardiovascular disease, stroke, kidney failure, and dementia.[6] Most of these conditions are a result of our poor lifestyle and behaviors, including poor nutrition, lack of exercise, stress, environmental factors, and an inadequate emphasis on prevention, wellness, and health. A third of Medicare's coffers is spent on the consequences of poor health and lifestyle in the last two years of people's lives as a result of multiple hospitalizations, countless diagnostic tests, and unnecessary procedures. One percent of the population accounts for 20 percent of the health care costs, and 5 percent account for nearly half of all expenditures. The average per capita health care costs for individuals in their 80s is more than $50,000 a year.[7]

Spending does not translate to good outcomes. People who live in big cities and who obtain their medical care at major academic medical centers are more likely to be hospitalized, spend more days in the hospital and the intensive care unit, see more specialists, and have significantly higher costs.[8] So one would intuitively expect better outcomes, but this is not the case. Data show that these patients get more unnecessary care, have higher rates of hospital-associated infections and increased drug reactions, and have higher ratings of dissatisfaction with the health care experience. All that and they don't live any longer than their counterparts. These data are even more dramatic when looking at patients with end-of-life hospitalizations. Patients admitted to New York University Hospital or Cedars-Sinai in Los Angeles (both major academic teaching institutions) can expect to spend nearly twice as long on their last hospitalization than counterparts in rural and nonacademic hospitals.[9]

What explains these disparities? Some of it occurs because in areas with high specialization there is less emphasis on primary care, on holistic issues of health care, and on a doctor–patient relationship that delves into the human person rather than that person's numbers.

For instance, those individuals with advance-care plans (health care proxies/living wills, etc.) who have had discussions with their loved ones regarding end-of-life wishes are much more likely to choose a less aggressive hospital course. Those that have better access to primary care are also more likely to have had these discussions, and appropriate advance-care planning discussions have been proven to decrease end-of-life spending and increase patient and family satisfaction.[10] But in our Flexnerian system, primary care has been displaced, and spending money on one's health through tests, drugs, and procedures is often seen as the best path to wellness.

The amount of money we squander on ineffective health care in this country is astronomical. Estimated to be as much as a trillion dollars a year, much of that waste is spending on unnecessary tests and treatments, the very cornerstones of the Flexnerian approach to care.[11]

Hospitals and physicians do not have reliable access to previous diagnostic and therapeutic interventions. To this day, many electronic health record systems do not communicate with each other, which is a major obstacle to care. This lack of cooperation leads to the needless repetition of diagnostic tests and procedures and risks patients' exposure to medical harm, even if insurance pays for these wasteful services and doctors earn more money. A recent patient in my faculty practice went to an urgent-care center for chest pain. She was 45 with no risk factors for coronary disease. The center was affiliated with one of our major health care systems whose electronic health records are not compatible with the rest in the city. She ended up with a referral to a cardiologist and gastroenterologist and a battery of needless tests – all normal. She then presented to the emergency department of another hospital for the same complaint and received the same bundle of needless tests because her health record information was not readily available. The patient was scared, never questioned the medical care, and agreed to all of the testing in her vulnerable state. She had recently lost her mother to COVID-19, was having marital problems, and lost her job, but no one ever asked. She is doing well with counseling, yoga, and meditation. Of course, all that spending enriches many members of the medical-industrial complex, and thus there are few in power who seek a solution.

Other areas of waste include the administrative complexity of our health care system, reliance on unproven guidelines and quality metrics, but also fraud and abuse. Doctors are often not incentivized or financially reimbursed to keep people healthy and out of the hospital. Even the primary care doctor makes more money when she sees patients in the hospital or emergency department rather than in her office. Our system, which is mostly fee-for-service, incentivizes doctors to see more patients in a short bursts of time. Sometimes doctors have only 10 to 15 minutes to address a complex medical issue, leaving little or no time to address prevention, wellness, and the social determinants of health. And if doctors see the patient too frequently, or bill at too high a level of service that falls out of some fabricated norm, they may be audited and financially punished or, even worse, lose their patients to a "more efficient" practice. Insurance companies have the right to dismiss any doctor they want off their plan if they think they are not "efficient and cost-effective" providers.

Data are starting to show that primary care physicians are now spending half of their working time on what is now referred to as "desktop" medicine. Desktop medicine is the time spent to document encounters, meet insurance company requirements and metrics, and deal with prior authorizations, denials for necessary medical services, and other insurance company hassles. A recent study in *Health Affairs* investigated how physicians split their time between patient visits and computer tasks.[12] On average, physicians spent 3.08 hours on office visits each day and 3.17 hours on desktop medicine each day.[13] I can tell you that this is true for ourselves and our colleagues (except for most of us, the daily hours are double those in this study). Many practices are required to add more nonclinical staff, further adding to the escalating costs of medical practice.

Many doctors now view the health insurance industry as one of their major barriers to delivering quality medical care. What was once a not-for-profit industry is now one of the most lucrative financial giants in our country, with projections for tremendous and continued growth. The big five for-profit health insurance companies – Aetna, Anthem, Cigna, Humana, and UnitedHealth Group – cumulatively grossed more than $4.1 billion in the first three months of 2017 alone. Their profits continue to rise. The average salary of a CEO of a major insurance company is more than $25 million a year, more than 300 times what their employees earn.

The highest paid, David Wichman of UnitedHealth Group, had a 2017 compensation package of $83.2 million.

Hospitals and insurance companies can feast from Flexnerian care, but when insurance is limited, the opposite tale is true. I recently had a patient with multiple myeloma (a type of blood cancer) who was admitted to the hospital after he fainted during chemotherapy. He had afib, a pulmonary embolism (blood clot in lung), and broke five bones in his back when he fell down. The insurance company denied his admission to the hospital. I was asked to do what is known as a peer-to-peer evaluation to discuss the case, meaning I was required to make an appointment with an insurance company medical director to discuss the case. I presented the scenario to the doctor on the phone, and he agreed with me, but unfortunately he could not approve the admission because it was past the time for verbal approval, and would require a formal written appeal. The time had passed because the insurance company did not notify me that the admission was denied until I received a letter a week after the patient was discharged from the hospital.

Primary care doctors often need to have their staff spend hours on the phone to get an authorization for a needed test for a patient, only to have them spend more time fighting for payment of a denied $60 office visit. Insurance companies make even more money by delaying payment or never paying if the doctor's office is inefficient or simply overwhelmed with bureaucracy and red tape.

A 2017 report in the *Annals of Internal Medicine* estimated that more than 34 percent of the health care dollar, or $2,500 per person, is being spent on the overhead of the insurance industry and physician/hospital staff needed for insurance-related issues – more than twice the amount Canada spends.[14] In addition, clinicians must fight for every penny of their income. We spend countless hours in front of the electronic health record clicking boxes to document what we have done so we can get paid, time better spent speaking with patients about important medical issues. Doctors must prove that they have satisfied a rigid set of "quality metrics," which are essentially report cards to assure that this test or that has been ordered, or that whatever numbers our overseers deem to be important to our patients have been fixed.

The price of medications has already spiraled out of control, and the pharmaceutical industry profits are in the range of $500 billion a year. We have discussed how pharmaceutical companies, in concert with many doctors, have fed the Flexnerian dictate to use drugs and to aggressively fix everyone's numbers, be it blood pressure, sugar level, cholesterol, bone density, and so much else. Big Pharma has higher profit margins than any other industry in the nation. The United States makes up less than 5 percent of the world's population yet accounts for almost 50 percent of the pharmaceutical industry's profits.[15]

CEOs of the major pharmaceutical companies average more than $25 million in annual income, with some executives earning as much as $100 million a year. John Martin, the former CEO of Gilead Science, which makes HIV and hepatitis C medications, made nearly $100 million in 2016. Some of these medicines are necessary and valuable; others are not, but are sold anyway, even by "respected" agencies. We will see, for example, how these companies worked with the Centers for Disease Control and Prevention (CDC) to increase the market for hepatitis C treatment. Why are the costs of these medications hundreds of times the cost of the same medications in other countries throughout the world? In our country, the pharmaceutical companies control most research; we will also see the strong influence they have over the CDC, Food and Drug Administration (FDA), and the US Congress. All of this leads to outrageous cost, and deceptive advertising convinces Flexnerian-educated doctors and patients that their medicines are worth every penny because they are so good at fixing numbers and thus clearly save people's lives.[16]

Recent evidence has highlighted that many diabetic patients have to ration their insulin because of the exorbitant costs associated with both long- and short-acting insulin products, leading to increased complications, hospitalizations, and numerous deaths. The average price of insulin increased 300 percent in the years 2002–2012.[17]

Other recent highlights include the EpiPen fiasco, a lifesaving drug for severe allergic reactions, which is only now becoming somewhat more affordable after it was out of reach for most Americans, costing more than $700. The EpiPen is an auto-injector medication that can be self-administered, even by children, and costs pennies to manufacture. How many children and adults with food allergies or asthma may have died because of the inaccessibility of the drug is unknown. The CEO of Mylan, Heather Bresch, the EpiPen's manufacturer, told Congress that the 400 percent increase in the price was justified based on improvements in its delivery system. Mylan has subsequently agreed to pay the US Department of Justice $465 million to counter allegations it overcharged Medicaid for the EpiPen. Bresch just happens to be the daughter of US senator Joe Manchin (I-WV).[18]

And who can forget Martin Shkreli, the convicted felon and founding CEO of Turing Pharmaceuticals. Shkreli obtained the license to manufacture a rarely used antiparasitic drug; he proceeded to raise the price from $13 a pill to $750, leading to his denotation as the "most-hated man in America." Nirmal Mulye, CEO of Nostrum Pharmaceuticals, raised the price of a bottle of a common antibiotic, nitrofurantoin, from $475 to $2,392 a bottle. He praised Shkreli, telling the *Financial Times* that Turing was the only company making Daraprim at the time, so "he can make as much money as he can. This is a capitalist economy and, if you can't make money, you can't stay in business."

Pharmaceutical companies are entitled to a fair profit, especially those that are truly investing in the research and development of new medications. However, the costs will only continue to rise for medications, many of which are marketed as being "necessary and lifesaving" by dubious Flexnerian barometers, few of which are actually necessary and lifesaving. Numerous shortages exist in generic medications, which can lead to delays in patient care and even death. Many of these shortages are only corrected after the prices of medications rise by hundreds of percent. This occurs even as we subsidize the pharmaceutical companies, allow them to conduct their own research, and allow them to advertise and promote useless drugs while gouging consumers with those drugs that are actually helpful and should be cheap.

The hospital system must take its fair share of the blame in our health care crisis. For years, hospitals drove the health care market. Mergers and acquisitions have consolidated the systems in many communities where the option of choice and competition has evaporated. Many academic health centers in our nation are training the next generation of students to become the most sophisticated specialists in the world.[19] They then order the most expensive procedures and perform the most expensive surgeries, which add to their bottom line. Profits in the hospital are not from taking care of simple infections, but rather from performing complex surgeries and procedures that generate the most profit and are justified in purely Flexnerian language.

What is often not discussed is that the cost of care in academic centers is 20 percent or more than that in comparable institutions. These expenditures are attributable to the high cost of training students and residents, who often order tests and procedures for "educational purposes." In addition, the strict supervision and educational requirements to train residents cost the system millions annually. So many in academic medicine will say that their exceptional care is worth it. Unfortunately, the facts do not support this. In fact, many of these centers have higher hospital-acquired-infection rates and more medical errors. The financial and clinical outcome data are even worse for the hospitals that are for-profit. Studies reveal that they have higher costs than their not-for-profit counterparts – and increased mortality rates. Most of us really do not believe there is a difference between for-profit and not-for-profit status anyway. Walk through the prestigious halls of our nation's top not-for-profit institutions, which are now rivaling many top-quality, five-star hotels, and tell me that they are a nonprofit organization. Look at the annual list of the earnings of the top CEOs of our nation's hospitals, which can be in the range of $10 to $25 million, and try to tell me again that they are a not-for-profit organization.

Doctors are not exempt from blame in our health care crisis because they are in fact the drivers of our Flexnerian orgy of care. There are many reasons physicians add to the costs of our health care. Many often blame defensive medicine on the overuse of diagnostic testing and treatments, and unfortunately a significant portion of this is justified because of our current malpractice mess. The United States has 5 percent of the world's population and nearly 50 percent of the world's lawyers (sounds like our pharmaceutical system).[20] There are nearly 30 percent more lawyers in our nation than doctors, and it is estimated that the cost of defensive medicine is nearly $125 billion a year.[21] Many of us feel the need to order useless MRIs or CT scans to cover our butts. It is well known that the vast majority of CT/MRI scans ordered in our nation's doctors' offices and emergency departments for headaches are unnecessary.[22] Doctors are ordering millions of dollars of useless tests simply to protect themselves from a malpractice case, and hospitals and radiologists encourage such behavior because it feeds their financial appetite. So much of this leads to overdiagnosis, overtreatment, needless worry, stress, subsequent complications, and even death. Data show that states that have had malpractice reform actually have better doctor–patient relationships and satisfaction with medical care and medical practice.

Our federal health care apparatus has also bought into the Flexnerian script, and it drives large swaths of the medical-industrial complex. By controlling reimbursement for a significant portion of our population through the Centers for Medicare and Medicaid Services, the US federal government manipulates reimbursement in such a way as to encourage tests and procedures. Most private insurers adapt the federal reimbursement formula. Through the FDA, the federal government also regulates the medications and devices that are manufactured and regulates how our hospitals function and are paid. The lobbies for the hospital, insurance, and pharma industries are among the richest and most powerful groups in the country. It is no wonder that so many politicians are indebted to members of the medical-industrial complex to fund their campaigns and influence their policies. The Affordable Care Act (2010) did a lot to bring health care to millions more Americans, but did nothing to reform the power of health care's masters to affect how the government spends its money.

Physician specialty organizations, such as the American Medical Association and the American College of Cardiology, are wealthy organizations that promote their constituents: doctors. Many of them represent the richest doctors, such as interventional cardiologists, neurosurgeons, and orthopedic surgeons. Specialty physicians often make two to three times more than primary care providers, with salaries often between $500,000 and more than $1,000,000, compared with primary care physicians, who average in the low to mid- $200,000s. These are the groups of physicians most reluctant to endorse significant changes to our Flexnerian spending spree. Primary care physicians don't have a powerful lobby, and thus are typically left without a voice.

Primary care doctors are getting burnt out or just simply fed up with the system. Few enter the field, and many older physicians can't keep up with the escalating metrics and regulatory demands, and they are struggling to maintain their incomes by simply pushing folks through the door. Physician extenders, such as nurse practitioners and physician assistants, may lighten the burden somewhat as their experience grows. However, many do not have the level of training necessary to provide comprehensive primary care, and their increased use will likely be associated with overreferral to specialists, leading to overtesting, overdiagnosis, and subsequent overtreatment. The ultimate result will be higher health care costs and worse outcomes. ✗

Patients must take a small part of the blame because they are just as intoxicated by the Flexnerian credo of doing a lot of tests and finding and fixing a lot of problems. Folks come in regularly wanting MRIs and CT scans after they read on the internet that they might have cancer, or simply want to know why they have low-back pain. I listen to patients every day telling me that they pay a lot of money for their insurance and that they are entitled to every test or treatment they deem to be necessary. Every day, I am forced to spend a significant amount of my time trying to explain to a patient why they do not need a test or why they do not need an antibiotic to treat a viral infection they have. I explain why the test is not necessary and will often lead to overdiagnosis and overtreatment. But most patients persevere, and often it is easier for a doctor just to give in. Clinicians who do not comply with their patients' needs will receive poor report cards from their insurance companies, which can threaten their livelihood. Many providers simply make the patient happy by ordering copious tests rather than spending time they do not have to make appropriate person-centered shared decisions. Even in primary care, it is better to get tests and fix numbers so our report card is stellar and our patients remain happy.

We are training not Oslerian healers but technicians who follow protocols, put their faith in the test-diagnose-treat formula of care, and adhere to quality metrics in a robotic way that often diverges from what a patient wants and needs. Osler sought to create an army of physicians capable of taking care of their nuanced and complex patients with a mix of humanism and science. Our convoluted wasteful and dysfunctional health care system, fueled by Flexnerian doctors, does just the opposite. We have let corporate America take over a field that was once dominated by independent doctors who care about and spend time and provide individual attention to each patient. We have let our nation's health care mega complex industry of pharma, device manufactures, hospitals, specialty societies, and the for-profit health insurance industry take our profession away from us. We as physicians let this happen because we were imbued by Flexnerian dogma and threatened by the ramifications of turning away from it. But it is not too late to stop it if we take time to understand what makes it run.

CHAPTER SEVENTEEN

Our Medical Education Quandary

Every medical student should remember that his end is not to be made a chemist or physiologist or anatomist, but to learn how to recognize and treat disease, how to become a practical physician.

– William Osler[1]

We all remember our medical school interviews: "Why do you want to be a doctor?" "To use science to help people" was what most of us said and, we hope, believed. Then we entered a medical education system that put everyone on a rollercoaster of competitive classes that doled out information with no relationship to the art or science of medical care, administered one-right-answer, multiple-choice examinations that were often tricky and thoughtless, and gave us very little patient contact for the first two years. It was grueling and demoralizing; many who entered for idealistic reasons left burnt out, depressed, or simply bent on earning money. We memorized copious information and were tested on minutiae – a lot. But we didn't learn how to be critically thinking physicians who care for complex human beings.

Both Flexner and Osler insisted that medical students complete four years of undergraduate education (which was not the case before the Flexner Report) and have some mastery of science. Both believed that students should be broadly educated in humanities. These changes by both Flexner and Osler greatly improved and formalized educational standards, established an improved medical education system, shut down subpar schools, and moved toward improved overall medical care. However, it was at this point that their paths diverged and Flexner's road to dogmatic science took hold.

Osler especially emphasized the need for students to exhibit both humanistic and critical-thinking skills. Medicine is not black and white; the exceptional physician must be able to apply basic science knowledge and evidence-based guidelines to the patient in front of them. To do this, the good physician must analyze the facts, synthesize them into a diagnosis, and put together a plan that is appropriate for the individual patient, not rely on a cookbook algorithm. Osler believed that throughout training, patients and practicing physicians must be a source of pragmatic wisdom that students could integrate with the newest science.

The current state of medical education has drifted far from Osler's dream. Most students obtain a scientific or premedical type of degree that does nothing to prepare them for the sound clinical judgment, empathy, and humanistic approach needed to become a physician. I still do not understand how calculus and physics have anything to do with being a decent doctor. Those who can best memorize scientific facts are the ones most likely to gain acceptance to medical school, and once in medical school the orgy of science – severed from patients and from doctors who see patients regularly – is shoved at students, who are required to memorize and regurgitate minutiae in a one-right-answer, multiple-choice format.

Getting into medical school is a grueling process; fewer than 40 percent who apply make it. Most who do get into medical school have wonderful memorization skills and a very narrow breadth of education. Most come from the top of their class, and at least half of them will be in the bottom half of their class when their training is complete, something that is difficult for many overachievers, and something that creates an atmosphere of competition and grade-obsession among students.

The major requirements to get into medical school are college grade point average and MCAT scores. The MCAT is a multiple-choice examination designed to "assess your problem solving, critical thinking, and knowledge of natural, behavioral and social science concepts." The MCAT – the most important eight hours of a future doctor's life – carries extraordinary weight in selection, more than virtually anything else. And yet, it does nothing to assess critical thinking and humanism. It is more a gauge of a student's ability to memorize and regurgitate huge quantities of detailed information, skills only helpful in assessing students who will be good at taking tests and memorizing protocols during their careers, the very doctors who inhabit our Flexnerian universe.

Studies indicate that the MCAT does not predict which students will become good doctors or even who will do well in medical school.[2] It is simply an onerous hoop to jump through, and likely deprives medical schools of the thoughtful, smart, and personable students it should be targeting.

Most medical schools spend more than 90 percent of the first two years of education teaching the basic sciences of medicine. The common theme, entrenched since the days of Flexner, is that students spend two years learning basic science in a classroom, followed by two years of clinical rotations, mostly in a hospital. There is a sharp divide between these two components of medical education, and rarely is the basic science component integrated into the clinical component. For one thing, the first two years of basic science are mostly taught by PhD and MD research scientists who have never applied the basics of the discipline to clinical medicine and the care of a human being. In the second two years, students are sent to various hospitals and have distinct rotations in medicine, surgery, and pediatrics. There is no cohesive or standardized education that each student receives and little continuity of care. The result is a group of passionate young physicians unprepared for the residency training programs they are about to enter. In the Oslerian system, students were introduced to clinical care from day one; the science of medicine and art of patient care was always seen as a continuum.

I have spent more than 30 years in medical education in a hospital, and I can tell you that today, most students enter their third year of clinical medical school training bereft of the skills needed to provide patient care. Many can barely do a basic history and physical examination, rendering them unable to apply clinical skills to formulate a diagnosis, let alone a treatment plan. They have little or no knowledge of basic communication skills. I ask all students who rotate with us on our family medicine or palliative care service if they have ever had training in communication skills, such as delivering bad news. Unfortunately, the answer is overwhelmingly "no."

The ability to deliver bad news, such as telling someone that they have cancer, is an essential skill for every physician. Too bad for the patient that our system recruits test-takers rather than caregivers. Our medical schools expect to turn out great practitioners, yet they don't prioritize professionalism and communication skills. Poor communication is associated with lower patient compliance, lower satisfaction with care, higher rates of medical errors, and increased medical malpractice. Patients who love their doctors do so because of the human touch, empathy, and compassionate communication they receive. These same patients are the ones who also have the best clinical outcomes and are most satisfied with their care and the health care system.

Many competent third-year medical students can quote scientific articles from the prestigious *New England Journal of Medicine* or the *Journal of the American Medical Association*. But ask them to tell you about a patient they saw, and to consider possible diagnoses and treatments for that patient's condition, or to assess whether these journal articles apply to the patient sitting in front of them, and they look at you with blank stares. This lapse results from two years of memorization and multiple-choice testing of information that is severed from the clinical reality they are now seeing. Schools are rated on the scores their students receive on these examinations, and residencies use these scores to rate candidates for their training programs. Higher scores get you into the toughest and most competitive of specialties, such as dermatology, orthopedics, and neurosurgery, and into the most prestigious of academic institutions. So, the better the multiple-choice test-taker you are, the "better" the program you get into and the better your school looks. No wonder our students are pushed to be more robotic thinkers than critical thinkers.

And when they cite articles, protocols, and expert advice, today's medical students are ignorant of the origins and meaning of the "facts" they tout. They do not understand the bulk of what we explored in part 1 of this book, from pharmaceutical control of medical research to the difference between absolute and relative benefit, to how studies are gauged to produce predetermined results. This gap in education leads them to advocate for a Flexnerian dogma that they simply do not comprehend.

Most students enter medical school to see and care for patients, but what they discover is a continuation of the competitiveness and mindless memorization that they faced in college. It is a buffet of basic science courses, tests (many of which are virtual now), and endless studying. Osler's vision of a patient-oriented curriculum has no place in the rigid Flexnerian system that has barely changed since 1911. I recently had to refer a fourth-year medical student for counseling because she felt broken, battered, and mostly unprepared for clinical medicine because the COVID-19 pandemic essentially eliminated a year and a half of her practical medical training. The pandemic turned many young clinicians to technicians running from one crashing COVID-19 patient to another. There was no time for study, reflection, thinking, or the care of "regular" patients, who were scared to seek care. The pandemic has exacerbated the decline of a failing educational system and will create a generation of underprepared doctors, but this is simply an exacerbation of the process that has been plaguing medical schools for a century.

Making it to the third year and actually getting to use your stethoscope for the first time is exciting for most. The third year consists of clinical core rotations, mostly conducted in hospitals, including medicine, surgery, pediatrics, obstetrics and gynecology (OB/GYN), and psychiatry, with minimal exposure to primary care or office-based practice. The fourth year of clinical training exposes students to more choices of specialty rotations and subinternships; these are the rotations where you need to show your worth to the specialty and hospitals at which you want to continue your residency training. Students often focus more on how they will do on the multiple-choice exams that constitute the majority of their grade than on developing clinical skills (which are not as important to the grade). They also must decide which path to take. Should I become a primary care doc, a surgeon, or an emergency medicine physician? These are some of the toughest decisions a medical student must make, and unfortunately their exposure to specialty fields and their life in a bubble of specialty-trained teachers pushes most away from primary care. The other driver of a student's decision comes down to dollars and cents.

The average cost of four years of medical school in a public school is now about $250,000, without room and board. The costs at some of the private schools are much higher. Many students are now graduating with student loan debt of $300,000 or even $400,000 or more.[3] Is there any wonder that students choose higher-paying specialties to pay off this debt? It is again amazing to many of us in primary care that specialists who perform technical procedures are paid so much more than primary care physicians who must treat a total patient in a complex way. But this reality forces some of the brightest young physicians to enter technical specialty fields rather than primary care. Until we change how we pay for health care appropriately, this dysfunction will continue, and we will have a dearth of quality primary care providers and a surplus of specialists. Exactly the situation we have today.

Some of the nation's prestigious medical schools are now giving free tuition to their students. These are the most elite of the medical schools that have the most money through endowments, grants, the ability to perform expensive procedures, and pharmaceutical payment of medical studies. These are the same institutions training our elite specialists and not primary care providers, adding to the divide between primary and specialty care and helping to further our nation's shortage of primary care doctors. Free tuition would do a lot to help alleviate our nation's primary care shortage, but it is being used in a way to encourage just the opposite.

After completion of medical school comes residency training programs, the main ones being medicine, surgery, pediatrics, OB/GYN, emergency medicine, psychiatry, and family medicine.

You must begin to make a career choice early in your third year of medical school, without the benefit of having completed all of your clinical rotations and without any benefit of actually seeing patients in the ambulatory setting where the majority of today's medical care is delivered.

At the beginning of the fourth year of medical school, students enter what is called "the Match," essentially a lottery system that determines where and in what specialty a student will enter. The more competitive the specialty, the harder it is to match. The top programs will not consider interviewing a candidate who is not a good multiple-choice tester and who has not done a fair amount of bench research, once again propagating a system that encourages rote memorization and a basic science focus rather than the skills of critical thinking and compassion. The Match is announced on what is called, obviously enough, Match Day. Schools hold big parties and advertise what prestigious hospitals and specialty fields their students match in. Most do not advertise how many of their students enter the less prestigious primary care field or show pictures of their students who do not match and have to enter what is called a "scramble" to find a residency position. Can you imagine going through four years of medical school, having hundreds of thousands of dollars of debt, and not having a job? It does happen.

Some of the prestigious hospitals in our country still do not have departments of family medicine and do not afford the opportunity for all of their students to have clinical family medicine training or even any exposure to a family doctor at all. According to the American Academy of Family Physicians, the schools without family medicine departments include Harvard, Columbia, Cornell, George Washington, Johns Hopkins, New York University, Stanford, Vanderbilt, Washington University in St. Louis, and Yale. Schools without family medicine departments send fewer graduates into that specialty despite the fact that about 40 percent of primary care visits in the country are to family physicians.[4] This is counterintuitive to what is needed for the health of our nation and our patients. A recent student of mine from a prestigious NYC medical school was ostracized by her dean for choosing primary care for a residency. She quoted her dean, "You are ruining our reputation as a prominent institution that trains the world's greatest physicians and scientists for the lowly field of family medicine, and you are an embarrassment and should become a real doctor."

Alan is a family physician who also practices and teaches hospice and palliative care. After college, he completed a one-year program called a rotating internship (medicine, surgery, pediatrics, OB/GYN, emergency medicine, and psychiatry), followed by a three-year residency in family medicine. About 50 percent of the training in a family medicine residency program is in the outpatient setting, including hospital-based clinics, community health centers, and private doctors' offices. Family physicians are trained to be primary care providers for people of all ages.

Andy is an internist and geriatrician. He completed three years of residency, just as Alan did, but in an internal medicine residency program. The adult primary care provider who completes an internal medicine residency program is referred to as an internist. An internist completes their four years of medical school training and then a three-year residency in internal medicine, also mostly in a hospital setting. After completion of the three years of residency, they have the choice of entering clinical practice as an internist or completing further training to become a medical subspecialist (cardiology, endocrinology, etc.) or a hospitalist. Unfortunately, fewer than 10 percent of internal medicine graduates are entering the primary care field, the vast majority going on to hospital medicine or specialty care, which provides either greater salary or enhanced quality of life.[5] This trend has been worsening for many years and is currently a significant contributor to today's shortage of quality primary care providers.

Internal medicine residency programs place little emphasis on training in the ambulatory care setting, furthering the divide between inpatient and outpatient medicine. Is there any wonder that so few students choose primary care as a specialty when they have little exposure to real primary care? No wonder that today's doctors are less concerned with patient wellness and holistic health when all of their training is in high-tech Flexnerian specialty care.

Some medical schools support primary care as a career choice, but many do not. City- and state-run medical schools, and schools of osteopathic medicine, graduate most of our country's primary care providers. Wealthy and prestigious private medical schools – those associated with academic medical centers – produce most of our nation's specialist physicians. Most of the major academic medical schools find it more prestigious for their students to enter specialty fields. I came from a school that actually supported primary care, but throughout my third- and fourth-year rotations, every time I said I wanted family medicine, I was told to be a real doctor and make some money. My residency was affiliated with a major NYC academic program where students were dissuaded from entering primary care: "You are too smart for that. That's the field for those that can't get into the best specialty programs at the best academic institutions. Don't embarrass our institution." Given that the funding of most of these schools is corporate-derived, and that the goal of the Flexnerian marriage between medical education and industry is to create specialization and research, it's no wonder that primary care and clinical medicine take a back seat to the science-based emphasis born from the Flexner Report.

Many graduates who do not specialize become hospitalists, that is, physicians who spend all of their time taking care of patients admitted to the hospital. They have no continuity relationship with the patient and do not provide follow-up care after they are discharged. Hospitalists are experts on the medical care and procedures that are necessary for the management of a hospitalized patient. They are there simply to admit the patient, form an assessment and a treatment plan, and refer them for tests and specialty visits that financially benefit the hospital. This system has nothing to do with what is best for the patient; it's about efficiency and money.

Why are so many graduates of medical school and residencies considering becoming hospitalists? Because they get paid more than primary care providers and can set predictable hours. When they are done with their shift, they are done, no further work, no follow-up on testing and consults, no handling patient phone calls. It is somewhat perplexing why a hospitalist is paid more than a primary care physician who must care for the complexity of a patient over time, but as with much in the Flexnerian universe, continuity of care takes a back seat to the primacy of testing and treating and specialty referral, something that medical students and residents are trained to do, and something that rewards the hospitals in which they work.

Unfortunately, we are also losing some of the brightest and best primary care physicians to jobs at urgent-care centers. Urgent-care centers and telehealth programs, like hospitalist positions, offer higher pay and better working hours. Most urgent-care centers offer three 12-hour shifts per week, a scribe to complete medical records, robust support staff, and someone else to do the necessary follow-up on testing and labs. Most of today's urgent-care centers are owned and operated by major hospital systems and for-profit medical corporations. Once again, higher pay, less stress, more home time, and a simple diagnose-and-fix scope of care; it is no wonder graduates are choosing these positions.

Patients who use this type of care often miss appropriate screening and other primary care services and may have critical delays in the diagnosis and treatment of cancer and other chronic medical illness, whereas in other arenas they are overtreated, overtested, and referred to too many specialists.[6] This is another example of disjointed medical care; patients go in for a quick fix to their problem but avoid the issues that often create the problem, such as diet or poor lifestyle choices. This is again complicated by the lack of communication between all of these centers and the primary care provider. I recently had a patient who went to an urgent-care center three times over a four-month period only to subsequently find out he had kidney cancer, which had spread to the bone. Comprehensive patient-centered medical care with continuity of care by a primary care provider is what leads to better health, higher patient satisfaction, and lower costs.

Urgent-care centers have been associated with increased use of antibiotics and testing, referral to specialty care, and cost.[7] They are another fork leading down the wrong road to poor health care, increased utilization and costs, and further fragmentation and degradation of our already dysfunctional health care system. But given that their providers are trained with a Flexnerian playbook, it is no wonder.

The Osler approach of bedside teaching died with the Flexner Report and is only now getting attention, more than 100 years too late. Some schools are finally implementing training programs in communications skills, integrative approaches to wellness and health, and palliative care. Others are bringing students to the bedside and clinics earlier so they can better apply the basic sciences they are learning. New training programs such as these are welcome additions but are woefully inadequate to meet the radical reform that is needed. The major problem is that most elite academic medical programs think they are doing a fabulous job, and there is no need for change. Based on their own metrics of matching their students to the most prestigious specialty residency programs in academic hospitals, and garnering corporate funding, they need not change. However, this is not helping the physical health and wellness of our patients or our economy. It is, however, adding to their profits and status as "America's Best Hospitals."

It's hard to become a physician: the competitiveness, the hoops to jump through, the time, and the financial burden are tough. It's even harder to stay true to your values and enter the realm of primary care, sacrificing money and prestige to be a broadly trained doctor. Many say it's not worth it, but when I look back at the differences I have made in the lives of many patients and their families, I do think it was. I have had multiple four-generation families in my practice, and little is better than watching the babies you care for become parents, doctors, lawyers, essential workers, politicians (okay, maybe not so good), artists, athletes, and writers. Great primary care providers become part of a patient's family; we celebrate the achievements of life and grieve pain, suffering, and death together. What can be more satisfying, intimate, and noble as a profession?

But students chosen and trained using the template that Flexner provided for our system will never understand that side of medical care. To Osler, the marriage between science and compassion, the unassailable need to know one's patient and to understand science through their lens, died with the Flexner Report. Now students become more like technicians, measuring and fixing numbers, focused on specialization and procedures, and losing all interest in the continuity of care that is so crucial to the care of the patient. Patients take a back seat.

Medical education in this country is a mess both in medical school and after in residency and fellowship training programs, where we are training some of our nation's smartest kids to become protocol-following drones more interested in numbers than people. Tests supplant human beings in our medical education framework, and little has changed in that process for more than 100 years.

It is crucial for us to recognize the flaws and dangers of continuing with our Flexnerian training process. It is producing doctors that would even have appalled Flexner, who too believed in the importance of primary care and critical thinking skills. Unfortunately, the system he orchestrated accomplished just the opposite. Osler had education figured out before Flexner even published his report. We have a model and template upon which we can base a new and exciting system that will enhance the skills and satisfaction of tomorrow's doctors. Osler's road is an easy place to start.

CHAPTER EIGHTEEN

The Dangers of Flexnerian Overspecialization in Medical Care

A radical error at the onset is the failure to recognize that the results of specialized observation are at best only partial truths, which require to be correlated with facts obtained by wider study. The various organs, the diseases of which are subdivided for treatment, are not isolated, but complex parts of a complex whole, and every day's experience brings home the truth of the saying, "When one member suffers all the members suffer with it."

– William Osler[1]

We simply get too much medical care in this country. Much of it we get from doctors we don't know. Worse, from doctors who don't know us. The personal relationship between a doctor and her patient is a special one based on communication, trust, and empathy. This close bond is developed by creating an open and honest professional relationship that grows with time. Evidence clearly shows that these partnerships lead to better patient care, better clinical outcomes, higher levels of satisfaction with care, and decreased utilization and costs.

"It's more important to know the patient who has the disease than the disease the patient has," Hippocrates said. Osler repeated a similar line in his many lectures.

But in our Flexnerian cloud, where digging into the body with technological precision is the modus operandi of our health care system, it is natural to have a doctor for every organ with their own array of tests, drugs, and procedures to fix the manufactured abnormalities that befall us.

Though accurate data are lacking, the overuse of health care services in this country probably costs more than a trillion dollars each year out of the $4 trillion that Americans spend on health. Estimates for unnecessary health care expenditures related to overuse range from 10 to 30 percent of total health care spending; this expenditure does not add value to a person's health.[2] Excessive care often flows from overabundant referrals to specialists or patients who seek specialists for every aspect of their medical needs, bypassing primary care physicians in the process.

A report, in the proceedings of the 2017 American College of Physicians International Forum on Reducing Overuse and Misuse in Medical Care, cited the major contributor to overuse as "misaligned financial incentives encouraging physicians to do more tests and procedures, while encouraging hospitals to promote services associated with higher levels of reimbursement. This theme of rewarding volume, not value, was identified as a problem by a clear consensus of participants."[3] In other words, overuse is caused by the very precepts built into Flexnerian practice. Other reasons cited include poor coordination of medical care (including lack of interoperability of electronic health records) and lack of a strong primary care infrastructure.

We see too many specialists; have too many tests, too many procedures, and too many surgeries; and take too much medicine. We see specialists at a greater frequency than in any other country in the world. Specialists do not know who we are as a person; they are most often treating an organ, a limb, or a disease process and not the whole person. Specialist physicians may do the appropriate things based on some clinical evidence or a clinical guideline. They may fix errant numbers or measurements as pertains to their organ of interest, but it may not be the right thing for the patient. Fixing one thing may make five other things worse, and, most important, may make you worse. Specialists perceive their interventions through a myopic focus. If the drugs and procedures they give you push other measurements out of line, or cause you to feel poorly, then they will often refer you to another specialist, but they'll never back away from thinking that whatever helps their organ is necessary and lifesaving, your complaints be damned.

I often laugh when my patients come back from certain specialists and describe their encounters. Last night an elderly patient with severe chronic lung disease on constant nasal oxygen described her latest encounter with her pulmonologist. He started pressuring her to walk to evaluate if the oxygen level in her blood falls while she's walking. The patient is confined to a wheelchair and can, with assistance, get up from the chair to get into bed, sit in a chair or couch, or go to the bathroom. But she cannot walk more than two to three steps. It amazed her that the doctor did not know this because he has been "taking care of her lungs" for almost five years. The pulmonologist is world-acclaimed, an excellent clinician, and a truly good person. It was not his lack of medical knowledge or empathy; it was his inadequate knowledge of his patient as a person.

Overuse of medical procedures and care is defined as the provision of medical services that are more likely to cause harm than good. On average, doctors estimate that 22 percent of prescription medications, 24.9 percent of tests, and 11.1 percent of procedures in their specialty are unnecessary.[4] Rarely are informed, patient-centered decisions made where people are given clear and convincing evidence about what they are doing or taking, and whether it is really necessary. Much of this number-fixing and excessive treatment occurs in a specialist's office, where organs are treated at the expense of the patient.

Two years ago, I began care of a frail 98-year-old woman who had a heart attack in her early 50s, but no subsequent events. She came to me for care because she had outlived her doctor. Mrs. X was on nine medications for blood pressure, cholesterol, and diabetes. She needed to walk with a cane, was at severe risk of falls, and already had several with minor injuries. Over a six-week period, I tapered her off all of her medicine except for one of her blood pressure meds. Her cardiologist called me, furious that I had stopped most of her meds. "You're killing her," he said. I responded that HE was killing her with all of his deleterious medications. He had no idea she was suffering from frequent falls, fatigue, and weakness; he probably never asked. Likely those minor complaints were unimportant in his mind compared with the necessity of his heart drugs.

Two years later, she is still alive, feels better than ever, and is no longer falling from low blood pressure. I recently attended her 100th birthday party. Since being off many of her medications, she has felt the best she has in years. We can debate the art versus the science of medicine forever. Specialists rely on the science of protocol and number-fixing; thank you, Flexner. Oslerian primary care providers rely on evidence-based science combined with a person-centric approach to care that relies on listening, communicating, and coming to an informed, shared decision for all medical care; thank you, Dr. Osler.

I recently admitted an elderly man with gastrointestinal bleeding secondary to being on too much Coumadin (blood thinner) that he was taking for his afib and abnormal heart valves. The cardiologist insisted the patient stay on the medication because he was at high risk of stroke, which is not the case. I called the cardio many times, saying that I could not control his dose of Coumadin because he was confused at times, failed to take the medication correctly, and failed to follow up for regular blood tests to monitor his drug level. But the cardiologist kept prescribing, and the patient came to the hospital for bleeding from an ulcer.

We have explored the newer and more expensive meds used for the treatment of afib, Xarelto and Eliquis among them. These drugs are among the most marketed drugs to cardiologists and to the public. Yes, they do help many people, but they also kill many from their complications. To the Flexnerian cardiologist who is prescribing the medication, he is treating his one area of interest without looking at the total picture, the human picture. To the Flexnerian cardiologist there is only one right answer – the patient must take a blood thinner or he will have a stroke. The bleeding is not his concern, death from the drug is not his concern, and so he minimizes the risks to the patient and insists that it is safe and necessary, no discussion allowed. Specialists are not bad people and they are certainly not bad doctors. Their focus is on only one thing, and thus they miss the big picture. They miss the whole person.

There is a saying in medicine that you should not do a procedure or a test if you are not going to do something with the result. Specialists are the least likely to understand whether a particular test, procedure, or a particular medication will help a patient with whom they do not have a close relationship. It is the specialists who, in proportion to their numbers, order far more invasive and noninvasive diagnostic tests and procedures than any other doctors.[5]

One of the classic examples of overtesting is the utilization of MRIs for back pain or joint pain, something done with great frequency by specialist doctors.[6] Patients pressure doctors every day to get MRIs for all of their ailments. Some patients simply just want to know what their diagnosis is or why they are in pain and to ensure they do not have something bad, such as cancer. Other patients have been falsely brainwashed into thinking that if they have a problem and there is a procedure for it, they must have the procedure whether it will help them or not. Most patients will not benefit and do not want surgical procedures for herniated discs in their backs or torn cartilage in their knees, which may sometimes hurt as many as they help. And especially in elderly patients, abnormalities are the rule even in people without pain. All this testing does is add to the costs of medical care without improving clinical outcomes or patient quality of life and satisfaction in many who undergo them. The vast majority of chronic back pain without significant neurological signs and symptoms should be treated symptomatically and with heat, ice, physical therapy, and other integrative modalities, such as yoga, which has been shown to be extremely effective in relieving pain and increasing mobility.

CT and MRI scans of the brain are ordered by providers and overrequested by patients. The cure for all headaches and head trauma is not a diagnostic test such as a CT or MRI.[7] The use of CTs for head trauma with no loss of consciousness and a normal physical exam is simply not indicated or appropriate. It is rare that I ever see a patient discharged from an emergency department with a head injury or even a simple headache without having a brain CT, which exposes the patient to needless radiation and potential false-positives. It is even rarer for me to send a patient to a neurologist for a headache and not have them order an MRI; in fact, I can never recall that happening. Specialists should assist the primary care provider in the appropriate evaluation of a patient. We are not referring to specialists just to order tests; we could do that on our own. But that often is the knee-jerk response in the specialty model of care, which seeks data points despite their irrelevance and potential harm.

"Choosing Wisely" is an initiative of the American Board of Internal Medicine Foundation that seeks to advance a national dialogue on unnecessary medical tests, treatments, and procedures.[8] Each medical society has compiled lists of tests, procedures, or medications that are overused or can be avoided. The mission of the Choosing Wisely campaign is to promote conversations between clinicians and patients by helping them choose care that is supported by evidence, not repeats of tests or procedures already received, free from harm, and truly necessary. It may be hard to gauge the success of such an enterprise, but it has at least made each medical society aware of what it is doing. We have stated many times in this book that overutilization of medical care is not without harm. Overtesting leads to overdiagnosis, which leads to overtreatment, which can instigate significant medical harm and unnecessary stress and worry.

Specialists often have an unfair advantage over primary care doctors when it comes to meeting quality metrics. Most insurance companies grade primary care providers on how many tests they do, how many referrals they make, how many times their patients go to the emergency department and hospital, and even how many antibiotics they prescribe. The same is not true for cardiologists who order diagnostic testing on the vast majority of patients they see or for the neurologist who orders an MRI of the brain with regularity. In fact, many neurologists own the MRI machines they use. Likewise, the cardiologist may own the echocardiogram and stress test machines, dramatically augmenting their incomes by self-referring. A large proportion of medical cost and harm derives from such self-referral, which feeds the cognitive biases of patients and is paid very well by our Flexnerian system.

The contrary is true for the primary care physician, who receives ratings from insurance companies based on use and cost. Insurance companies are now known to rate their doctors and then to steer patients to their lower-cost providers. In fact, if a cardiologist orders a stress test, echocardiogram, and carotid ultrasound every year in their office – tests of little to no value but very expensive and profitable – and gives patients expensive medicines, hospitalizes them, and refers them to other specialists, it is that patient's primary care doctor who will be punished for the high cost of patient care, while the cardiologist and other specialists enjoy the bounty of their self-serving plunge into Flexnerian health care.

So, let me continue to pick on the cardiologist because that is where a huge chunk of the health care dollar is being spent. In cardiology, an estimated 11 percent of stents are delivered to inappropriate patients.[9] Patients appropriate for the procedure include those having an acute heart attack and those with symptoms showing they are about to have a heart attack, known as "unstable angina." Some stents are inappropriate because the evidence shows that medical management of stable coronary artery disease is the same or better with appropriate medications, diet, and exercise. At some hospitals, that rate is closer to 20 percent. Inappropriate use of noninvasive cardiac testing, such as a nuclear stress tests (injecting radioactive material to assess cardiac tissue during a stress test) is even more rampant. The American College of Cardiology's number one recommendation in the Choosing Wisely initiative is to avoid performing annual stress cardiac imaging or advanced noninvasive imaging as part of routine follow-up in asymptomatic patients.[10] What this means is that if you have a patient with stable coronary artery disease, or one who has had a previous heart attack, you should not order a stress test unless there are symptoms. In my world, annual cardiac testing – on machines owned by the cardiologist – is the norm. Given the escalating cost of these tests – $100 billion a year – without any improvement in outcome, it is in fact the norm everywhere. And yet, because these tests are ordered by specialists, nothing is done to curb their use. After all, in Flexnerian logic, we need to find problems if we are going to fix them.

Cardiac catheterization is one of the most widely performed cardiac procedures, with more than 1 million cardiac catheterization procedures performed annually in the United States. Any invasive procedure has risks, and the same is true for cardiac catheterization, where the risk of major complications is about 1 percent, and the risk of mortality is 0.05 percent just from the test.[11] The risks are far higher if they decide to "fix" a blockage and put in a stent. With millions of people getting these tests unnecessarily, tens of thousands die and are harmed every year. Cardiologists are paid very well for such tests, whether the outcome is good or not, whether the test is necessary or not.[12]

Once you see a death as the result of a cardiac catheterization, you will not forget it. A patient of mine with a prior history of coronary artery disease went to see her cardiologist at a major academic center for her annual evaluation. She had no symptoms, but the cardiologist said it would be prudent to do a stress test. Thus began an unfortunate spiral that did not have a good ending – something we call the "Swiss cheese explanation model."

It was James Reason, professor emeritus of psychology at the University of Manchester, England, who proposed this metaphor to describe how a series of barriers put in place to prevent poor results (in this case a medical error) can actually bring about the very outcome that is feared. Because each barrier to a bad out-come will have unintended holes – hence the similarity to Swiss cheese – harmful effects can get through when those holes are aligned. In the medical world, tests and interventions are pur-ported to be in service to the patient. Unfortunately, the sheer number of procedures carried out in our system can actually make a patient more susceptible to a bad outcome. There are just too many specialists, too many tests and interventions, and no one to oversee the process. Tragically, it often starts with an intervention that's not even necessary in the first place. Proce-dure 1 leads to perceived numerical abnormalities that lead to more tests that lead, in turn, to procedures 2 and 3 and so on, and then more medicines and more side effects, which lead to more medicines and more specialty visits.

The elderly woman did have a previous history of coronary disease and a heart attack 40 years ago, but had no symptoms, and was subjected to a stress test because her cardiologist just wanted to be safe. The next event in the Swiss cheese model was an equivocal result on the stress test, meaning it was not normal, but not abnormal either. So, this asymptomatic woman underwent a cardiac catheterization in one of our nation's top academic centers. She got through the test "well" and then came to us two days later with pain in her foot because the insertion of a catheter cut off blood supply to her leg. She went to have the clot removed and unfortunately suffered a major stroke. Mrs. X died one week later in our hospice unit. She died from a test she never should have had in the first place, one that a Flexnerian specialist believed to be necessary because he was looking for something he could fix in a patient who was feeling well. Tests done this way are as dangerous as any disease. And sadly, they are common occurrences in our specialized medical society.

Unnecessary surgery – a hysterectomy, an orthopedic procedure, or the removal of the gallbladder – can similarly cause
harm when not indicated. The truth is, the body has many "broken" parts that are perfectly fine if left alone and do not impair
our health. It's "fixing" them that can cause great harm.

Most people are under the impression that the more testing
and the more advanced technology we use, the better. But testing done to "see if something is wrong" often leads to incidental
abnormalities that are not dangerous but that specialists often
feel the need to fix. With the advancement of radiologic screening
and its increased unfettered use, more subtle and insignificant
abnormalities are being discovered. These incidental findings
lead to more tests, more procedures, and more risk of harm. And
the data clearly show that specialists order most of these kinds
of tests. If the specialist does not find a reason for a symptom
related to his organ system, he may order tests or refer the patient
to another specialist who will order more tests until either nothing is found, or – all too commonly – something is found completely unrelated to the symptom.

One of the barriers to fixing the overutilization of specialty
care is the belief by some, including doctors, that seeing a specialist leads to better results. If your knee hurts, go to an ortho-
pedist. If you have diabetes, go to an endocrinologist. If you
don't want a heart attack, get a checkup with a cardiologist.
Many of my patients see so many specialists that each of their
organs is carved up into tiny slices; they end up getting excessive testing and are on copious amounts of medicines that rarely
help them and often make them feel horrible. But they still think
they are getting the best care possible. Their organs are getting
"fixed" one by one, but no one is taking care of *them*. Evidence
to support the misplaced idea that specialty care produces better results simply does not exist, but the evidence for effective

comprehensive primary care is abundant. A specialist will perform certain tests that are routine for them to look for anything that may be wrong in their narrow realm, will fix those things, and will keep seeing you and trying to convince you that you will be dead without all this stuff. You can't blame them for doing what they were trained to do and for what most think is the right thing to do. It's what we were all told to do in medical school, it's how we are judged as physicians, and it leads to the highest payment. But it is not helpful to human beings or to our bloated medical system.

I highly respect the specialists with whom I work. I have chosen the ones who are willing to work with me in taking care of my patients holistically. I have stopped referring to many specialists over the years who refuse to acknowledge my crucial role in caring for our mutual patient, who test and treat too much, and who can't look beyond their organ.

The current culture of overuse is driven by many forces: defensive medicine by doctors trying to avoid lawsuits and financial incentives to overtest, overtreat, overprescribe, and perform too many needless procedures and surgeries. Flexnerian physicians are trained from the beginning to do more and more for their patients, using flimsy, often industry-scripted, evidence to support it. The current fee-for-service payment structure incentivizes us to have as many visits, tests, and procedures as possible, and the Flexnerian mantra provides a rationale for this orgy of care. Self-referral is normal and acceptable. We live in a society where there is a cultural preference for technological solutions. Test-diagnose-fix is our creed, rather than eat healthy, exercise, and take good care of yourself. The results of this are quite apparent.

The solution is not to eliminate specialists, who are crucial cogs in the success of our health care system, but to limit their engagement with patients by paying them appropriate fees for procedures, training fewer of them, and placing an emphasis on primary care. Then they can be the type of doctors that Osler perceived them to be: consultants when primary care doctors need some help, which, despite the prevailing lore otherwise, will not be very often.

CHAPTER NINETEEN

US Insurance Companies: Bankrupting Our Nation One Sickness at a Time

To combine in due measure the altruistic, the scientific, and the business side of our work is not an easy task. In the three great professions, the lawyer has to consider only his head and pocket, the parson the head and the heart, while with us the head, heart, and pocket are all engaged.

– William Osler[1]

The insurance industry in the United States is unlike anything else in the world. No other country in the world allows the profitability of the insurance industry to dictate "appropriate medical care" at the expense of the wellness of patients and dissatisfaction of providers. In both its administrative inefficiency and its willingness to finance our leap into Flexnerian care, the insurance industry has escalated cost at the expense of quality. In fact, the overhead of the insurance companies accounts for almost 25 percent of health care spending. This is in contrast to less than 2 percent overhead on Medicare spending and spending in other nations. Doctors feel the sting of this: we are put through so many hoops just to take care of our patients, from preauthorizations to quality indicators to the many petty requirements tossed at us, that we squander almost half of our time. But insurance is needed to keep the wheels of our Flexnerian machine moving, to assure that money is funneled to those who profit most from excessive care, to demean the role of primary care, and to pass all cost to the consumer under the veil of necessity.

What was the origin of health insurance after the Flexner Report, and how did it evolve to finance our current plunge into a sea of largely unnecessary and excessive care at high cost?[2]

The first insurance plans started in the 1930s to cover the costs of more expensive hospital care. The original Blue Cross policies were not-for-profit. At that time, more than 95 percent of premiums were spent on patient care and 5 percent on administrative costs. As the system evolved and more money could be found by insuring more people, employer-provided health plans became the norm, something unique to our nation. In fact, large percentages of Americans under the age of 65 are still covered by employee-based plans.

Because the landscape of health care before the 1960s was not cluttered with copious drugs and tests and procedures, the Flexnerian system seemed to be working. Without so many available medical interventions, care costs were not high, and doctors had no incentive to overtest or overtreat. The hospital at that time was more of a place to recover from illness than it is today, and thus it was low cost and not focused on tests and procedures. Also, many doctors did specialize, but even those tended to practice general medical care because there was little that specialists could do that differed much from that of a primary care doctor.

Flexner himself went on to work at both the Carnegie and Rockefeller Foundations and helped to finance some of the medical programs his report produced. But he became increasingly frustrated by the specialization of health care and the lack of creativity and diversity that his report instigated. In later years, as he talked about the need to include poorer people in health care, and to train more general practitioners who were not imbued with rigid scientific principles but rather more broadly and holistically trained, he sounded a great deal like Osler.[3] But by then it was too late; the American Medical Association (AMA) ruled the roost, and the top-down, protocol-based German model of education and care prevailed.

As the AMA orchestrated a physician-directed medical establishment that grew and prospered, few complained. Overall, the Flexnerian system proved more reliable and scientific than the mess it replaced. And doctors were both respected and financially thriving. But some kinks began to show in the late 1940s and 1950s. At that time, it became clear that not everyone could afford even basic health care and some of the emerging drugs and technologies. Health insurance started to emerge, mostly financed by employers who sought to reduce the burden that illness placed on their business, and these plans (starting with Blue Cross) covered catastrophic care, such as surgery and operations. The AMA negotiated with these organizations to assure that doctors maintained their autonomy to order any tests, drugs, and procedures that they deemed appropriate, and that doctors could set their own fees. Again, given the low cost of hospital stays and of most tests and procedures, they were not onerous to insurance carriers, and thus could the Flexnerian system persevere and be woven into health insurance policy.

But following the lead of many European countries, some reformers in the United States advocated national health care, something that climaxed with President Truman's National Health Insurance bill in 1945. By this time, health care costs had increased by 15 percent over the past five years because of increased physician services and fees, and because more drugs and tests were available. It is estimated that at some point in their lives in the 1940s, 25 percent of Americans went into debt trying to pay medical bills for these increasing services. The Truman bill would impose a 3 percent payroll tax to pay for all care for 80 percent of the population, excluding only the very rich, who could afford such services, and the very poor, who received charity care.

The AMA fought hard against the Truman bill, using Flexnerian language to defeat it, claiming that through this piece of "socialist legislation" the government would replace doctors as the arbiter of health care provision, and that doctors alone had the capacity to know what was best for their patients. Morris Fishbein, MD, editor of the *Journal of the American Medical Association*, denounced the National Health Act as "the kind of regimentation that led to totalitarianism in Germany and the downfall of that nation." The AMA hired a PR firm and ran an advertisement declaring that the scientific acumen of properly trained physicians would be replaced by robots programmed by the government, warning of long lines and lack of access to care. In its widely disseminated, 24-page brochure, *Showdown on Political Medicine*, the AMA portrayed the bill as "an unusual crisis of great peril" that would "establish a core of collectivist control under which freedom of enterprise in any form could not long survive."

As a compromise, the AMA advocated an increase in state-directed funding for charity care – which would be controlled by local medical societies affiliated with the AMA – and an expansion of private health insurances, which already complied with AMA policy. Essentially, the AMA would only accept a program that placed no restrictions on the tests, drugs, and procedures that doctors could order, or the fees that they could charge.

The AMA won the battle, but over the next 20 years the number of medical interventions increased, more specialized doctors emerged, new and expensive drugs hit the landscape and were perceived to be necessary and lifesaving by the doctors who prescribed them, and hospitalization became more complex and expensive.

This pushed the AMA to the brink because many started again to clamor for government-controlled health care. President Johnson heeded the call by introducing Medicare and Medicaid in 1965. Once again the AMA fought back, decrying this new assault on the integrity of the physician, labeling the bills as socialized medicine. AMA president Donavan Ward wrote about Medicare, "Look only at the intrusion of Government in the field of medicine, which cannot be avoided if this measure is adopted. With the quantity of care thus restricted for the sake of controlling costs, the quality must deteriorate. The patient is the ultimate sufferer."[4] In other words, the battle cry of doctors had grown to echo a Flexnerian truism now firmly planted in the minds of many Americans: doctors alone, through their unrestricted ability to test and treat patients, could assure the safety and health of their patients. Any interference in physician autonomy would be catastrophic.

The AMA's massive publicity campaign did not defeat Medicare but carved out accommodations that granted even more power to it and to the nation's doctors and hospitals. And, after 1965, as technology exploded, so too did the health care industry. Medicare sanctified fee-for-service in all aspects of health care delivery, which thus incentivized doctors to do more.

With Medicare's coffers failing to keep pace with the price tag of medicine, with doctors having no restrictions on what they could charge and order, and with private health care feeling the strain and passing that onto both private policyholders and employers, the Nixon administration supported the inception of strategies to rein in cost. Writes health historian Paul Starr, "The need now was to curb its insatiable appetite for resources. In a short time, American medicine seemed to pass from stubborn shortages to irrepressible excess, without ever having passed through happy sufficiency ... The system needed fewer hospitals, more primary care incentives ..., and better management and organization."[5]

Books such as *Doing Better and Feeling Worse* shot an arrow right at the Flexnerian myth that gained a strong foothold in the public mind after Medicare. Mostly, these books demonstrated that as doctors ordered more interventions, as they hospitalized more patients and fixed every aberrant number in their body, people were feeling worse. This was Osler to its core.

The Nixon administration's prescription was the health maintenance organization (HMO) movement. HMOs are health insurance agencies that rely on primary care and curtail medical interventions for which there is no proven benefit. They, in essence, remove the AMA from its central leadership role, and place barriers in the way of Flexnerian health care.

The result was disastrous. Americans, who were now wedded to the myth that more is better and that every abnormality must be found and fixed, rebelled against HMOs. They did not want anyone preventing them from getting whatever medical interventions they or their specialist doctors wanted. People overwhelmingly grasped the implications of spiraling costs of the system, but few wanted to restrict their personal appetite for unending care. As a result, HMOs fizzled, and the AMA – which fought yet another pitched battle against them – preserved what it had inaugurated in 1911 and what now had won the hearts and minds of most. Flexner, it seemed, could not die.

Paul Starr's iconic book on health care, *The Social Transformation of American Medicine* (1982), demonstrates the medical landscape after the AMA's victory in both the Medicare and HMO challenges to institutionalized physician autonomy and Flexnerian philosophy. When one reads Starr's conclusions today, it is as if, 42 years after it was written, nothing substantive has changed. He writes,

> The dynamics of the system in everyday life are simple to follow. Patients want the best medical services available. Providers know that the more services they give and the more complex the services are, the more they earn and the more likely they are to please their clients, because doctors are trained to practice medicine at the highest level of technical quality without regard to cost.

Without saying so, Starr defined the ramifications of the Flexner Report on physician and patient beliefs and behavior now codified into health care.

If we look at just a few tests/procedures that were either not extant at the time Starr wrote his book or were used only on a limited basis, we can see how much the cost of Flexnerian care has expanded in the past 40 years. These interventions have become standard of care and largely endorsed by both insurance companies and the public, despite their less-than-proven benefit and their high cost. Because they achieve Flexner's promise of finding and fixing problems, few will question their efficacy. And yet each of these tests is deeply flawed and often used in a way that is not beneficial to patients.

As of 2020, approximately 8 million nuclear stress tests are performed in the United Stated a year, at a cost of $28 billion.[6] Cardiologists also perform approximately 8 million echocardiograms annually, at a cost of $24 billion.[7] To fix the blocked vessels found on some of these tests, cardiologists and cardiac surgeons place approximately a million stents a year, at a cost of $35 billion, and perform a half million coronary bypass surgeries, at a cost of $45 billion. Doctors also order 40 million MRIs a year, at an average cost of $3,000 per test. Orthopedic surgeons perform about 750,000 arthroscopic surgeries just of the knee each year, at a total cost of $3 billion – all costs that insurance willingly pays. And that's just a start.[8]

Small businesses suffer the most from the current insurance structure because they end up having to pay the highest premiums and then pass the expense off to their employees or customers. Many people are forced to accept generic plans through their work with benefits that they may not need and that may not be the best plan for them. Some people in low-paying jobs receive no insurance at all or plans they cannot afford, usually with very high deductibles, rendering them useless for most medical needs. According to eHealth's data, 7 percent of the population pays for their own health insurance, with an average monthly cost of $440 for an individual and $1,168 for a family in 2018.[9]

Why do insurers fight the little stuff and pay for the big stuff? It comes down to who will complain more when insurers try to appear as though they are cutting costs, something that their employer-clients and shareholders expect them to do. When insurance does not cover certain services, often touted by doctors as being necessary, this drives patients and employers to change plans.

I once spoke with a medical director of a large health insurer. I asked him why he continued to pay for so many stents in people who did not need them; surely his company would save money, and would be able to lower premiums, if they cut back such high-cost, low-value procedures. He laughed. "You don't mess with the cardiology lobby," he told me. "They'll beat you every time." Cardiologists are among the highest-paid physicians, and they exert great influence on Congress. In fact, every specialty group sends powerful players to Capitol Hill to assure that Medicare maintains high payment for procedures, and because Medicare sets the prices that most private insurers follow, this lobbying trickles all the way down to the consumer.

The insurance industry, it turns out, garners the most profit and least amount of reprisal from the public and medical establishment if they endorse and finance our bloated medical system as is, making small cuts here and there, but not stamping on Flexner's well-entrenched footprints. It is not in their interest to push for reform, cut costs, lower reimbursement, or advocate the type of patient-centric program Oslerians seek. They can make more money if they spend more, as backward as that may seem.

If you want to understand the self-serving and often base nature of our private insurance industry, listen to someone who spent his career concocting lies and deceptions for that very industry. Wendell Potter, who was the head of public relations for CIGNA until he resigned in 2009, wrote *Deadly Spin*. Potter on the industry's spin: "Health care costs are out of control because new treatments and technologies are more expensive than ever, the population is getting older and sicker, too many people are seeking care they don't really need, and health care providers are all too willing to provide this care that people don't really need."[10] In other words, it's not the fault of insurance that premiums are escalating; it's the fault of the system.

Potter says that the industry does best by raising premiums rather than cutting costs. And, as it turns out, that posturing has also helped the industry become very profitable. The more they can spend on health care, the more they can pay their shareholders and executives.

There are many reasons insurance companies are willing to pay big bucks for interventions they know don't work or that could be provided at a far lower cost. It comes down to the medical loss ratio. The more an insurer pays for patient care, the more it can keep for its stockholders and executives. In Medicare, 97 percent of all money goes toward health care. In many private insurances, that number is much lower. Under the Affordable Care Act (2010), insurers are required to spend at least 80 percent of premiums for health care, and no more than 20 percent for other costs, namely, executive compensation. So, how do insurers increase executive compensation while adhering to this restriction?

The answer is simple. Since profits are limited to 20 percent of the premium, the only way to escalate profits is for the insurance company to spend more. Let's say that a certain insurance company spends $1,000 for the medical costs of all its members. Under current law, the most it can allot to its own executives and shareholders is 20 percent of that, or $200.

Let's say the same insurer above pays $10,000 for its health care expenses, citing the rising cost of technology, the aging population, and their desire to not get between doctors and patients. Now that it's spending so much more, the 20 percent it can give to itself is now $2,000. Spend more, keep more, and blame the system.

Hence, when insurers pay for everything and keep payments high, when they accept and finance Flexnerian medical care rather than trying to educate patients and doctors to be more sensible, they make more money for themselves. It's a win-win situation. Consumers' demands appear to drive care, which Potter said is spun into the palatable *consumer-driven model of care*. Who pays for the extra cost of care? Policyholders of course, in the form of high premiums. Everyone makes money, and consumers and businesses pay the price. But those same consumers think the insurance companies are being generous to pay for all their stuff.

The insurance industry, rather than being an ally in promoting patient-centric, high-value care, is a bulwark against change.

Insurance companies, like specialist doctors, hospitals, and so many others, champion the current system in its full-spending mode. It's been a bonanza for their industry.

There is a deep-seated and long history of the insurance industry's stealth campaign to undermine health care reform, from its assault on Truman's health bill to its labeling of Medicare as "socialized medicine," to its effective maligning of President Clinton's health care reform as a "government take over of health care." All along it hinges its position on a basic Flexnerian creed: that anything getting between doctor and patient, anything that prevents doctors from leaping into a measure-diagnose-fix spending spree, is detrimental to patient care. That's why we can't have federal health care plans, single-payer, or even federally directed regulation. Potter on the Clinton plan: "It was clear the voters were frightened away from [Clinton's reform bill] by the specter – conjured up by the insurance industry and its business and political allies – of government bureaucrats coming between them and their doctors. What Americans got instead was private insurance companies doing exactly the same thing."[11]

Very often the insurance industry will create front groups, such as community groups and patient disease advocacy organizations (which are partially funded by pharma and insurance companies), allegedly speaking for the common people to demand that insurers pay for everything that the good doctor orders.

When Michael Moore's *Sicko* (2007) was released – a movie that critiqued the bloated health care industry in the United States – the insurance lobby pounced immediately by promoting fabricated consumer outrage under the umbrella of a group called Health Care America, a fabricated group "funded by money from the health insurance industry and other special interests ... for the sole purpose of attacking Moore and his contention that people in countries with government-run systems spent far less and got better care than people in the United States."[12] The industry created similar groups to assail the public option under President Obama's plan. The message is always the same: "Don't let anyone come between you and your doctor and don't put any curbs on our measure-diagnose-fix mantra or else we will all suffer."

Hence, today's health insurance industry finances the most egregious leaps into futility – such as paying high prices for ineffective tests and procedures ordered by cardiologists, radiologists, and other procedure-oriented specialists – while devoting few resources to primary care and other more effective and undervalued services.

The insurance companies will also do everything they can to cherry-pick their patients. Recruiting in higher-income communities amid higher-end employers, they do everything they can to avoid high-cost and sicklier patients. Insurance company recruiters from Medicaid plans put up booths outside bodegas or churches in underserved communities, while the private insurers hold dinners in restaurants or camp outside upscale communities to find more "desirable" patients. A *STAT+* health article (July 2018) talks about this extensively: "The companies are tracking your race, education level, TV habits, marital status, and net worth. They're collecting what you post on social media, whether you're behind on your bills, what you order online. Then they feed this information into complicated computer algorithms that spit out predictions about how much your health care could cost them."[13]

Once the insurance company signs you up, they will do everything they can to make everything as complex as they can. This creates the illusion that they are conscious about cutting costs, but its sting is felt most strongly in primary care offices. Doctors' offices and hospitals are required to hire copious employees to handle this process, leading to a 25 percent administrative cost of working with the insurance companies. Each insurance company uses different criteria for approvals and denials, and each insurance company has a different formulary. Each year the medication formulary may change, requiring physicians to change people's medications, even if those medicines are effective.

The insurance companies will then do everything they can to deny or delay payments for the care doctors have already provided. A recent study revealed that almost 15 percent of initial claims are indiscriminately denied by insurance companies. Eighty percent of these denials are eventually paid after being proven to be appropriate, but at a tremendous cost to our health care system and burden to our providers and their practices. For non-Medicare patients, a large number of admissions to hospitals are denied after the fact.

Under our current insurance mess, patients receive care they don't need and have to fight for care they do need. Their insurance is often tied to their workplace, which impedes their ability to change jobs. The more an insurance company pays for expensive care, the more it spins the illusion that it is helping its patients, but, in fact, the more it is earning for its executives. Doctors' offices are overwhelmed with needless complex tasks that detract from the quality care of their patients, while being judged by meaningless metrics with which insurance companies can "prove" they are endorsing quality care. Even Flexner himself could not have anticipated this.

CHAPTER TWENTY

The Power and the Influence of the Pharmaceutical Industry

For generations the people of the United States have indulged in an orgy of drugging. Between polypharmacy in the profession, and quack medicines, the American body has been saturated ad nauseam.

– William Osler[1]

The global pharmaceutical market is worth more than $1.2 trillion.[2] Escalating costs, rising profits, drug shortages, and a lack of integration with the rest of the system define a cog of the medical-industrial complex, whose job it is to produce what we have been led to believe are necessary and lifesaving drugs. There has been a recent lack of innovation, with much of medicine development focused on producing expensive copycat drugs that do more to fix numbers than to help patients. Simply changing the delivery system, duration of action, or dosing schedules can add years to a drug's patent and millions to the pharmaceutical company's profits. It's a brilliant marketing scheme – with little investment in research dollars – because patients want the latest and greatest drugs they see on TV, which are no better than or the same as what they are already taking.

Predictably, these companies speak in a Flexnerian language – "Our drug can dramatically drop cholesterol" – that appeals to patients and doctors alike. And with the Food and Drug Administration (FDA) allowing companies to tie benefit to an improvement in surrogate markers, more drugs are flooding the market that offer no real value to the patients who are buying them, to the tune of billions of dollars a year.

The United States is the world's largest market for pharmaceuticals. Through Medicare, the United States is also the only nation in the world that does not negotiate prices with the pharmaceutical companies. Simply by negotiating the costs of medications, we could save our nation billions of dollars in health care and pharmaceutical costs. The reason we don't is based in a statutory prohibition on government drug price negotiations. Medicare, through its part D plan, covers the costs of medications for a large number of our older population. Despite the ability of Congress to change this policy, it has not.

A 2019 report by the US House Ways and Means Committee titled "A Painful Pill to Swallow: U.S. vs. International Prescription Drug Prices," compared drug prices in the United States with drug prices in the United Kingdom, Japan, Ontario (Canada), Australia, Portugal, France, the Netherlands, Germany, Denmark, Sweden, and Switzerland. It concluded that Americans pay significantly more than the other countries, and that the United States could save $49 billion annually on Medicare part D alone by pricing drugs similarly to the other countries studied.[3] The average prices in most countries were 24 to 30 percent lower than those in the United States. This report by the Ways and Means Committee showed that we pay on average nearly four times more for prescription drugs than 11 economically similar countries. Why does this occur? A huge part is lobbying by the industry to Congress. In 2020, the pharmaceuticals and health products industry in the United States spent more on lobbying efforts than every other industry, totaling about $300 million.

The pharmaceutical industry often touts the need to charge more money so that it can finance its research and development programs, programs they promise are necessary if the country is to create the next wonder drug. This claim lacks all credibility. The billions of dollars the industry makes is not being spent on research. In fact, research and development for most major companies is the smallest part of their expenditures. Most spend more than double the research expenses on marketing and administration costs. A 2020 *Journal of the American Medical Association* study, which included 63 of 355 new therapeutic drugs and biologic agents approved by the FDA between 2009 and 2018, estimated that the median cost to produce a new drug was $985 million.[4] This is easily offset by the tens of billions of dollars in profits that are made by many drugs, including Eliquis and Ozempic, which earn their companies billions annually. The Campaign for Sustainable Rx Pricing, using global data, conducted a 2019 study that revealed that pharma spends on average 22 percent on research and development, 22 percent on production and operations, 19 percent on marketing and advertising, 18 percent profits, 10 percent taxes, and 9 percent overhead and administration.

The bar is very low for drug companies to get their drugs approved. The requirements of the FDA for drug approval have plummeted over the past few years – the companies themselves participate in and fund the approval process. The recent FDA approval of the dementia medicine aducanumab (Aduhelm) was based on surrogate data, even though the drug had no meaningful benefit. The FDA ignored its own advisory group in approving this medication, based on influence from the pharmaceutical company and the Alzheimer's Association, at a cost of more than

$60,000 a year, not including the costs of testing and monitoring, which may be another $40,000 a year.[5]

The pharmaceutical industry provides up to 65 percent of the FDA's budget. Drug companies need to show that the medication is *likely* effective and *unlikely* to inflict significant harm, even if it is effective in a purely Flexnerian way, that is, it fixes a surrogate number. Pharmaceutical companies design drug studies in ways that almost always assure that their new drug will be shown to have remarkable benefits and virtually no side effects. What's more, they rely on numeric success rather than clinical benefit, and will use statistical methods that magnify benefit and minimize risk. If the drug company does not get the result it wants, it won't publish the study.[6]

In addition to direct-to-consumer advertising, practicing doctors are the other targets of pharmaceutical marketing. Doctors are paid millions of dollars and given copious medication samples to dole out to patients. In most clinicians' opinion, including mine, there is a clear conflict of interest when a physician who is providing medical care has any financial interest in a medical product or its research and development. Physicians who receive payments for products prescribe these products more than their peers. But many doctors don't see it that way, believing that they are helping their patients to endorse new medicines to fix all those errant numbers.

ProPublica – a nonprofit newsroom that investigates abuses of power – has for many years exposed the obscene amount of money that pharma pays to clinicians as consultants, researchers, or speakers for their products. In 2019, ProPublica stated that "more than 2,500 physicians have received at least a half million dollars apiece from drug makers and medical device companies in the past five years alone, and that more than 700 doctors received at least a million dollars."[7] These payments do not include monies paid for research or royalties from inventions. Most of this money is spent on the same products that most viewers know from TV ads, such as the anticoagulants for afib Xarelto and Eliquis. Diabetes drugs come next in payments, for such medications as Ozempic, Tresiba, Trujeo, and Farxiga, to name a few. The TV ads all tell you to ask your doctor if these medications are right for you. What you should first ask your doctor is if they are receiving payments for promoting these medications, or if the doctor has read any studies not designed and financed by drug companies that demonstrate meaningful clinical benefit.

Many of these drugs are extremely expensive and used for rare conditions, others are fairly expensive and used for common conditions, but what unites all of them is scanty proof of benefit compared with older and cheaper drugs, along with a massive marketing campaign involving advertising directly to patients and more subtly to doctors. These drugs can also be promoted by authority figures, from university hospitals, government agencies, and consumer advocacy groups, which receive the flow of money from the pharmaceutical industry.

The pharmaceutical industry spent $6.1 billion in 2017 on direct advertising of prescription medications to the consumer.[8] The United States and New Zealand are the only nations in the world that allow this costly practice. Proponents for advertising state that consumers are given important information about diseases and their treatments that they can discuss with their doctors. The facts are that these advertisements disseminate misinformation, increase costs, and are a barrier to the physician–patient relationship. If only doctors could serve as the buttress between the ads and their patients, then it would not be of concern, but our Flexnerian-trained doctors have not proven themselves worthy of that task.

The Physician Payments Sunshine Act (2010) was designed to increase transparency about the financial relationships among physicians, teaching hospitals, and manufacturers of drugs, medical devices, and biologics.[9] The Centers for Medicare and Medicaid Services fulfill the law's mandate via the Open Payments Program. ProPublica now has a website, https://projects. propublica.org/docdollars/, where you can enter your doctor's name to see if they are receiving pharmaceutical and device manufacturer payments.[10] It's simple to navigate the website, and I highly suggest that everyone enter every physician they see into this website to determine if they have any significant financial disclosure that could cloud their medical judgment. I now routinely enter any new physician specialist to whom I refer patients to ensure there is no bias they may have based on financial incentives. Of course, doctors are rewarded in other ways that will not put them on this list, such as receiving research funding from drug companies, working on a drug-company-designed study, or being paid by a foundation that is financed by the drug company.

Despite the attention that the Sunshine Act has received, the law's reporting requirements have made no dent in payments made to clinicians. Osler said that physicians are not immune to corporate greed, and sometimes their medical judgment is clouded by financial incentives. I must admit that as a young physician I was guilty of this in a very small way. I never received payments, but I did invite pharmaceutical representatives into my office to give me samples of their newest drugs.

Providing samples of drug products to a doctor's office is a simple way for a pharmaceutical company to market its products. Drug companies send an often young and attractive marketing representative into doctors' offices to teach them about their products, provide skewed graphs about the drug's marvelous effects, and sometimes offer a lecture with lunch by a community or university doctor to tout the drug's benefit, and then say, "Give it a try, it's free, we'll give you a lot of samples."

First of all, what truly educated physician wants to learn about a product from a marketing representative (probably right out of college, with no medical training whatsoever) who works for a company trying to sell medications? Pharmaceutical company representatives are often reimbursed by how much of their medication their doctors prescribe, and they can track a doctor's prescribing pattern so that next time they come back they'll guilt the doctor into prescribing more, always with some perks in their pockets, usually with a big smile and a few compliments. As a young doctor, when I went into the sample closet to help a patient out with free medication samples, I thought I was doing a good thing. If I had a choice of, let's say, two similar antihypertensive drugs, I would go to the closet, give the patient a sample and see them in a month. If it worked and there were no side effects, I would continue to prescribe it. Not a bad scenario, and I was not paid or given any financial incentive to do this, so it felt guiltless. However, over the years I did see how it affected my prescribing of medications, something confirmed by multiple studies. What it does is convince us to prescribe the newest and most expensive medicine for free via samples until the closet is emptied, after which we write a prescription for long-term use. Without samples, most of us would use older, cheaper medicines from the start, such as antibiotics, antihypertensives, and diabetes medications. Suffice it to say, we have no samples in our offices now.

ProPublica reports that between 2014 and 2018 the industry paid approximately $2 billion to doctors for speaking, consulting, meals, travel, and gifts.[11] Federal prosecutors are now looking at some of these deals as kickbacks. In a sense, these companies use willing Flexnerian doctors as their most potent salesmen, and the result has been a flood of new and unproven drugs that are tossed into patients because doctors are led to believe that they work because they are shown to be better at improving numerical outcomes.

By 2018, 250,000 Americans had died during the two preceding decades from overdoses involving legal drugs that were produced by pharmaceutical companies and prescribed by doctors.[12] Purdue Pharma, the maker of OxyContin, has generated more than $21 billion in US sales and earned between $12 billion and $13 billion in profits since 2010, but it filed for Chapter 11 bankruptcy in 2019. When the drug was introduced in 1996, the company touted OxyContin as a safe alternative to other, highly addictive opioid painkillers, such as Vicodin and Percocet. In 2007, the company and some of its executives were convicted of charges that they had misled regulators, doctors, and patients about the drug's risk of addiction and its potential to be abused. The bankruptcy decision is the center of the company's efforts to shield itself and its owners from more than 2,600 federal and state lawsuits. The drug is being blamed for helping to start the opioid crisis.[13]

Sadly, again, Flexnerian doctors themselves fell for this trap. They did not look at studies that would have shown them the lack of clinical efficacy of these drugs. Some pharmaceutical companies concocted a pain scale – yet another classic Flexnerian innovation that rates pain by a measurable number that doctors can put in their charts and try to "fix" with opioids – and said it should serve as another vital sign. Doctors asked patients about their pain using this untested numerical scale and then flooded patients with narcotics to "fix" the number. The drug companies certainly knew how to play their Flexnerian card and appeal to exactly what our doctors most value.

As the opioid crisis and the pharmaceutical deception became big news, the government had to act. Instead of educating doctors, their answer was to make it difficult for all doctors to prescribe opioids, even those who were using them responsibly in a palliative way or for patients who literally could not tolerate any other medicine and who were not likely to abuse these medicines. In a classic one-right-answer approach, now doctors are punished for using these medicines in any capacity; there was no nuance or patient-centric approach taken – it was all or nothing. Regulation and scrutiny have led many of my colleagues to stop prescribing these often medically necessary drugs, forcing many people to buy narcotics on the street. The utilization of potent street medications, such has fentanyl, has fed the crisis and led to countless overdose deaths of good folks who were innocently prescribed pain medication for legitimate use, but then denied.

Sadly, many of my patients, many of whom are old and impaired by arthritis, either are now afraid to take these drugs or find it difficult to get them, leading to unnecessary disability. The one-right-answer approach of our medical community hurts people on both ends of the spectrum: the ones who abused the drugs when that was the right answer, and the ones who are suffering from not having a medicine that helps them when the drug became the wrong answer.

In addition to being dangerous, the prolific use of new and expensive drugs has led to a skyrocketing medication cost in this country. As doctors and patients crave the "necessary and life-saving" medicines advertised to them, the cost of medications has been climbing so steeply as to rank it as one of the main drivers of our health care system's financial strain. This has not led to anything more than a massive dose of number-fixing; real health outcomes have not improved. But doctors keep prescribing and patients keep taking, and in the end the pharmaceutical gamers have proven how successful and unassailable an old-fashioned Flexnerian rulebook can be.

Many in the pharmaceutical industry are shifting the blame for the high costs of medications to pharmacy benefit managers (PBMs). According to the American Pharmacists Association, "Pharmacy Benefit Managers are primarily responsible for developing and maintaining the formulary of insurance companies, contracting with pharmacies, negotiating discounts and rebates with drug manufacturers, and processing and paying prescription drug claims. PBM's manage commercial health plans, self-insured employer plans, union plans, Medicare Part D plans, the Federal Employees Health Benefits Program (FEHBP), state government employee plans and managed Medicaid plans." PBMs are supposed to lower the costs of medications for patients by negotiating for lower prices and passing these savings onto the patients.

There are three large PBMs – CVS Caremark, Express Scripts, and UnitedHealth's Optum – that now account for more than 70 percent of claims volume. The Pharmaceutical Care Management Association is the national association representing PBMs in the United States. According to their website, they save the average patient $941 annually on prescription costs. PBMs who run prescription drug insurance programs can make more off a higher-priced drug, because they negotiate percentage rebates. The entire system lacks transparency. As per a *STAT News* (2018) investigation, PBMs sometimes charge more for generic medications in a practice known as "spread pricing," failing to pass on rebates from bulk buying and deceiving insurers and patients into thinking they are saving them money. So essentially what happens is the pharmaceutical companies increase the price of the drugs to compensate for higher rebates to PMBs.[14]

Because formularies of each insurance company constantly change, as do costs of medications, physicians often do not know the cost of the medicines they prescribe. So, physicians constantly change a patient's medications, often at the request of patients, to keep up with shifting costs. These formulary changes have nothing to do with good patient care and have everything to do with corporate profits over patient well-being. In actuality, what has been created is a middleman that simply adds another layer of bureaucracy and cost to an already bloated system.

Generic drugs are manufactured after the patents for the branded products run out. For the vast majority of medications, the ingredients are the same with the same strength, dosages, safety, clinical efficacy, and side effect profiles. The FDA generic drugs program conducts a rigorous review to make sure generic medicines meet these requirements, yet patients often request products with the branded logo, which doctors willingly prescribe, at a higher cost to the system. In fact, about half of all generic medications are manufactured by the same company that makes the brand-name drug.

Because the pharmaceutical companies have produced so few new drugs in the past decades, and because so many of their drugs are becoming generic, they are fighting to keep people using brand names. One way to do this is to extend a patent on the drug, citing need, or even paying the generic companies to delay production of their medications. Another is to invent a copycat drug that works the same as a current generic drug but that is marketed as superior. Common gimmicks to promote copycat drugs include changing the delivery system, applying for new indications for medication use, and combining two old products into one new drug. A change in the delivery system could be as simple as a liquid formulation, a different kind of inhaler device, or a longer- or shorter-acting medicine. These offer little or no benefits except for prolonging the patent for the drug and adding to pharma's gross profits. Most drugs marketed by drug companies are copycat drugs, very often touted to "fix" some abnormality in a new way – "lowers cholesterol," "dramatically reduces sugar levels," "controls your blood pressure" – that is "fixed" just as well by older drugs, which have been far better studied.

Common examples of copycat drugs include the class of drugs called proton pump inhibitors, used for gastrointestinal problems, including acid reflux and peptic ulcer disease. Well-known drugs include Prilosec, Prevacid, Protonix, and Nexium, to name a few. Except for small differences, these medications all do the same thing as their over-the-counter and generic equivalents, but by convincing doctors and patients of their new uses, these drugs have contributed to profits of the pharma industry by the billions. I remember when Prilosec – called "the purple pill" – was touted as being the best of all acid-reducing drugs. That was until its patent ran out. Then, suddenly, a new drug – Nexium – was found to be better, and it was colored purple and called the new "purple pill." It is estimated that substituting one of the generic equivalent medications for Nexium would have saved Medicare alone more than $870 million in 2013.[15]

A similar substitution of Crestor, a lipid-lowering statin, with a generic equivalent statin would have saved Medicare $1.2 billion in the same year. But for some reason, doctors and patients are convinced that they must use Crestor. Crestor has no proven benefit in outcomes, its sales pitch relying instead on its ability to lower cholesterol numbers more than some of the other drugs.[16] This direct appeal of Flexnerian logic swindles doctors and patients, but it led to a plethora of lawsuits against the company for deceptive advertising, all of which were settled for a few hundred million dollars. These settlements are small fries for AstraZeneca, which earned $6 billion in 2013 alone from this copycat drug. Doctors are vulnerable to the appeal of these companies that tout benefits in a number-lowering language they understand.

Another game of the drug industry is the repeated shortages of many medications we have been using for years and that are actually necessary and safe. In fact, the FDA has an entire website dedicated to drug shortages, https://www.fda.gov/drugs/drug-safety-and-availability/drug-shortages. The major cause of drug shortages has been attributed to manufacturing and quality issues, and fewer companies making medications that are the least profitable. I have not seen any shortages of branded products lately; most drug shortages have been in older generic medications, the ones industry makes the least money from.

As of 2019, the FDA had more than 150 products on the list, including antibiotics (azithromycin), blood pressure medication (losartan), antiarrhythmic medication (beta blockers and calcium channel blockers), local anesthetics (lidocaine), and pain medications (morphine).[17] It is estimated that drug shortages are associated with increased patient deaths in the inpatient setting and an annual cost to the health care system of more than $13 billion.[18] The end result of these shortages is the necessity for prescribing more expensive medications, which is exactly what the pharmaceutical companies are trying to do.

The high price tag of the old and generic drug insulin is one of the major contributors to the high cost of treating type 1 diabetes (insulin-dependent). The average annual per-patient spending on treatment for type 1 diabetes increased from $12,467 in 2012 to $18,494 in 2016.[19] NovoLog, a short-acting insulin preparation, increased its price by 353 percent from 2001 to 2016. A bottle of Levemir or Lantus (long-acting, once-daily insulin drugs) can cost more than $400. Each unit of the medicine can cost as much as 40 cents. Because the average dose of this drug is about 30 units a day, diabetics spend as much as $360 a month on this medication alone.

Diabetics are required to test their blood sugar, so then add the cost of testing supplies, and many diabetics are spending more than $1,000 a month on medications and supplies. Type 2 diabetics typically don't need insulin (but many are on it) and can treat their condition with inexpensive oral medicines (or even cheaper lifestyle changes), but now they are receiving the "newest and best" drugs, which meet the Flexnerian criterium of lowering A1c without necessarily being clinically helpful. Some such drugs and their monthly costs (via GoodRx) are Januvia, $455; Trulicity, $760; Victoza, $921; Tresiba, $512; and, of course, Ozempic, $773.[20] "O, what a bargain!" The ironic thing is that there is little evidence that any of these products help you live longer or better, and exercise and diet are much more effective at addressing the cause of diabetes instead of just fixing a number. We are selling these drugs to people who don't benefit, and are denying insulin to type 1 diabetics who will die without it. That's our system.

The Right Care Alliance, a Boston-based advocacy group, has made it a crusade to bring attention to our country's escalating insulin prices.[21] The prices are so high for many that they are forced to ration their insulin, which is extremely dangerous, sometimes leading to a condition called diabetic ketoacidosis. It is known that at least 10 people died in 2017–19 from not being able to afford their insulin. What is not known is how many others died from and how many will suffer the long-term complications of undertreated diabetes, such as heart attacks, strokes, kidney failure, and death.

Unless you work for the pharmaceutical industry, receive "gifts" from them, or own their stock, you are probably a victim of their perfidious influence on our medical society. Still, despite that clear knowledge, nothing is done to curb their deception and abuse. Pharma companies spend countless dollars lobbying Congress and advertising to the consumer. They essentially pay off doctors through inappropriate marketing, consulting, and speaker programs to influence their prescribing of pharma's medications. They finance our research and have an army of university physicians to do their bidding. They have their tentacles in our federal watchdog agencies, including the FDA and the Centers for Disease Control and Prevention, and finance consumer advocacy groups.[22] But despite all of this, without a nation of Flexnerian doctors willing to fall for pharma's bait and write prescriptions for their drugs that do nothing other than fix some surrogate endpoint, these companies would not be dangerous at all. To fix the problem, we must repair our system, so that our doctors become not the agents of the pharmaceutical industry, but rather their most potent adversaries, as Osler hoped they would.

CHAPTER TWENTY-ONE

In Medical Societies We Trust

Despite the agency's disclaimer, the CDC does receive millions of dollars in industry gifts and funding, both directly and indirectly, and several recent CDC actions and recommendations have raised questions about the science it cites, the clinical guidelines it promotes, and the money it is taking.

– Medical journalist Jeanne Lenzer[1]

Last month, my state medical board received a complaint about me from a patient's daughter, who was upset that we were being lax in treating her mother's diabetes. Her mother was in hospice and lived in the dementia unit of an assisted-living facility, but the daughter demanded strict diabetic control, citing (erroneously) American Diabetes Association (ADA) recommendations for monitoring and treating this disease. I disputed her conclusions and stated that I don't sheepishly follow ADA recommendations because the ADA is in the pockets of the pharmaceutical industry. The complaint that she filed with my state medical board asked, How can a doctor who rejects ADA guidelines be considered competent?

The ADA is a trade group that purports to educate doctors and patients about diabetes, craft clinical recommendations about treatment, and advocate for patients. Its very veneer is that of being an unbiased, informative, and patient-centered organization. But is it? We have discussed earlier how the ADA helped to create the "disease" of prediabetes and promote testing and treatment for this phantom condition, which now afflicts millions of Americans. Thanks to the ADA, the United States has the most expansive definition of prediabetes in the world. Currently, 10 drugs are being developed to treat this condition, which is neither dangerous nor predictive of who will get diabetes,[2] but which certainly will generate profits for the medical-industrial complex.

The ADA is one of many patient advocacy groups dependent on pharmaceutical funding to survive. In 2015, it received $26.7 million from drug companies,[3] and, according to the *New York Times*, "is now a fixture in [pharmaceutical] marketing strategy," typically emphasizing drug therapies rather than lifestyle changes. Often the ADA executive committee is led by, or has significant participation from, pharmaceutical company employees or doctors tied to the drug industry. It accepts advertisements by the drug industry in its journal and promotes new diabetes drugs at its convention.[4]

The ADA's strong ties to industry – and its self-declared authoritative perch from which it can influence doctors and patients, not to mention craft policy – is endemic to many of today's medical organizations we have come to trust. Under Flexner's umbrella, doctors and patients are equally beholden to large organizations. Flexner's revolution was spearheaded by the American Medical Association, which in subsequent years achieved hegemony and unbridled power over medical education, medical practice, physician licensing and salaries, and federal health care policy. Flexner's report and medical school reform were themselves funded by private corporate entities, and such corporations provided money in subsequent years to influence and shape the direction of medical education, practice, and research. Today's medical research is almost exclusively controlled by industry. Moreover, industry-sponsored organizations and foundations drive much of what we think and how we act. All of this is a direct legacy of Flexner.

Few can dispute the sway that the Centers for Disease Control and Prevention (CDC) holds over medical care and our willingness to accept certain "truths" about disease, prevention (especially immunization), and treatment. As we write, the CDC is scripting our nation's response to COVID-19, and most local health departments and doctors are forced to heed its word. But the CDC is not the neutral and scientifically driven organization that many of us assume it to be. Its endorsement of such treatments as Tamiflu and Prevnar are not scientifically validated, and both industry donations and industry-affiliated members of its board swayed its positions on these and other recommendations.

In 2015, Jeanne Lenzer wrote a muckraking article in the *British Medical Journal* (*BMJ*) that shook my confidence in the CDC.[5] Lenzer, author of *The Danger within Us*, discusses how in 1983 Congress approved the CDC to seek external gifts to bolster its budget, and how, nine years later, Congress created the CDC Foundation, whose purpose was to accept drug company money and funnel it to the CDC. Lenzer went on to show how the CDC's campaign to endorse testing for hepatitis C and treat the flu with Tamiflu was tainted by drug company contributions to the foundation. In the case of hepatitis, the CDC Foundation created the benign-sounding Viral Hepatitis Action Coalition to look into hepatitis C testing and treatment, accepting $26 million in donations from industries that would benefit from such testing and treatment. Lenzer states that such contributions have been influential in CDC policy. A year later, she wrote an article in *BMJ* citing an anonymous letter by CDC scientists: "It appears that our mission is being influenced and shaped by outside parties and rogue interests. This 'climate of disregard' puts many of us in difficult positions. We are often directed to do things we know are not right."[6]

The CDC's actions mirror those of many organizations that helped drive health care policy during the early days of Flexner's revolution. They may appear benign, but these organizations, including the Carnegie and Rockefeller Foundations, financed a health care agenda that benefited them. Now many self-serving companies have infiltrated the CDC and have persuaded it to endorse testing and treatment that are not scientifically validated, but that are beneficial to their own self-interest, much in the Flexnerian vein.

Let's talk about the antiviral drug Tamiflu. The CDC's "Take 3" campaign to educate people about preventing and treating influenza recommends the use of Tamiflu for all cases of flu. Roche, the company that produces Tamiflu, has contributed significantly to the campaign.[7] The CDC has stockpiled billions of dollars worth of Tamiflu in case of an influenza pandemic.

A 2020 article describes the efforts by scientists to ascertain the actual efficacy of Tamiflu.[8] Only two studies showed that Tamiflu worked; both were sponsored by the drug companies making the antiviral drug, but eight studies of Tamiflu had not been published. When (after international pressure) Roche released the unpublished studies in 2014, Cochrane, in its Cochrane Database of Systematic Reviews, concluded that Tamiflu did not prevent complications of influenza, did not reduce the transmission of influenza during outbreaks, and was more dangerous than originally thought. Despite these facts, the CDC continues to promote Tamiflu, recommending prolific prescribing to the tune of billions of dollars.

According to Peter Doshi of the *BMJ*, "The original rationale for pandemic use was that randomized controlled trials showed [Tamiflu] reduced complications. When we showed that wasn't true, they turned to observational studies that found reduced complications, but they didn't mention other observational studies showing the opposite, and they don't mention that the observational studies they rely on were funded by Roche."[9] Why would the CDC be so fixated on ignoring science and pushing drug treatment that has been shown to be more harmful than helpful?

Roche contributes significant money to the CDC Foundation, and many administrators and scientists with ties to Roche sit at the highest level of the CDC. The marriage of industry, policy, and trusted medical organizations is very clear.

Hepatitis C screening recommendations also reveal how the CDC is influenced by industry when scripting policy decisions. Hepatitis C is a viral infection that can fester in the liver and sometimes cause serious adverse outcomes. Because of this, the CDC recommends testing for hepatitis C for everyone born between 1945 and 1965 (among whom is it most common) and treating any people found to have the disease. The cost is approximately $84,000 per treatment; the companies that develop testing and treatment have donated $26 million to the CDC's Viral Hepatitis Action Coalition. After the CDC endorsed this policy, testing increased, and the incidence of newly discovered hepatitis C jumped by almost 50 percent, with billions of dollars of antiviral treatments then prescribed.

In fact, only 6 of 1,000 people infected with hepatitis C will get severely ill from the disease, and most of those fit into easily identified categories: they are drug users, alcoholics, or obese, or have HIV. The preponderance of studies showing benefits of testing/treatment for hepatitis C are drug-sponsored and observational, and rely on surrogate markers (improvement in lab tests rather than in survival) to demonstrate the value of the CDC approach. Treatment can be far more harmful than some studies suggest. One combination of medicines causes a 4 percent increased risk of death, which is far more dangerous than the disease itself. The authors of a *BMJ* study conclude that "given the uncertainty about the validity of the surrogate markers, the lack of evidence regarding clinical outcomes of treatment or of screening strategies and the adverse events caused by the newer regimens, screening may be premature." But the CDC continues to push for screening and testing. Why?[10]

The marriage between industry and the CDC answers that question. Not only does the CDC Foundation receive copious industry dollars from companies that benefit from generalized hepatitis C testing and treatment, but CDC executives and doctors making these decisions often have direct ties to these industries themselves. For instance, members of the CDC Advisory Committee on Immunization (ACIP) "receive direct financial returns when more vaccines are added to the current schedule" because they own vaccine patents or receive pharmaceutical funding for their work. A list of patents held by ACIP members is public and extensive,[11] showing why a push for immunization by the CDC enriches many of the CDC scientists making those decisions.

Shannon Brownlee of the Lown Institute states, "Government-chartered foundations exist in part because they allow industries to directly fund and thus control the work of agencies that are either supposed to regulate them or conduct research that help or hurt their business."[12] Thus, the crucial role of the CDC is muddied by its ties to industry, ties that drive it to promote ineffective and often dangerous medical interventions.

Another trusted government health agency, the Food and Drug Administration (FDA), has even more direct ties to the drug industry. In 1992, because of the FDA's deliberately slow policy of new drug approval, Congress passed the Prescription Drug User Fee Act (PDUFA), which forces drug companies to pay fees to the FDA for reviewing their drugs during the approval process. This solved two problems: helping the government to finance the very expensive drug-approval process and speeding that process. Three-quarters of FDA money used for drug approval is paid directly to the agency by the very companies whose drugs are being reviewed.[13] The ramifications of this policy were exposed by the Project on Government Oversight (POGO) in 2018.[14] Every five years, the FDA and drug companies meet to iron out the rules of their collaboration, and as the years have gone by, industry has made it easier and easier for the FDA to approve drugs: "This arrangement gives the pharmaceutical industry extraordinary influence over its government overseer. It leaves the regulator beholden to the regulated."[15] No kidding. Before the deployment of PDUFA, the FDA approved 36 percent of drugs on the first try, but by 2015 it approved 95 percent of all new drugs.

According to POGO, because of agreements with industry, the FDA is now more willing to use surrogate markers, paid patient testimony, and "real-world experience" (a vague term to mean that people in the community like the drug) to enable drug approval in lieu of good clinical trials with meaningful endpoints. Both the Institute of Medicine and a *New England Journal of Medicine* study point out major safety concerns with drugs approved by the FDA through this collaborative process.

In addition, as with the CDC, many FDA members who are involved in the drug approval process are paid by the drug industry. A 2018 study in *Science* "found widespread after-the-fact payments or research support to panel members" of FDA physician advisors who review new drugs.[16] What this means is that although FDA physician advisors can claim to have no ties to industry while approving a drug, that very drug company will pay them either directly or for their research after the approval is complete. Of 107 physician advisors in the study, 40 received funding of more than $10,000, 26 received funding of more than $100,000, and 6 received funding of more than $1 million – typically after the review process ended – by the very companies whose drugs were being reviewed. According to Vinayak Prasad, "The people who are asked to weigh this evidence importantly often stand to gain tremendously in their future professional careers from a positive relationship with the company ... It's in their best interest to play nice with these companies."[17]

Again, the marriage between industry and a crucial federal watchdog organization is deeply embedded in our medical system. This has caused both the CDC and FDA to approve drugs, policies, and vaccines that are not scientifically valid but that – because of the authoritative pretense under which both agencies exist – they have pushed on doctors and the public with direct backing by, and profits for, the drug industry.

Health care lobbying – by organizations linked to industry or medical professionals – is another driver of tests and treatments that benefit the industries doing the lobbying, often through the creation of clinical guidelines and recommendations. A 2017 National Public Radio report showed that two-thirds of medical advocacy groups receive industry funding and tend to hold positions in line with those industries.[18] For instance, new statin guidelines authored by the American College of Cardiology and American Heart Association use a flawed calculator to push people to take medicines of unproven benefit. Almost half of the guideline authors have ties to cholesterol drug manufacturers. Two-thirds of committee chairs and 90 percent of co-chairs have conflicts of interest in the same vein.[19] Overall, outside groups spend $555 million each year in lobbying for medical issues.[20]

Many clinical guidelines scripted by professional societies are self-serving on a number of levels. Guidelines – which are often adapted by health insurance, such as Medicare, and disseminated to doctors and patients as being standard of care – frequently do not use good data in reaching their conclusions and are written under a cloud of collusion between their authors and ties to industry. In cardiovascular clinical guidelines, for instance, more than half of the authors have a direct conflict of interest by being linked to the industry whose products, such as medical devices, or drugs they are promoting.[21] The American College of Cardiology spends more than $2 million a year lobbying Congress for self-serving policies,[22] and scripts many clinical practice guidelines (such as optimal treatment parameters for cholesterol and blood pressure), even though only 10 percent of its recommendations have scientific validity. The American College of Radiology had, as of 2017, 14 lobbyists and spent $2.4 million a year[23] promoting high salaries for radiologists and copious use of expensive X-rays that often have dubious clinical utility. The list goes on and on. No wonder so many of our clinical practice guidelines differ sharply from sound medical practice and have a strong Flexnerian taint that promotes number-measuring and aggressive treatments for almost every "discovered" medical condition.

Perhaps the most egregious conflict of interest occurs in the least scrutinized and most venerated arena: patient advocacy groups. These groups, from the American Diabetes Association to the American Cancer Society and the Alzheimer's Association (AA), posture themselves as being impartial groups whose goal is to help patients make good decisions and to disseminate accurate information. Sadly, much like the Rockefeller and Carnegie

Foundations, they are often the tools of industry and shape health care policy in Flexnerian directions, with a test-treat agenda hidden under a thick coat of altruistic intent.

Drug companies spend about $63 million a year lobbying Congress to promote new tests, drugs, and treatments, and they donate $116 million a year (2018 data) to patient advocacy groups. Many advocacy groups use pharmaceutical funds for 20 to 50 percent of their entire budgets, and, according to the *Washington Post*, "Six drug makers, the data shows, contribute a million dollars or more to individual groups that represent patients who rely on their drugs."[24] ClassAction.com states that 80 percent of patient advocacy groups accept industry money.[25] Its website (and a 2019 article) list advocacy groups that accept the most money, showing that almost half of advocacy groups have a pharmaceutical executive on their board.[26] This infiltration of industry into these groups has pushed many of them to endorse tests and treatments that are not always clinically appropriate.

Just as the ADA's ties to the drug industry – $26 million in 2015 – may well encourage aggressive testing and drug treatment, many other advocacy groups similarly echo the talking points of the companies that finance and help govern them. Included on this list are the Arthritis Foundation, the Crohn's & Colitis Foundation, and the AA, which promotes early detection and treatment of dementia, despite a total lack of evidence that these interventions help patients live longer or better. Certainly, as a recent report shows, people who are tested early and think they have the disease will be more likely to accept treatment, especially if that treatment is endorsed by AA and by the patient's doctor. The AA accepted $20 million from drug companies that make dementia drugs between 2012 and 2016 (a full list of AA "donations" can be found on its internet site)[27] and has drug representatives on its board. Psychiatrist Susan Molchan:

"They sell the sickness using fear, and they also create false hope for cure." Because of AA's drug-directed philosophy, many local dementia societies have split off from the AA.[28] We have shown that drugs touted to improve dementia – a multibillion-dollar industry – work no better than placebo, but they are sold and prescribed at least in part because of nebulous data and advocacy by AA and other groups that purport to be unbiased despite thick industry entanglement.

The American Heart Association (AHA), according to a recent *Huffington Post* report, receives about $1 million a year from statin manufacturers. In line with new AHA guidelines – which employ the flawed calculator we discussed in chapter 10 – 44 percent of men now are instructed to take statins, or 13.5 million more than for previous recommendations. Half the authors of these guidelines have direct ties to the statin industry. The AHA's "Go Red for Women" campaign, designed to educate women about statin use, heavily pushes women to take these drugs. According to the campaign's website, "If your doctor has placed you on statin therapy to reduce your cholesterol you can rest easy – the benefits outweigh the risks." You can't get more Flexnerian than that.

Statin maker AstraZeneca sponsored an AHA learning council about statins in 2010, and in that year the AHA defended the controversial drug Vytorin (a combination of a generic statin with an expensive and ineffective drug called Zetia), whose manufacturer "donated" $2 million to the AHA. "How did we arrive at a place where conflicted parties get to make semi-official pronouncements that have so much impact on public policy?" asks Dr. Jerome Hoffman of the University of California, Los Angeles.[29]

Perhaps that says it all. Once Flexner and his cronies constructed a health care system that melded private foundations, drug manufacturers, and medical societies into the highest echelons of medical policy and practice, we were destined to have a culture that mirrored the wants and needs of industry. Despite uttering a language of science and patient advocacy, these organizations – from the FDA and CDC, to professional societies, to well-respected patient advocacy groups – support a Flexnerian agenda that promotes aggressive care in the test-diagnose-treat mold, feeding our bloated and expensive medical system to the detriment of many patients. Rather than rein in cost, rather than help doctors and the public to understand best medical practices, rather than being advocates for the science-based, patient-centered medical philosophy echoed by Osler, these groups have a self-serving agenda that does more to deceive than to educate, with an eye more to profit than to patient care.

CHAPTER TWENTY-TWO

The Metric Mess of the Health Care System

Various degrees of probability we may attain to and do reach daily but in the very busy round of teaching and practice we are apt to forget that positive certainty until we have a rude awakening and a useful lesson in the folly of over-confidence.

– William Osler[1]

The vast majority of health care providers enter the field for altruistic reasons – and yes, to make a decent living. Good intentions aside, no one disputes that they must be held accountable to accepted standards of practice, or that as the health care system grows increasingly complex, the need to accurately measure the quality of care becomes even more important. Unfortunately, the measurement of quality of care – and the standards that characterize it – has morphed from adherence to clinical guidelines and patient safety initiatives into a numbers game that impedes good patient care and increases wasteful spending.

There are simply too many metric programs that physicians must follow. I call them the alphabet soup of metrics. Healthcare

Effectiveness Data and Information Set (HEDIS) is a group of quality indicators developed by the National Committee for Quality Assurance (NCQA). Others include the Agency for Healthcare Research and Quality (AHRQ), the Institute of Medicine (IOM), Institute for Healthcare Improvement (IHI) and, of course, Centers for Medicare and Medicaid Services (CMS). These agencies develop and monitor metrics, which are in the thousands and range from hospitals to nursing homes to doctors' offices. They cover every conceivable aspect of care, from cost to quality to utilization, morbidity and mortality, and satisfaction with care. But how do these groups measure quality care?

In a Flexnerian worldview, all health can be measured and tabulated. There are discrete numbers that equate to good health, and our goal as providers is to assess and "fix" any abnormal measurements. Hence, there are certain tests that we must do on all patients, and certain results that we must achieve for all patients if we are to be considered quality doctors. It is from this philosophy that our clinical metrics sprout. Osler did not believe that there is always one right answer for every patient. People are complex; numbers can be misleading. Metrics, though, push doctors further down the Flexnerian wormhole of a uniform focus on numbers and not on patients by tying quality report cards and even physician pay to the achievement of rigid numerical endpoints.

According to CMS, "Quality measures are tools that help us measure or quantify healthcare processes, outcomes, patient perceptions, and organizational structure and/or systems that are associated with the ability to provide high-quality health care and/or that relate to one or more quality goals for health care. These goals include: effective, safe, efficient, patient-centered, equitable, and timely care."[2] Sounds good, but the devil is in the details.

On October 30, 2017, CMS administrator Seema Verma announced a new approach to quality measurement, called "Meaningful Measures."[3] The Meaningful Measures Initiative involves identifying the highest priorities to improve patient care through quality measurement and quality improvement efforts. And yet, despite attempts to "reform" our metrics, little has changed.[4] Metrics help fuel spending, drive tests and treatments, encourage specialization, and feed the medical-industrial complex. No wonder they are difficult to stamp out.

Currently, there are more than 2,500 quality metrics being studied and used. Who scripts them, how they are utilized, and how well they correlate with outcome are all problematic. Most metrics are robotic; for example, all people under the age of 85 must have a systolic blood pressure reading below 140. What if a patient does better over 140? What if their pressure in the office is always artificially elevated because of the stress associated with a visit to the doctor? What if blood pressure drugs fix the number but make the patient dizzy and confused? None of that matters; a metric is absolute. It is the one right answer, Flexnerian at its core. A doctor who views his or her patient as a complex individual, one who may need a higher blood pressure, is deemed to be practicing low-quality care and is stamped as such. His pay and quality scores will suffer.

Metrics in medicine include measures such as 30-day hospital readmission rates and emergency department visits. Some of this can be controlled by quality medical care and more access to after-hours care to cut down on emergency department visits, but much of this is totally out of control of the provider. There is no accounting for patient demographics. Working in underserved communities where patients may not have access to quality food, be able to afford their medicine, or have strong family or social support is not considered.

Sometimes people go to the emergency department because they have no choice.

Hemoglobin A1c, the surrogate measurement of the control of diabetes, is one of the most discussed metrics. We can instruct our patients on the importance of diet, exercise, and the appropriate use of medicine, but we cannot control what they do when they leave the office. Yes, we contact patients, send them to nutritionists, and educate them on the importance of diet and exercise, but their compliance is not up to us. So essentially, if our diabetics have a poor A1c (the surrogate metric on which we are graded), we are scolded (and financially punished) for poor quality because our quality report card will invariably be lower than that of a doctor who sees compliant patients. In addition, what constitutes a "normal" A1c for one patient may not be normal for another; sometimes dramatic lowering of this number causes harm, and yet if a doctor lowers her patient's A1c so low that she faints and breaks a hip, she will be rewarded as practicing quality medicine. Moreover, getting an A1c down from 13 to 10 in a poor, noncompliant patient is a very worthy accomplishment, but because the A1c is over 9 the doctor will fail the measure.

To be effective, metrics must be evidence based and measure quality, *clinically relevant* care, not just surrogate measurements, and they must be patient-centric. If someone with heart disease cannot tolerate or does not want to take a statin after a discussion of the risks and benefits, the doctor cannot fail that metric. Patients' satisfaction with their care – measuring what matters to patients – is more important than a raw number. Thus, metrics must afford the provider ample room to customize treatment to the individual patient. Metrics that are uniform and number based do not meet these requirements, and yet, in our Flexnerian world, our metrics are scripted in this narrow and ineffectual way. They transform doctors into robots.

In an attempt to formalize metrics and enhance the quality of care, a system has been developed called "pay-for-performance" (P4P). P4P ties physician pay to metric-defined outcomes. The measures that are being used don't enhance the care of patients and patient choice. They constitute both generic numerical measurements (that doctors are compelled to "fix" so they fall into some preordained range of normal) and mandatory screening tests (to which all patients must submit without any discussion of risk/benefit and preference).

The problem with many of these quality metrics and P4P programs is that there is little or no evidence that they have led to any significant improvement in patient outcomes. In actuality, what has occurred is the proliferation of tests and treatments to "fix" errant numbers that may be as harmful as they are helpful, and an incentive not to talk to patients lest they refuse to comply with the quality standards doctors are forced to push on them. The burden currently is placed disproportionately on the primary care provider more than the specialist physician, who often has to pass only one or two metrics to meet their quality scores and receive their full payment for the care they provide.

Primary care providers must pass a huge menu of quality and satisfaction metrics in order to get their full payment. This problem is exacerbated by the disparity of metrics across various insurance carriers. A patient may have a Blue Cross plan, for example, but there may be 10 or 20 different plans, from health maintenance organizations to personal provider organizations, exclusive provider organizations, point-of-service plans, health spending accounts, and on and on, each with different metrics. Most physicians' offices require at least one employee whose job it is to decipher the metrics so the doctor can get paid. This adds to the cost of providing care, does little or nothing to improve patient outcome, and interferes with shared decisions between doctors and patients. Rather than caring for patients and discussing important issues with patients, doctors spend most of their time checking boxes and assuring that they comply with often irrelevant standards.

Not all metrics are useless, not by any means. Take for example screening for tobacco use and cessation. Asking patients for smoking status and implementing programs to help them stop is a good thing. Check the box in the electronic health record that they smoke; offer counseling, medication, mindfulness techniques, or referral; and check another box that you did it. Not a complex or bad thing to do. Getting someone to stop smoking will decrease the risk of heart disease, stroke, lung disease, and many cancers. Unfortunately, clicking the box for smoking status or a smart phrase that states "we have counseled our patients on the importance of smoking cessation" has never been shown to have any meaningful benefit on smoking cessation rates.

Metrics for many cancer screenings are not as good. We can't generalize who needs, wants, and would benefit from a screening test. We have already discussed that cancer screening is often more dangerous than lifesaving. Good examples are mammograms for women who may be at low risk and decline the test, or who want to get it at a frequency less than required by a specific specialty group, society, or insurance company. If we speak with our patients about the pros and cons of a mandatory screening test, such a mammogram, and if they elect not to get the test, then we as the doctor get dinged and are told we are not practicing quality care, further risking our reimbursement and quality report card. If a patient, after a shared decision-making discussion, declines a test, why should a physician be penalized? Perhaps the best quality measure in terms of screening is not whether a patient gets the test, but rather whether the doctor and patient discussed it.

A good quality measure should enhance a patient's care and quality of life, make them live longer or better, lower cost, improve satisfaction with care or life, and most important matter most to the patient by providing the care that they want. Unfortunately, most measures focus on specific disease states, screening tests, and other interventions and do little or nothing to measure overall wellness, health, or satisfaction. All are generic; none are patient-specific. Many have no scientific basis to back their prolific use, especially in certain demographics that are being forced to comply with them. They are an appendage of Flexnerian absolutism that has no ties to scientific scrutiny or to concern for the patient. They are, in fact, a snake oil approach that appeals to cognitive biases, delineates normal and abnormal in a binary and inflexible fashion, and deludes the patient into thinking she is receiving quality care.

Many quality metric programs create a distinct disadvantage for physicians who care for poor, elderly, diverse, underserved, and other vulnerable populations. There are limitations to a physician's ability to influence an outcome for any patient, but this is more pronounced when dealing with impoverished patients with limited access to many medical services, quality food, and exercise and other wellness initiatives. A patient's socioeconomic status and the social determinants of health greatly affect their health care outcomes and transcend the control of their provider. It is not the doctor's fault if a patient cannot afford his prescription or lacks access to healthy food options. And yet, none of that reality is factored in.

We must also recognize that many of the quality metrics, though seeming reasonable and benign, are often not. Many people are forced into testing they do not want or understand, or drugs or procedures that they may not need and that could be harmful. They may end up with serious medical complications, side effects, and even death from the metric-mandated intervention.

Once again take my least favorite example, the hemoglobin A1c test that measures the three-month average of someone's blood sugar. I am not saying it is a useless test because it is not; it helps guide treatment of diabetes in those patients who benefit from appropriate interventions. The problem is that a good number for one person may not be good for someone else. Some younger patients with type 1 or insulin-dependent diabetes benefit from tight glucose control to prevent the long-term complications of diabetes. Other patients with type 2 – or what was known as "adult-onset" or "obesity-related" diabetes – may not benefit in the same way; many elderly people, especially those with dementia or high fall risk, may be harmed if their sugars are driven down into the "normal" range. To me, the best way to treat the disease is with diet, exercise, and mindfulness interventions that improve a person's overall health far more than prescribing expensive medications simply to fix a number. But this metric drives overprescribing.

There is evidence that the drug approach to treating type 2 diabetes is more expensive and can expose the patient to the complications of the medications, along with significant drug–drug interactions and kidney, liver, or heart damage. Yes, medicines are easier to prescribe and are more likely to lower sugars quickly enough to allow doctors to pass their metric score; taking time to work with my patients to treat the underlying cause of the disease rather than mask it with a drug that is simply treating a number will get me a demerit from the insurance company. The same is true for blood pressure control, congestive heart failure medication use, anticoagulants for afib, or lipid management, to name a few. Each of these conditions can and are treated with multiple medications that can have copious side effects and drug interactions, not to mention morbidity and mortality. Unfortunately, the quality metrics do not measure what really matters to an individual patient. It is the relationship of the primary care provider with her patients and shared decision-making discussions that are most important when evaluating quality.

Flexnerians measure and set numbers in a fixed and uniform way. Oslerians care for their patients, who they acknowledge are complex individuals, with an understanding that all measurements and treatments are plagued by nuance and uncertainty. Our quality metrics, being of purely Flexnerian design, only reinforce the detrimental medical philosophy that puts numbers over patients.

Again, quality care that is efficient, patient-centric, and proven to derive beneficial patient outcomes is important to all physicians. Getting there in a smart and effective way is essential. It must be in a way that does not lead to overtesting, overutilization, overdiagnosis, and overtreatment, all of which generate increased costs and harms and are not associated with improved patient survival or quality of life. What these measures are associated with is a useless burden on our health care providers and a desecration of the doctor–patient bond that is so essential to quality medical care.

CHAPTER TWENTY-THREE

Hospitals: The Epicenter of Patient Care

A place where new thought is materialized in research – a school where men are encouraged to base the art upon the science of medicine – a fountain to which teachers in every subject would come for inspiration – a place with a hearty welcome to every practitioner who seeks help – a consulting centre for the whole country in cases of obscurity.

– William Osler[1]

Hospitals used to be a place of last resort. This has all changed over the past decade as hospitals have evolved to become the epicenter of medical care. Hospitals promote their own self-interests through their grants, philanthropy, research interests, and academic programs – often at the expense of the patient. Both academic and community hospitals are moneymaking machines that drive a large sector of the economy, feed an army of doctors and administrators, and cope with regulatory and legal loopholes in order to stay in good standing. These are their main concerns, not their patients.

The evolution of hospitals from a place of last resort to the epi-center of medical care has been influenced by a number of social and cultural developments, including the changing meanings of disease, economics, religion, ethnicity, socioeconomic status, scientific growth, and the perceived needs of populations. But it was the Flexner Report that did more than anything to desig-nate the hospital as the anchor of our new medical system. By devaluing the doctor–patient relationship and focusing on large teaching hospitals, Flexner made it possible for these monolithic institutions to flourish. Tellingly, primary care has vanished from the hospital setting. It is now a place of technology and number management, not one of patient-centric caring. The result of this, sadly, has been catastrophic.

If you are having a heart attack or have suffered an unfortunate accident, the hospital is the place to be. The health care system in the United States excels at sick and emergency care. But hospitals are also very dangerous and expensive. They treat patients more as commodities than as people, and in the most Flexnerian of ways, test and treat nearly everything, often exposing patients to unnecessary risk.

Yes, hospitals are businesses, and they are the most expensive locations to get health care, a fact only apparent to patients after they return home. Middle-class people are the ones who often suf-fer the most from hospital care, with hidden costs, lack of trans-parency, high copays, and huge deductibles, all of which are the leading causes of medical bankruptcy in our country. The most affluent and well-insured can likely afford their medical bills, but the poor and underserved either have Medicaid or are covered by a governmental pool of money called "bad debt and charity care." Many in the middle class are squeezed. But the financial strain of hospitals is often the least of the worries faced by trusting souls who are brought into their doors with the promise of cure.

Medical errors contribute to more than 250,000 deaths in the United States each year, according to a 2016 Johns Hopkins study, making it the third-leading cause of death after heart disease and cancer.[2] Other studies put the figure as high as 440,000, but calculating this number is extremely difficult. Many feel that these data are inaccurate, fabricated, and grossly overestimated, that they are used to unjustly assail our nation's hospitals. Others will tell you that the numbers are much higher and that many errors are cleverly concealed. These figures also do not include deaths from overtreatment that occur in hospitals, that is, people who are assaulted with tests, drugs, and procedures that they don't need and that kill them. Nor does it include the 100,000 people who die every year from hospital-acquired infections. We can tell you (from collectively spending 65 years working in hospitals) that we have seen countless deaths from medical errors, needless procedures, hospital-acquired infections, medical malpractice, and negligence. Much of this goes undetected or unreported unless the victim or family speaks up or initiates a malpractice suit. And this happens not only in safety-net hospitals in poor communities, but also in our nation's top hospitals.

Our own stories are copious. Sometimes they are subtle, like a healthy patient of mine admitted to the hospital by her cardiologist for afib – not life-threatening and something I usually treat in my office – who suffered a series of misfortunes caused by the hospital. She became confused and was treated with potent drugs. When she didn't eat, she was fed forcefully and given intravenous fluids. She then aspirated fluid into her lungs and developed pneumonia. After that a catheter was placed in her bladder and that led to another infection. My patient was put in the intensive care unit for a week until she died, at a cost of more than $100,000. And these weren't even medical errors. Just the ramifications of aggressive Flexnerian specialized treatments.

Countless others arrive at the hospital for minor issues and acquire infections in the hospital that either maim or kill them. Health-care-associated infections (HAIs) – infections people get while receiving health care for another condition – can occur in any health care facility, including hospitals, ambulatory surgical centers, and long-term care facilities. HAIs can be caused by bacteria, fungi, viruses, or other, less common pathogens. A significant cause of illness and death, they can have devastating emotional, financial, and medical consequences. At any given time, about 1 in 25 inpatients have an infection related to hospital care. These infections lead to the loss of between 50,000 and 100,000 people a year and cost the health care system billions of dollars each year.[3] The causes of these infections are multifactorial and are often related to zealous overtreatment, including the use of intravenous catheters, endotracheal (breathing) tubes, and urinary catheters, and often unnecessary broad-spectrum antibiotics. Some of these procedures may be necessary to help save your life, but many – too many – are more a reflection of zealous Flexnerian overtreatment.

Hospitals are often not properly cleaned and disinfected, which means communicable diseases can easily be passed between patients and health care workers. This lack of hygiene was highlighted during the COVID-19 pandemic. A team led by researchers at the University of Cambridge analyzed data and found that patients were a large source of COVID-19 spread, exacerbated by overcrowded emergency departments.[4]

Other common causes of hospital death include missed or delayed diagnoses, medication errors, technical errors, and poor or even absent communication between providers. These errors can include the misidentification of patients, leading them to have the wrong test, wrong procedure, or the wrong medication. With the use of electronic health records (EHRs), new breeds of medical errors have been created from entries in the wrong chart dosage miscalculation, and improper documentation of allergies. The challenges, complexities, and time requirements of using an EHR combined with the number of alerts and warnings are simply overwhelming and unmanageable, leading to "clicking errors" that can be fatal.

I had a patient who was allergic to a medicine, but that allergy was not listed in her EHR, and so she was given the medication, with disastrous results. It turns out that it was listed in my medical record, but not in the hospital's EHR, which was more than five years old and did not communicate with mine. The failure of hospitalists and hospital specialists to communicate with primary care physicians is a common cause of error and leads to disability and death in my patients on a regular basis.

Competency issues are another common cause of medical errors, from the simplest procedure to the most complex surgery.[5] I often tell my patients who are considering a surgery or procedure that "tomorrow someone is going to undergo a surgical procedure from the worst surgeon in our nation. How do you know it's not going to be you?" The easiest way to cut down on medical error and hospital-acquired infections is to go to the hospital only when absolutely necessary and have only those procedures or surgeries that are absolutely crucial.

All of this is exacerbated because primary care docs who know the patient well are often now not allowed in the hospital because hospital-paid "hospitalists" run the show, not knowing their patients at all, and are incentivized to call in copious specialists and order a plethora of tests.

Specialization is a salient predictor of hospitalization. Specialists, not primary care physicians, rule the roost in the hospital. It's a place where they have captive patients on whom they can perform many lucrative tests and procedures, and capture more willing patients for their practice. Studies show, and our experience confirms, that specialists are far more likely than primary care doctors to hospitalize patients, even for minor ailments that can be treated in a primary care doctor's office. Once admitted to the hospital, patients are treated to a Flexnerian orgy of test-diagnose-treat.

But perhaps the biggest hospital-related scam is the so-called not-for-profit hospitals in our nation that give the impression they exist to care for the poor and underserved. The fact is that most nonprofit hospitals have higher profit margins than for-profit hospitals when taxes are taken into account. More than 60 percent of hospitals in the United States are nonprofit, meaning they pay no property tax, no federal tax, no state income tax, and no sales tax.[6] If you look at cities such as New York or Los Angeles and add the taxes that hospitals avoid paying, you can calculate what they actually earn.

Many of these prestigious "not-for-profit" institutions decorate their lobbies and rooms with marble, steel, and glass, boasting hotel-like amenities and paying their executives millions of dollars. Ironically, many of our prestigious, not-for-profit hospitals advertise the high-end amenities they provide as they fight for our country's wealthiest patients with other nonprofit institutions to reap the awards of our Flexnerian system that allows them to test and treat everything with huge profits as their reward. Even those institutions that provide some free care, education, and community service earn hefty profits from their paying customers. Their huge profits are invested in salaries, equipment, hotel-like amenities, and infrastructure. And yet they pay no taxes and deceive us that they are altruistic nonprofit institutions existing only for the good of society.[7]

Hospitals have many tricks to prove that they are spending more than they are earning. One such ploy is to inflate the cost of care that they provide to the few underserved and uninsured they are willing to admit, then write off these charges and list them as charitable care. For example, what Medicare is charged for a service and paid to the hospital could be inflated by 8 to 10 times the allowable costs for uninsured patients. According to a 2021 NPR report, a colonoscopy might cost you or your insurer a few hundred dollars – or several thousand, depending on which hospital or insurer you use.[8] It is estimated that nonprofit hospitals are subsidized by more than $30 billion a year through this and other tricks. If these dollars were truly going to the care of the poor and underserved, it could be understandable. But the sad facts are the money goes to exorbitant CEO salaries, fancy facilities, and technology investments so they can bring in more revenue. More technology leads to increased utilization of high-cost and often unnecessary care, which leads to profits and harm. These are the ironic ramifications of care in Flexnerian hospitals.

Top 82 U.S. Non-Profit Hospitals: Quantifying Government Payments and Financial Assets, a report published in June 2019, clearly demonstrates that the nonprofit hospital schemes are a multibillion dollar scam and that reform will save our nation billions.[9] These are some of the most powerful and profitable systems in our nation, and they spend freely on lobbying and public relations campaigns. According to the report, the average CEO salary for these top 82 hospitals was $3.5 million a year, with the top five earning between $10 and $22 million.[10] Not bad for a nonprofit salary.

Hospitals and nursing homes spent nearly $100 million lobbying in 2018, according to the Center for Responsive Politics.[11] The organization of our nation's hospitals, the American Hospital Association, spent $23.9 billion in 2018.[12] A large portion of this spending comes from our nonprofit hospitals. Why are these hospitals spending so much? The answer is simple: to preserve their tax-exempt status and to ensure massive profits.

Pharmaceutical companies pay millions of dollars to hospitals and specialty societies to fund research and develop treatment guidelines that will help their products be the standard of care for hospitals. This is also supported by the health insurance industry, with many plans demanding that doctors have hospital privileges. Why are insurance companies strong advocates of the centrality of hospitals when hospitals are the most expensive places to deliver care? You would think that insurance companies would prefer care to be provided in a better, more economical way. Medicare and Medicaid pay hospitals for their services at set regional rates. Insurance companies also negotiate rates, with some of them paying more than three to four times the Medicare rate. Why on earth would they agree to this? Certainly, in order to attract patients, insurance companies need to be affiliated with top hospitals, so it may make some sense to pay more for certain top centers, but three to four times the amount? As we noted in chapter 19 on insurance, the reasons are counterintuitive: the more insurance companies spend for high-cost care, the more their executives can earn, the more effective their spin can be, and the more they can justify increasing premiums.

This method of negotiating costs is also forcing many smaller hospitals to merge with larger hospital systems so that they can negotiate higher rates. This, in turn, has led to fewer hospital systems and decreased competition, further escalating the cost of care and decreasing choice, especially for those in rural and inner-city, underserved communities.

Perhaps the most obvious victims of our hospital system are poor and underserved patients who are often covered by Medicaid. Many doctors simply do not accept Medicaid, either because it reimburses too little or the patients are "too difficult." Poor patients are often less compliant with medical treatment and are severely affected by social determinants of health. The result is patients flocking to our nation's emergency departments to get medical care. Funded by the federal government and administered by state governments, Medicaid is meant to cover our nation's most vulnerable populations. Unfortunately, the way our system is designed often limits access to primary care and preventive services, mostly because of inadequate supply. Our nation continues to train an army of specialist physicians at the expense of primary care, especially in poor urban communities. Thus the poor are dependent on hospitals and their emergency departments, which are open 24/7 with no appointment necessary, no copays or deductibles for most, and an acceptable standard of care. So, our nation's inner-city institutions are unfortunately overwhelmed with routine viral illness, medication refills, wound-dressing changes, and other routine care, rather than taking care of what they were designed to, acute medical illness and trauma.

As we see with much of our nation, where the income gap continues to increase, there is a sharp disparity between rich and poor hospitals. Many rural hospitals are struggling financially and closing. According to a 2018 Government Accountability Office report, 64 rural hospitals closed between 2013 and 2017, and more than 100 rural hospitals have closed since 2010.[13] Reasons for closure include financial loss, complex patient populations, and difficulty attracting and retaining doctors in rural areas. University of Washington researchers examined these closures and found they were associated with a 5.9 percent increase in mortality rates because patients have had to travel farther and farther to get the necessary health care emergency services, and many more may die from a lack of primary care services.[14]

A safety-net hospital is a facility that by legal obligation or mission provides health care for individuals regardless of their insurance or ability to pay and whose patient population includes a substantial share of uninsured, Medicaid, and other vulnerable patients. Safety-net hospitals make up about 5 percent of our hospitals but provide up to 20 percent of uncompensated care, totaling nearly $40 billion annually and up to 23 percent of all charity care, which added up to almost $6 billion or more in 2019.[15] When the government does not provide care for these patients, the safety-net hospitals must provide care to these uninsured patients who cannot afford to pay their medical bills. Safety-net hospitals must write off these bills as charity care or collect low sums of money from governmental charity pools, called "disproportionate-share hospital payments." These payments have been cut and do not cover the costs of hospital care. It is estimated that between bad debt, charity care, and low reimbursement from federal payers, these hospitals recoup less than 50 percent of the loss.[16] Is it any wonder that many of these institutions have closed and that many more are on the brink of closure?

I talk about the rural hospitals and the safety-net hospitals to highlight that not all institutions are rolling in the dough. These institutions are not the recipients of significant National Institutes of Health grants and philanthropy, they do not cater to insurers who pay them four times the going rate, and they cannot gouge patients with their Flexnerian quest to find and fix everything. The rich get richer and the poor get poorer, and the same is true for our nation's hospital systems. Sadly, it is the wealthy nonprofits that are running the show.

In any business transaction or purchase, we agree to terms before committing. At the very least, we consider and discuss the estimate of costs. Transparency is essential for a competitive and well-functioning health care system. In hospitals, there is nothing further from that. Patients enter a hospital, may have a procedure and diagnostic tests, and see specialists. They may be fully covered, but have surprise billing with exorbitant copays, deductibles, or coinsurances. In addition, some of the providers they see may not even be covered by their insurance plans, such as an anesthesiologist during a surgical procedure.

Hospitals are required by law to post their charges online. If you look at such a posting, it is impossible to evaluate and even more impossible to understand what your costs will be. Congress is currently evaluating bills to ensure price transparency in health care. Those few hospitals that are becoming transparent are showing increased satisfaction with care.

ProPublica has been bringing attention to hospital costs and the abuses of hospitals. In some of the poorest communities, hospitals are harassing patients, suing them, and even having them arrested for not appearing in front of court for unpaid bills or failing to participate in a "debtor's exam,"[17] even though some hospitals are among the richest in the nation.

Hospitals have the ability to care for the sick and injured but do little or nothing to prevent disease and promote wellness. They are often very dangerous as a result of errors, overtreatment, and infections. They are cash cows willing to subject patients to any number of tests and procedures, to have them see a copious number of specialists, and to dispense powerful drugs with substantial harm, all in the interest of profit and all justified in Flexnerian language. Flexner's report elevated hospitals to the center of care, doing so at the expense of the community primary care physician, whose role is the most significant in helping people stay healthy, but who is largely excluded from the Flexner-on-steroids world of the hospital. Before you think that the hospital is the safest place to go, think again. It's not, most of the time. It is very costly, and very dangerous. Just like the Flexnerian system as a whole.

CHAPTER TWENTY-FOUR

The Case for Primary Care

There are, in truth, no specialties in medicine, since to know fully many of the most important diseases a man must be familiar with their manifestations in many organs.

– William Osler[1]

I have heard many times throughout my career that everyone should have a primary care physician. I have heard that mantra sung at hospital meetings, and I've read in hundreds of articles and governmental or not-for-profit foundation reports that our health care system should be based on a strong primary care foundation, that every American should have a primary care provider. This is, in fact, one of the few points on which both Flexner and Osler agreed.

So why is our medical society doing all it can to put the primary care physician out of business?

It's simple: the specialty medical model does not want it to happen because it will diminish their profits and erode the Flexnerian model. Making people healthier will lead to fewer invasive procedures and hospitalizations, less testing, less prescribing of medications, and lower utilization of all nonpreventive medical services. Too bad for the medical-industrial complex. Too bad for us, though, that most medical organizations, the lobbyists they fund, and the politicians they influence script health policies that are invested in a Flexnerian system bereft of primary care. That's why investment in primary care and prevention – an investment that will make us healthier again and save our nation billions of dollars – always hits a roadblock when it comes to reform. Our system of copious testing and drugging and fixing is anchored in the sea of specialty care, because it is there where most of our money is spent and most of our tests and procedures are done. To have a system based on primary care would discredit our Flexnerian assumptions and pose a severe threat to the medical-industrial complex.

Fifty years ago, more than half of the physicians in the United States were in primary care. We had one of the highest life expectancies in the world, and one of the highest patient levels of satisfaction. Today, fewer than one-third of all providers practice primary care; the majority are involved in specialty care and hospital medicine. Primary care is the most efficient and effective way to deliver care, yet primary care physicians provide a fraction of our nation's care and get only 2 to 6 percent of the funding.[2]

We have 2.56 primary care doctors per 1,000, Germany 4.1 per 1,000, and France 3.1 per 1,000. The vast majority of developed health care systems throughout the world rely on primary care. In most of these nations, 70 percent or more of the providers are primary care practitioners. These countries have longer life expectancy, lower health care costs, and higher rates of satisfaction with their own health care and their health care system.[3]

According to a recent article in the *Journal of the American Medical Association*, the supply of primary care physicians in the

United States decreased between 2005 and 2015 by more than 10 percent.[4] And because the supply of primary care physicians per capita is decreasing, we should expect a continued decline in the longevity and well-being of our nation, which indeed we are seeing. This will lead to reduced access to primary medical care and increased utilization of emergency departments and specialized doctors. This decrease comes at a time when the population of our nation is rapidly aging. Elders are harmed more than anyone by Flexnerian aggressiveness. Those who do not have access to a primary care doctor are less likely to have had a discussion about advance-care planning and are more likely to spend time in the emergency department and the hospital, to get more testing and procedures, be prescribed more deleterious medications, and to be dissatisfied with the quality of their health and health care.[5]

But even our young are hurt by the lack of primary care physicians. A 42-year-old patient of mine recently came to the office after an extensive work up for chest pain. She was at her job when she developed a racing heart and some pressure in her chest. She went to an urgent-care center near her office and presented her symptoms to the clinician, where she was seen by a physician assistant. Her physical examination was unremarkable, and her EKG was normal; nevertheless, the provider was concerned about the pressure in my patient's chest and called an ambulance to take her to a nearby hospital, commonly known in our community as "the heart hospital." Despite a normal initial evaluation, the patient was admitted to the hospital to rule out a heart attack, and a cardiologist was consulted and ordered a nuclear stress test. The stress test was equivocal in its findings – which is often the case in young women – prompting the need for further evaluation. The patient was subsequently referred to an interventional cardiologist and underwent a cardiac catheterization, the results of which were totally normal. The doctors told her that her heart was normal; they could not find a cause for her chest pain. They said it was safe to go home and that she should see a gastroenterologist because they thought the pain was possibly from gastroesophageal reflux disease.

Following the advice she had received at the hospital, the patient had a consult with a gastrointestinal (GI) specialist who performed an esophagogastroduodenoscopy to look in the esophagus, stomach, and duodenum. The tests were normal. Still not feeling well, she didn't know what to do next, so she scheduled a visit with me. She had not been in my office in a few years because she was well and had no cardiac risk factors (smoking, high blood pressure, diabetes, or family history) or other medical complaints. Her exam was normal, and when I asked her if there was any stress in her life, she began to cry. She had a recent separation from her husband and her mom was undergoing cancer treatment. She needed to work and had the burden of taking care of her two young children on her own. She had reached out for help from urgent care, Emergency Medical Services, a teaching hospital, and several specialists, all of whom worked up her heart and GI tract but did not treat her as a complex human being. All it took was a couple of questions to see that she was anxious and needed stress relief, not tens of thousands of dollars of potentially harmful tests, which only exacerbated her anxiety. This is by no means an isolated case. Emergency departments and urgent-care centers constantly send their patients to specialists with whom they have referral arrangements. Urgent-care centers often do not share the information of their visits with the primary care physician and often do not refer them back to us for continuity of care.

The utilization of mid-level practitioners – nurse practitioners (NPs) and physician assistants (PAs) – is becoming more and more prevalent as primary care physicians are driven to extinction.

The data on utilization and costs vary greatly in many published studies.[6] To become a PA you need a college degree and two or three years of classroom and clinical training. To become an NP the requirement is to first become a registered nurse and then receive an advanced degree. Some NPs graduate with as little as 700 hours of clinical patient care.

Compare this with the training of a physician, who needs a four-year college degree, four years of medical school, followed by at least three years of residency training. There is clear difference in the level and requirements for training. I work with and highly respect many NPs and PAs; in fact I (Alan) am a PA. I clearly understand the difference in training and expertise. I went on to medical school because I wanted to be a primary care provider and felt I did not have the required knowledge and experience to deliver sufficient quality of care. I want to be clear that I admire NPs and PAs and work closely with them on a daily basis. But we have to acknowledge that there is a clear difference in the level of training and experience. To assume that NPs and PAs will fill the void left by evaporating primary care is a disservice to the crucial role that primary care physicians play in a vibrant health care system.

I recently had another case where a patient worked for a local urgent-care center as one of their information technology specialists. He was seen in their office 38 times for various conditions. He was referred to almost every specialist in existence, from cardiology to ear, nose, and throat to pulmonary, gastroenterology, and on and on. Not once in the 38 visits did anyone ask about the frequent visits, the reasons for the frequent visits, or if he had a doctor taking care of him. The patient was exposed to useless testing and risked overdiagnosis and overtreatment, not to mention the stress of exorbitant and unnecessary costs. The patient clearly had an anxiety disorder leading to multiple somatic (physical) symptoms. He needed counseling and an integrative approach to his health care, including stress-reduction and relaxation techniques, not referral to multiple "ologists."

The system we have created exacerbates an already dysfunctional and overly costly mess, which adds to overutilization, poor medical care, poorer health, and lower satisfaction with care. It is the very antithesis of an Oslerian system in which a broadly trained physician who knows his patient well is best poised to treat the patient.

Specialists regularly refer their patients to other specialists in return for the referrals of other patients back to them. It is rare in my experience that if a patient complains to a specialist about a problem not related to his particular area of expertise (i.e., his one organ of interest) that the specialist tells the patient to see the primary care doctor. I have seen specialists refer patients of mine to up to eight other specialists – leading to more tests, drugs, and procedures – for problems I could have handled in a more comprehensive and holistic manner. It is a revolving door of hospital and specialty care that almost always could – and should – be handled in the office of the primary care provider.

Our system doles out money for specialty referrals and tests and procedures but fails to recognize that what is important is a careful history, including a psychosocial evaluation, and spending time listening to people. This is thanks to our Flexnerian educational system that focuses on regurgitation of scientific fact and not a reliance on human interaction. Listening is what often gets to the core of the patient's problem. This Oslerian approach leads to a more appropriate medical workup and is less likely to involve excessive testing and referral to specialty care. Once again, our insurance system and Medicare continue to pay well for procedures and surgeries, and fails to reimburse primary care providers adequately for the time needed to listen to patients, provide adequate preventive care to keep people well, and manage the complexities of chronic complex medical illness.

The millennial generation is a classic example of a group avoiding primary care. Almost half of millennials use urgent-care centers and virtual or telehealth visits for their primary care.[7] This may be adequate for a significant portion of healthy young adults, but this type of care is fragmented and not comprehensive, and it doesn't offer continuity of experience. Urgent-care centers overtreat with antibiotics and use increased numbers of diagnostic tests and specialty referrals. Whether these centers will be associated with delays in diagnosis of chronic medical conditions, such as cancer, cardiovascular disease, mental illness, and substance abuse, remains to be seen.

I recently had a patient come to me after a "virtual" visit to a specialist provider from a local orthopedic specialty hospital. The patient had a week of leg pain following a minor sports injury. The physician conducted a history and a "patient-assisted" physical examination via FaceTime. The diagnosis was leg pain, and the provider ordered an X-ray, MRI, and venous Doppler test to rule out a blood clot in the leg, all without touching the patient. If the patient had seen me in the first place, I would have diagnosed a muscle strain, prescribed ice, heat, and some ibuprofen, which I did. He got better in a week or two, the only residual issue being his large copayments and deductible. My patient truly thought he was doing the best thing by "seeing" a specialist provider. He very quickly found out he was wrong.

Too many easy tests are not a good thing; they need to be ordered in an intelligent and patient-centric way. A smartwatch can now diagnose afib, which can lead to the overdiagnosis and overtreatment of a condition that is likely harmless in the absence of symptoms. People may be unnecessarily scared, put on blood thinners that can cause harm, and be tossed forever into the lap of a cardiologist, where they will get more tests, drugs, and procedures. All because their watch told them they had afib. Our advances in technology are making us sicker and poorer, with no improvement in health care outcomes, subjective wellness, or satisfaction with care.

Hundreds of studies support the case for primary care, usually concluding that patients who have a continuing relationship with a primary care physician live longer and at lower cost and have higher satisfaction ratings both with their personal health and with their experience in the health care system.[8] The benefits of primary care, chronic complex disease management, and preventive services take years or even decades to prove, whereas the benefits of a coronary angioplasty or stent are immediately seen when we look at surrogate markers. A stent increases blood flow instantly, even if it never does improve someone's health or prevent heart attacks and death. A good diet, an exercise program, and a medical regime carefully prescribed by a primary care doctor will not improve any surrogate markers, but over time will actually prevent death and heart attacks.[9]

But we want instant, if meaningless, results, and specialty care makes them possible. A patient gets a stress test, is found to have a blockage, a stent is placed, and $40,000 later the blockage is gone. Never mind that we still didn't address why the patient developed the condition in the first place – and more important – what we're going to do to prevent other more minor plaques from breaking off and causing a heart attack. We have done nothing other than give the patient deceptive Flexnerian snake oil, fixing something that didn't need to be fixed while ignoring the more difficult but crucial aspects of the patient's health.

CHAPTER TWENTY-FIVE

An Overlooked Legacy: The Impact of Flexner on Racial Divisions in Health Care

What I inveigh against is a cursed spirit of intolerance, conceived in distrust and bred in ignorance, that makes the mental attitude perennially antagonistic, even bitterly antagonistic, to everything foreign, that subordinates everywhere the race to nation, forgetting the higher claims of human brotherhood.

– William Osler[1]

In 2008, the American Medical Association (AMA) issued a public apology to the preeminent Black medical association of the past 100 years, the National Medical Association (NMA), and subsequently has worked to repair the racial breach in health care. Ronald M. Davis, MD, then the AMA's immediate past president, stood before an auditorium of majority African American doctors: "Today, on behalf of the American Medical Association, I unequivocally apologize for our past behavior. We pledge to do everything in our power to right the wrongs that were done by our organization to African American physicians and their families and their patients."[2] What was the AMA apologizing for and, more important, what consequences did those actions have on both the physicians and the patients that they care for?

Sadly, much of it came down to Flexner.

The AMA cannot be blamed entirely for the wrongs perpetrated on African American physicians and their patients, but its powerful grip on the institution of health care after Flexner's report placed the AMA in a unique position to change the field's pervasive bigotry. Instead, it codified racism in both its own organization and across the entire medical landscape, forcing Black physicians to fend for themselves against organized institutional oppression.

A recent report analyzing the trauma suffered by Black physicians after the Flexner Report summarized Flexner's legacy this way: "The Flexner Report was a seemingly benevolent document with traumatic racial implications for African-Americans and their health experience ... Exclusion and violation experienced by Black medical students, physicians, and patients historically and in the present day are markers of trauma that not only made African-Americans vulnerable to institutional abuses but fostered distrust and marginalization."[3]

Although the AMA wielded little power over state laws regarding who could build a medical school, it utilized its growing political lobbying status to change the licensing processes for physicians. The AMA's political power eventually pushed many states to pass laws requiring licensed doctors to graduate from "a reputable medical school." It sought political power to lobby for more regulation of doctors, and in 1900 helped reorganize local and state chapters to standardize their regulatory rules throughout the nation and thus become a stronger lobby at state governments. The regulations and lobbying ability of the AMA triggered a decline in unorthodox practitioners entering the medical field, primarily through loss of licenses among nonorthodox schools and doctors.

Though many felt that consolidating medicine into the hands of educated professionals was a positive change, the AMA now had the power to exclude Black practitioners from orthodox medical licensure, thus barring them from reputable medical practice. Because the AMA sought to dignify the image of practitioners, and because many local medical societies in the South viewed white men as the only doctors worthy of such status, acceptance of Black physicians hindered the AMA's goals. The AMA's attempts to create a homogenous medical elite pushed Black practitioners to the periphery of newly defined medical professionalization.

Initially during the AMA's consolidation, Black practitioners, facing similar struggles to their white counterparts, attempted to join the professionalization movement within medicine. The most famous of these is the example of the Medico-Chirurgical Society of the District of Columbia (MCSD). This medical society was founded in 1817 and had permission from Congress to control the licensing requirements for DC physicians. In 1870, the society voted to admit three Black doctors. There was immediate and intense backlash, and the society's leadership passed a new rule requiring at least one year of practice and a Washington, DC, medical license. This regulation successfully barred the three Black doctors from MCSD.

These Black doctors and their white physician allies then appealed to Congress for relief. They formed a new medical society, the National Medical Society (NMS), with hopes that if Congress reined in the MCSD, the integrated NMS would become the main medical power in Washington, DC.[4] Many US senators, such as Charles Sumner of Massachusetts, were in support of removing MCSD's charter, but the bill did not pass in the four times it was brought to the floor of the Senate. The NMS then appealed to the AMA to be recognized as an AMA affiliate for Washington, DC, a request that was denied. The official reason for the denial was that the NMS recognized practitioners not licensed by the MSDC, but race was clearly a major factor. With this decision, the AMA set a precedent that racial exclusion was acceptable within its affiliate medical societies. This decision ended the four-year struggle for the three Black doctors to join the MCSD. It also ended the quest of Black practitioners to be accepted as equals into white medical societies, especially those affiliated with the AMA.

It should be no great surprise that the racism so prevalent in American society during the late nineteenth and early twentieth century tainted the practice of medicine. The story of John Edward Perry, MD, a Black physician originally from Texas, provides a telling example of the barriers that Black physicians faced as they attempted to traverse the medical field.

After attending Meharry Medical School in Nashville, Edward Perry practiced in the small town of Columbia, Missouri, which had 5,000 residents, approximately a quarter of whom were Black. When Perry tried to integrate himself into the town's medical community, the established town doctor told him, "The practice among your people is done by White brethren in the profession and it would be a might hard thing for a man of your age and especially your color to wring it from their hands."[5]

Undeterred, Perry moved to Columbia and, in the first months of his career, described himself as a "busy doctor with an abundance of work and limited income."[6] He could only recruit patients without the ability to pay in full or with diseases so dire that the other town doctors had already told them treatment was hopeless. In one account, he says that "a young lady of sixteen became ill but [she was] apparently of not sufficient significance to justify medical care." He was the only doctor willing to take care of her. She could not afford to pay him and so promised to work off her debt by sweeping his fireplace once a week.[7]

Such payment in kind prevented Perry from furnishing his living quarters or purchasing the latest medical journals, creating a broader image in Columbia's medical community that he was failing as a physician. His reputation plagued him constantly as his fellow doctors questioned his competency and spoke of him with disdain.

When he relayed his struggles to an established man in town, the man replied, "The time has not yet come for a colored doctor in Columbia."

"When would it ever come?" Perry asked.

"When some of the prejudice among the Whites and ignorance among the colored dies."[8]

Needless to say, Perry decided that something must be done to remedy his predicament. He began to believe that he could dispel the notion of his inferiority only through higher education, and thus he applied to the postgraduate medical school in Chicago.

After Perry was accepted in 1898 and moved to Chicago, the superintendent approached him and said, "Dr. Perry, when we were corresponding with you we did not know you were a colored man. We cannot tell you that we will not take you because it would be a violation of the laws of the state, but I can tell you that we had rather not have you, and further, there is not much we can do for you."[9]

Perry, convinced that education represented his only path to professional respect, replied, "Well, I am going to stay and if you will not give me a loaf for which I am paying, I shall have to be satisfied with the crumbs."[10]

It was not just the administration that derided his presence; his fellow students "would sit in the library and smoking rooms for hours, reading, smoking, and discussing cases with each other, but would refuse to enter conversation with [him]."[11] But as the year progressed, people around him became accustomed to his presence and even allowed him to share in a few of their discussions about patients and other medical topics. Perry became optimistic, believing that they might have finally peered beneath his skin and acknowledged his medical talent.

But discrimination still permeated all facets of his medical education and practice. Approaching a sympathetic supervisor with complaints about his treatment and opportunities at the facility, he was told, "We would like to do more for you, but it is just impossible."[12] Perry left the school, and wrote, "For the first time, I began to see the other side of the picture. Large sums of money, no doubt, had been spent erecting a building and establishing an institution. In order to succeed in their endeavor, it was necessary for them to have and hold securely the commendation of a large number of men who hailed from the deep south and strenuously objected to the presence of a Negro."[13]

He realized that he could never fully surmount his second-tier status among the white students and faculty within this system. He left the educational facility humiliated and discouraged, realizing that Black physicians even in the best of circumstances were impeded by rampant discrimination. He confronted a hostile medical establishment his entire career, from the moment he entered Columbia, Missouri, during his time as a struggling physician, and throughout his training in Chicago. He knew that unless the system changed he could never complete the training necessary at a white-run facility or dispel the stereotypes of Black physicians as being uneducated and substandard.

The AMA's consolidation of power became complete with the publication of Flexner's report. And because the AMA spearheaded most of the report's objectives and conclusions, it became the primary organizational body overseeing health care, especially because it controlled the dispensing of medical licensing. Thus, whatever bigotry the AMA adopted during its rise to power – much of which affected the professional lives of people such as Perry who were not permitted to practice within the white-dominated medical society that the AMA built – gained traction with publication of the report and, in essence, became the new creed of health care.

Within his report, Flexner included a short chapter titled "The Medical Education of the Negro." It is in this 2-page section of a 346-page document that many ideas were expressed about what should be done about Black medical schools and the rising number of Black medical practitioners. Most of the ideas that Flexner espoused were not new – they were prevalent within the AMA, local medical societies, and among white doctors and patients – but by entrenching them in a document seeking to revolutionize medicine in the United States, he codified these ideas not just as scientific fact, but as a blueprint for the future. As medical education and the practice of health care evolved under the auspices of the AMA, in large part driven by Flexner's report, the recommendations he put forward in terms of race and Black medical schools have had enormous implications for the lives of Black physicians.

Flexner exemplified white medical thinking of his time: "The negro must be educated not only for his sake, but for ours. Not only does the negro himself suffer from hookworm and tuberculosis; he communicates them to his White neighbors."[14] "Self-protection not less than humanity offers weighty counsel in this matter; self-interest seconds philanthropy," said Flexner. He finished this line of thinking by declaring that the Black population "belongs to a potential source of infection and contagion." Flexner betrayed a prevalent stereotype of the time, that people of color, especially those rural and impoverished, exercised poor hygiene and suffered from more illness. Subsequently, the theory claims, the Black community spreads their diseases to white communities, making them a serious vector of disease to unsuspecting white people.

Building his case that Black people constituted a danger to whites, Flexner then proposed to utilize Black physicians: "The practice of the negro doctor will be limited to his own race," with the main task of the Black medical community being to teach the Black population to "practise fundamental hygienic principles."[15] In this way the "negro sanitarian [would be] be immensely useful" to the "White population."[16] Included in his proposals were the stipulations that Black medical practitioners could not poach white patients from white practitioners, and that Black physicians' ideal role was on the first line of defense against the spread of disease from the Black population to the white population. In other words, Black doctors would be trained to treat the diseases prevalent in Black people that most threatened the white population, Black doctors would not be permitted to compete with and practice with white doctors, and essentially Black doctors would be excluded from the white medical community.

What Flexner so obviously neglected is the systemic racism and oppression that caused Black communities to be more afflicted by illness and poor health care. The failure of the country's medical system to ameliorate the suffering of Black communities often stemmed from the very organizations within the health care establishment that Flexner touted as being part of the solution, primarily the AMA and its local medical societies. Such organizations marginalized Black physicians and ignored Black communities. Flexner had an opportunity to radically change Black health in this country by including Black physicians in its mainstream, but because of prevalent racist views at the time, and likely the strong hand that the AMA exerted over its content, his report perpetuated contemporary perceptions of Black physicians as inferior to white physicians, making it more difficult for Black people to be trained and licensed as doctors.[17] This missed opportunity left a legacy with which we are still living today.

Flexner's (and the AMA's) prime objective with the report was to eliminate "substandard" medical schools and to standardize the curricula and admission standards at those schools left standing. Perhaps more than anywhere else, this is where Flexner's report exerted its most enduring and devastating effect. Before his report, seven Black medical schools existed, producing far fewer Black doctors than would be needed to take care of the growing Black community. Recommending that five of the seven Black medical schools be immediately closed, the report then stipulated that the remaining two medical schools (Howard and Meharry) focus on producing health professionals who could focus on the hygiene of Black communities. One author states, "With only two Black medical schools in the country, Black physicians were produced in low quantities. Ironically, Flexner acknowledged that there would not be enough Black physicians to care for everyone in their race despite the fact that he believed Black physicians would provide better care for the African American community."[18]

Flexner may have been objective about the deplorable state of Black medical schools at the time, but he failed to recognize the institutional racism that precipitated such substandard conditions: "Black medical schools had less access to resources than many White medical schools and largely lacked funding because those with money (foundations and wealthy benefactors) did not choose to invest in Black medical schools as they did White schools." Rather than use his power and resources to help regenerate these schools and thus procure a class of well-trained Black doctors, Flexner reinforced a racialized structure of exclusion that had implications for many years to come. Especially because virtually no other schools would accept Black students, the ramifications of Flexner's consolidation of all Black medical education into two institutions meant that a lack of Black doctors persisted. The proportion of Black doctors to the Black population was 2.5 percent in 1910; in 2008, almost a century after Flexner, it had diminished even more, to 2.2 percent.[19]

To make matters worse, the Flexner Report codified an idea within the medical establishment that Black physicians were inferior and poorly trained. Before Flexner's report, most institutional bigotry emanated from local medical societies and state licensing boards; after the report, those prejudices became nationalized and standardized.[20] Black physicians found themselves on the defensive, having to fight being relegated to a hygienic role for the purpose of benefiting the white population, from having access to medical education curtailed, from being prevented from working in communities where they might "steal" patients from white physicians, and from being denied access to the broad profession medical society under AMA's umbrella. Flexner's report nearly decimated the entire Black medical professional class.

One consequence of marginalizing Black doctors was that they lacked a podium from which they could repel these injustices. This was destructive not only to Black physicians and patients, but also to the Black population at large. Consider the medical community's exploitation of the Black community with government-sponsored forced sterilization of Black women in the South, and the Tuskegee, Alabama, syphilis experiment, whereby the US Public Health Service infected 600 poor Black sharecroppers with syphilis to study the course of the disease. Because no one in the Black medical community could effectively protest these crimes, and because the white medical community and the AMA remained silent, these and other similar instances went unnoticed by the public: "Compulsory sterilization and the Tuskegee syphilis experiment are symptoms of an underlying problem – Black lives are not valued. The Flexner Report helped institutionally facilitate this issue through lack of representation of African Americans in medical institutions."[21] Clearly, Black physicians needed an organizational home of their own.

In stepped the NMA, founded a few years earlier than Flexner's report to combat the growing dissatisfaction among Black physicians over their limited access to patients, low pay, and disrespect from patients and the medical community. Because most local medical societies, and the AMA, barred Black membership and thus denied Black physicians a forum through which to advocate, the NMA would do for Black physicians what the AMA was doing for their white counterparts. Led by a fiery group of Black physicians, the NMA published articles, including "Report of Committee on Medical Education on Colored Hospitals," which came out the same year as the Flexner Report. This large survey showed that Black hospitals produced equal cure rates as did white hospitals, thus dispelling the Flexner Report's assertion of the inferiority of Black institutions and doctors.[22] Other NMA articles, including "Seeing Red," directly confronted the racism woven into American medical thinking. This article diagnosed white physicians with "Dementia Americana," whose symptoms included white male arrogance that led to stigmatization of the nonwhite population, while arguing that "poverty, disease and crime are not however race problem, but human problems."[23]

The NMA's growth led it to support an alternate system for Black health care. Partly through donations, and partly through the contributions of its own doctors, the NMA funded Black hospitals, established an academic journal (the *Journal of the National Medical Association*) that was germane to and written by members of the Black medical community, and helped the two extant Black medical schools surmount the restrictions imposed by Flexner by broadening educational opportunities and expanding admissions. Without their proactive intervention, it is likely that the Black physician pool would have dwindled to an even smaller number than those who practice today, and that the quality of both the education and career opportunities afforded to Black doctors would have been far inferior. Flexner's report pushed Black health care and the plight of Black physicians into a hole from which they have barely emerged. The NMA countered Flexner by fighting racial inequities experienced by both medical practitioners and disenfranchised patients, a fight that it continues to this day.

CHAPTER TWENTY-SIX

Why We Are So Unhealthy and What We Can Do about It

One of the most striking characteristics of the modern treatment of disease is the return of what used to be called the natural methods – diet, exercise, bathing, and massage."

– William Osler[1]

The United States spends more on health care than any other nation in the world – not by a little, but by a lot. In fact, we spend almost double the next highest-spending nation, almost $11,000 per capita. The US government spends more than $3.5 trillion and 18 percent of the gross domestic product on health care through Medicare and Medicaid expenditures.[2] This number is rising every year, with no decreases in sight. This wouldn't be so bad if we had the best system with the best outcomes in the world, but that's not the case. Life expectancy in our country is decreasing for the first time in a century, but it is increasing in the rest of the developed world. People in Japan, for example, live an average of six years longer.

We can make a lot of excuses for this sorry state of affairs. And we do. But there are two core causes of these problems, and until we address them, we are not going to improve our system. The first issue is the dysfunctional Flexnerian health care system, which focuses more on number-fixing than on health promotion. The second is the horrific state of personal health. To put it bluntly, we have become a nation of unfit and obese individuals. We spend too much time working, watching TV, and eating poorly, and we rely on doctors, medications, and quick fixes to make us healthy. We spend far too little time being fit and taking care of our bodies and our minds.

These factors are interconnected. By focusing on fixing numbers, we have moved away from fixing ourselves. We can lower cholesterol and open blocked blood vessels, but the underlying cause of heart attacks – high levels of inflammation that cause cholesterol to stick to our blood vessels and form plaque that is unstable – is not treated by such deceptive cures. Only by lowering inflammation through diet and exercise, and by avoiding pro-inflammatory factors, such as smoking and stress, will we keep our vessels clean. Making a number look good or opening a tiny piece of a plaque-riddled blood vessel lulls us into thinking we can sit around and smoke and eat potato chips because – thanks to our Flexnerian doctor's thorough care – we are taking medicines to lower our cholesterol and we have two stents that we were told will save our life.

Tobacco use, obesity, and physical inactivity are the greatest preventable causes of morbidity and mortality in the United States.[3] Alone they account for far more deaths than COVID-19 and many of our Flexnerian epidemics put together. Therefore, a better understanding of the genetic, social, environmental, and individual determinants of risk behaviors would contribute greatly to improved strategies for primary, secondary, and tertiary disease prevention. This, more than anything, should be our focus.

Smoking still kills 500,000 Americans a year; 40,000 people who don't smoke die from the smoke from others. All of these deaths are preventable.[4] Our Flexnerian system spends tens of billions of dollars trying to fix the ramifications of smoking, and billions of dollars on tests to try to detect lung cancers early. But how much do we invest in smoking cessation? The answer is, barely nothing.

The nation's obesity rate is approaching 40 percent, after holding at 35 percent between 2005 and 2012, according to data in *The State of Obesity: Better Policies for a Healthier America 2018*.[5] No state has had a statistically significant drop in its obesity rate in the past five years. Obesity rates are higher among Latinos (47 percent) and Blacks (46.8 percent) than among whites (37.9 percent). Women are more likely to be obese than men, 41.1 percent versus 37.9 percent. Adults in rural areas are more likely to be obese than those in metro areas, 34.2 percent versus 28.7 percent. Seven states now have the dubious distinction of having 35 percent or more of the population battling obesity: Alabama, Arkansas, Iowa, Louisiana, Mississippi, Oklahoma, and West Virginia. I personally know the food is amazing in these states, but unfortunately it is killing their citizen's one bite at a time.

Obesity is a complex health issue that results from a combination of causes and contributing factors, including behavior and genetics. The most lethal epidemic in our nation, it kills an estimated 300,000 every year.[6] Obesity causes us to be sick, depressed, and immobile, but because it doesn't fit nicely into the Flexnerian world of simplistic fixes, we spend a great deal more addressing the ramifications of obesity than on confronting obesity itself, despite new wonder drugs alleged to take the weight off without us having to exert any effort. It's much more profitable to measure and fix numbers with drugs and procedures than to do the hard work of addressing the causes of this disease.

The cost of obesity in the United States is sky-high. In 2008 dollars, it has been estimated to be $147 billion.[7] The annual nationwide productive costs of obesity-related absenteeism range between $3.38 billion ($79 per obese individual) and $6.38 billion ($132 per obese individual.)

We treat diabetes with medications used to lower the sugar number as measured by A1c. We don't address diet, exercise, or obesity because there are no incentives in our Flexnerian system to cure diabetes this way. It's easier for doctors to write a prescription than to do the intensive lifestyle modifications that are necessary and effective. The pharmaceutical companies advertise all of their wonderful drugs to treat this horrific disease, calling it an epidemic and demanding strict numerical repair. They promote medications to physicians in their offices and in their journals. Never mind that the efficacy of these medications are based on studies that have been mostly funded by the pharmaceutical companies themselves. Never mind that these studies measure surrogate endpoints (A1c) and not survival. These medications may lower blood sugar, but there is very little evidence that they make people live longer and better.

We are far off the mark in how we approach prevention, wellness, illness, and disease management. We need to take a more holistic, patient-centered approach to the prevention and treatment of disease. We must use all possible modalities and combine the best of traditional Western medicine with complementary therapies. In other words, we have to be more Oslerian. That means embracing a concept of integrative health that redefines the relationship between the practitioner and patient. We need to focus on the whole person and the whole community, to coordinate traditional healing practices along with complementary therapies. And we need health care that is patient-centered, science-based, and team-delivered.

Integrative health is the pursuit of personal health and well-being foremost, with the support of a health team dedicated to all proven approaches – conventional medicine, complementary and alternative medicine, and lifestyle/self-care.[8]

If a nonmainstream practice is used together with conventional medicine, it's considered "complementary." If a nonmainstream practice is used in place of conventional medicine, it's considered "alternative." Lifestyle medicine involves the incorporation of healthy and evidence-based self-care, as well as behavioral approaches into conventional medical practice to optimize health and well-being.[9]

According to a 2012 national survey, many Americans – more than 30 percent of adults and about 12 percent of children – use health care approaches not typically part of conventional medical care or that may have origins outside of usual Western practice.[10] Yoga, acupuncture, and massage, for example, have been well studied and recognized as nonpharmaceutical approaches to caring for patients with chronic back pain. With our nation's opioid epidemic killing many of our young people, alternative modalities are becoming more common and more necessary, yet they are slow to be covered by our insurance industry, despite significant evidence that they work.

We look for a quick fix for everything. I have a cold, give me an antibiotic. I am fat, give me a diet pill. I have diabetes, give me that new drug I just saw on TV. Classically Flexnerian. Unfortunately, life is not that simple, and being healthy is not simple either. Osler said that we are complex organisms and do better by living healthy lives than by flooding ourselves with snake oils.

It is estimated that longevity is based on genetics (30%), individual behaviors (40%), environmental factors (20%), and health care (10%).[11] We can't do much about our genes, but we can understand our genetic predisposition to illness and vigorously work to prevent those conditions we are predisposed to with appropriate diet, exercise, and mindfulness.

The fact is that we spend only 5 percent of the health care budget to pay for prevention, but spend hundreds of billions to treat the ramifications of poor health.[12] We would rather wait for people to get sick and fall into our Flexnerian trap of measure-diagnose-treat, flooding our patients with tests and pills and procedures, than address the causes of poor health.

The medical-industrial complex of hospital systems, pharmaceutical companies, device manufacturers, medical specialty organizations, and insurance companies make billions on people's illness and misfortune. Unless we redefine our focus on how we both deliver and pay for care, nothing will change. Major academic institutions and quaternary care hospitals make their money treating diseases that affect few individuals in comparison with our entire population. Hospitals that feast on interventional cardiac and neurological procedures will see huge reductions in their business if we prevent diseases rather than treat them. The market simply won't allow it, and there is little incentive for prevention for these huge medical corporations making huge profits on our sick folks. To fix the system, we must move away from a Flexnerian template.

Yes, only 10 percent of your health care outcomes are determined by all the tests and drugs and procedures you go through; 40 percent is determined by you.[13]

My surgical, emergency medicine, and interventional friends have come a long way in research and clinical care to save many lives, lives that should have never needed their interventions in most cases if we focused on prevention. How simple a fix that would be, and how radical: a medical system less focused on number repair and one focused instead on people.

CHAPTER TWENTY-SEVEN

The Path Forward

Nothing in life is more glaring than the contrast between possibilities and actualities, between the ideal and the real.

– William Osler[1]

We as a nation spend significantly more per capita on health care than any other industrialized country, but our results are significantly worse. The United States ranks 26th in the world in life expectancy and 37th in overall health care outcomes, yet spends twice as much per capita than the world's leading nations. Most countries in the industrialized world provide universal health care. Not here, where millions of people are either uninsured or underinsured, and so lack access to primary and preventive care services, causing them to use more expensive care provided in the emergency departments and hospitals, leaving them sicker than anywhere else in the world.

The United States is one of the few nations where most insurance benefits are linked to employers. This practice affects job security, hampers the ability to easily change jobs, limits insurance options, and significantly adds to the cost of health insurance coverage. It is estimated that there were more than 37,000 deaths in 2017 because of a lack of health insurance. These statistics make ours the most inefficient, ineffective, and costly health care system in the world. The COVID-19 pandemic has laid bare the harsh fact that our health care system is unfair, unaffordable, and unsustainable.

Health care has become a lucrative industry, where money is made at the expense of human life and individual suffering. Our medical-industrial complex is a huge for-profit industry that runs in collaboration with hospitals, the insurance industry, big pharma, medical device makers, and medical and specialty societies. Our system, predicated on the Flexnerian mantra of measuring and fixing numbers, of ascribing to its patients as many diagnoses as abnormal numbers allow, misinforms people about the real significance of those numbers and sells them deceptive fixes.

We pay for procedures and testing with little regard for quality or beneficial outcomes. We pay excessively to treat sick people and not to take care of well people who may become sick; in fact, 1 percent of patients spend 20 percent of the health care dollar; 5 percent account for half of all health care expenditures. If we would just invest our time and money preventing the diseases that affect this 5 percent, we would save billions of dollars and help people to live better and longer lives. That's what Osler taught us, and his wisdom is still valid, except to those who reap the benefits of our medical-industrial complex and the politicians they are funding.

One-third of Medicare is spent on health care in the last year of the patient's life. A significant portion of this cost is on a last hospitalization, where many spend as much as 10 days suffering in the ICU before having a horrific and often painful death. Adequate geriatric care with appropriate advance-care planning, including effective hospice and palliative care, would eliminate a significant amount of this expense while improving outcomes and increasing patient and family satisfaction. Instead of focusing on fixing numbers and adhering to protocols – the mantra of Flexner's system – we could go a long way to remedy this by focusing on our patients, their needs, and their wants.

It is estimated that a third of what is done to and for patients is medical waste, including needless tests, procedures, and medicines that don't work as advertised. This amounts to about a trillion dollars of useless and often harmful medical interventions each year. We also squander billions of dollars each year on the administration of our dysfunctional health care system, which requires an army of individuals to deliver care and to get paid, a second army that spends billions regulating the system and auditing the system, and a third army that develops and enforces meaningless metrics and guidelines that make doctors angry and disillusioned, all the while making patients sicker and poorer. These expenditures are useless and cumbersome. They don't improve care but instead place a significant burden on providers of care. The incentives to do things to patients rather than do things for them adds to needless costs and complications without improvement in quality or longevity of life. Osler's vision of taking care of one patient at a time is lost in the morass of administrative dictates that kills our ability to be caring doctors to our patients.

The Affordable Care Act (2010) was a step in the right direction, but it did not meaningfully address the problem of our health insurance industry or the health delivery system. It did not even come close to achieving its goal of health care for all. And it did nothing to dismantle or reform the basic infrastructure of our Flexnerian ethos, our Flexnerian institutions, and our Flexnerian incentives. Until we tackle Flexner, until we rediscover Osler, then merely expanding health insurance will do nothing to get us off this dangerous road.

An Oslerian health care system would be fought vigorously by those who profit by, and who are accustomed to, our current Flexnerian model. It would not, however, be difficult to assemble. All we need to do is reimagine the way we educate, reimburse, and grade doctors. We would have to build a strong primary care base, keep industry out of health care, and, above all, provide patient-centric care. It can be done.

Educating Doctors: We must move away from the one-right-answer, protocol-driven method of Germanic teaching that Flexner and his colleagues adopted in the early 1900s. What we need is to return to the humanistic patient-based teaching that Osler helped to construct at Johns Hopkins.

Students need to be exposed to the science of medicine and to patient experiences simultaneously. All education should start with the patient, and students should begin medical school at the patient bedside, not in a classroom. Medical students should be taught by physicians who have been caring for patients all their lives.

Osler did not minimize the necessity of a solid education in the physiology of the human body but found it crucial that such information be incorporated into the clinical experience. In other words, all four years of medical school should be a continuum whereby students learn from patients, from books, and from experienced doctors all at once. Only in this way can students understand the nuance and complexity of the human body, and that there is never one right answer or a single protocol that applies to everyone. Our suggestion for reform should include the following:

• The MCAT should be eliminated from medical school admissions, with an encouragement for students to broaden their minds in college with a liberal arts curriculum, delving into academic and creative pursuits. Medical students should be not be chosen based on their ability to answer basic science questions on a multiple-choice test, but on their broad humanistic, critical thinking, and scientific skills.

- Multiple-choice testing should be removed from medical schools.
- The medical school curriculum should be a four-year program of integrated medical science and patient care. Professors must have an understanding of both clinical and scientific skills and be able to tie the two together.
- Teaching should occur in the hospital and in the community, with clinical primary care physicians providing the bulk of the educational duties.
- Students should be encouraged to pursue research, quality improvement, patient safety, and clinical projects during their schooling.
- Education on humanism, communication, empathy, interpretation of data, critical thinking, and Osler's foundation of knowledge on the art of medicine must be infused into the entire curriculum.

Reimbursing Doctors: To change the culture of health care, we must reform our payment system. Osler believed that doctors were healers who came to know their patients, who were able to customize care based on specific patient needs and circumstances, and who were critical thinkers who could apply the newest scientific knowledge to the person sitting in front of him. He also stressed the importance of prevention, of promoting a healthy lifestyle, and of avoiding medicines and other interventions unless they were absolutely essential.

Unfortunately, when our system pays doctors more to do things TO patients and less to care FOR patients, it has drifted far off the Oslerian road and landed squarely on the test-diagnose-fix path paved by Flexner. If we continue to pay doctors more to put in a stent than to sit with patients and grapple with prevention and complex medical problems that will obviate the need for that stent, we'll have a lot of stents and a lot of sick patients, all at high cost. That's where we are today. Only returning to some basic principles of medical care will drive us back onto Osler's road:

- Payment for procedures, whether reading an X-ray or fixing torn cartilage, must be drastically reduced and be commensurate with payment for patient-centric office-based care.
- Payment for primary care has to be buttressed either with a direct payment model or with a patient-by-patient reimbursement system that rewards doctors for spending time with patients and addressing both preventive and holistic patient needs. Complex patients must elicit higher pay, as is being done now in certain accountable care organizations, Medicare Advantage plans, and Value-Based Purchasing Agreements.
- Primary care pay must be equal to specialty pay if our system is ever going to improve.
- Doctors can receive bonus payment by keeping overall costs down, reducing hospitalizations, and promoting preventive services. This is already being done to some extent in Medicare.
- Doctors should not be allowed to own or have interest in any diagnostic or procedural equipment, or facilities, to which they refer for their own reimbursement.

Grading Doctors: Our current system of protocols and quality indicators is as antithetical to Oslerian care as any other remediable element of our nation's health care system. Flexner's system of encouraging one-right-answer thinking leads to narrow definitions of disease based on numerical abnormalities that do not vary from patient to patient (definitions that are rigidly determined by groups and individuals who profit by making more people seem sick). This has led to the generation of protocols and quality indicators that reward doctors who test more, medicate more, and measure more – in other words, doctors who put numbers over patients; doctors who don't discuss the risks and benefits of interventions with their patients out of fear that their patients may make the "wrong" decision; doctors who believe that every patient is the same and must have the same normal measurements as defined by the protocol.

This reliance on Flexnerian absolutism detracts from patient care by squeezing everyone into the same mold. Osler spoke often about this. He believed that patients were complex and varied human beings whose range of "normal" could change based on circumstance and individual need. It was the job of the doctor not to follow a robotic set of rules, but rather to get to know his or her patient, understand the science of medicine, and inaugurate an appropriate patient-centric plan of care. As long as doctors are graded by how well they perform on generic protocols, the further we will drift from an Oslerian vision of good care. Thus, to reform our system, quality indicators need to be reshaped in an Oslerian mold. Quality should be assessed based on documented discussions of the following:

- various medical interventions (whether they have been initiated by a specialist or primary care doctor) using accurate and comprehensible patient education tools that can be quantified, *including the option of not testing and not treating*
- polypharmacy, diet, exercise, advanced-care planning, smoking cessation, and excessive utilization of emergency department and specialty care
- cancer screening and immunization

- disease conditions, such as hypertension, diabetes, and coronary artery disease, that may require treatment, with clear plans indicated

Ultimately all measures of quality must acknowledge shared decision-making between doctor and patient, and the variability of disease and its treatment between different patients.

Building a Primary Care Base: Both Osler and Flexner agreed that any viable health care system must rely on vibrant primary care. However, the Flexner system's emphasis on finding and fixing measurable diseases, its reliance on metrics and numbers, and its endorsement of procedures and drugs has helped to create a specialized medical society. Osler advocated an army of broadly trained physicians who know their patients well and can treat and manage all facets of their patients' health issues and interventions. Specialists, according to Osler, should be consultants seen for advice, for procedures, and for management of complex medical issues.

Unfortunately, today, specialists constitute 80 percent of health care providers. They see patients regularly, are incentivized to perform tests and treatments, and often refer their patients to other specialists. Our specialty-oriented medical system has led to more medicines, more tests, more hospitalization, and more procedures without an improvement in outcome. It has promoted care that is fragmented and wasteful.

How can we mitigate our primary care shortage and reenergize primary care so that it can become both an attractive field for students and a field in which providers have the time and the tools to care for their patients in the way Osler envisioned? Here are a few ideas:

- Reform reimbursement so that office visits are valued as highly or more highly than procedures, and the income of primary care doctors is on a par with that of specialists.

- Practice structure reform, whereby primary care doctors have the time and tools to care for patients, and the ability to design their practice in a way that enables them to meet the needs of their particular patient mix, to visit hospitals and long-term care facilities, and to coordinate with mental health and dietary services.
- Institute loan repayments that incentivize medical students to enter office-based primary care.
- Institute medical education reform so students have more outpatient experiences and more primary care role models who teach them.

Keeping Industry out of Health Care. Osler, more than anyone, believed that all industry, and most medical organizations, had no place in the education and clinical practice of physicians. He derided the pernicious seduction of the drug industry, fearing that doctors could be easily led back down the path taken by snake oil salesmen and patent-medicine doctors. Sadly, he was far too prescient.

Flexner invited industry and large top-down medical societies into his health care landscape, and they have ruled the roost ever since. Industry designs medical studies and develops clinical guidelines to promote its products. It lobbies Congress to assure payment to doctors and hospitals who are procedure-oriented, and it has a firm grasp on such agencies as the Centers for Disease Control and Prevention (CDC) and Food and Drug Administration (FDA) while being a primary payment source to medical schools, consumer advocacy groups, and the media. What's more, it pays money to patient education groups and medical societies to promote the use of drugs and procedures. The sponsorship and control of medical societies over the vast majority of clinical research makes the results of most studies suspect, and also ties academic doctors and institutions to their largesse. Drug advertising is just a start. The drug and device industry owns health care, and self-promoting medical societies seem to control who gets paid what and for what. We have devolved into a situation worse than that even poor Osler conceived, and likely even worse than Flexner could have anticipated when he invited industry and the American Medical Association in.

Even a nationalized health care system cannot fully eliminate the huge influence of industry on those who make the rules and determine reimbursement. But we must try, and it will require a national investment, one that will be paid back many times over through cost savings by cutting back on unnecessary drugs, tests, and procedures. Here is how to start:

- Clinical research must be financed and conducted by a national body, such as the National Institutes of Health, with pharma involvement completely eliminated.
- Medical schools, academic hospitals, and their employees can have no relationship with industry, even to finance one of their studies.
- The CDC and FDA must be purged of industry financing, industry meddling, and any employees who have had any industry affiliations.
- Drug advertising must cease, and pharmaceutical companies must be required to print the absolute risks and benefits of their products and be transparent about who was included in the studies promoting their products and who was not.

Providing Patient-centered Care: In the end, it will be the duty of our health care system to focus on the health of each and every patient, one patient at a time. Osler believed in this more than anything. He knew that only by training critically thinking, humanistic, patient-oriented physicians who were not tied down by the influence of medical societies and drug companies can we provide excellent care in this country. Osler wanted to train and nurture an army of scientist-doctors who could deflect the deceptive profit-making, drug-fixated medical world he so abhorred. Instead, down Flexner's road, we have done just the opposite. To reach the peak of Osler's mountain, we must focus on the patient first. That means doing the following:

- Provide patients with honest, transparent, and individualized choices based on the bedrock of medical science and their particular circumstances and wants.
- Eliminate calculators and other weapons of math destruction, and focus all our attention on the patient sitting in front of us.
- Reform malpractice so that doctors are not punished if they stray from the Flexnerian playbook.

We need to change our current reactive sick-care model of health care delivery, which looks for and finds numerical abnormalities, into one that is proactive and focuses on wellness, health, a strong primary care foundation, and patient choice that both Osler and Flexner would have endorsed.

William Osler paved a path forward to exactly the humane and scientific model that we lay out in this chapter and throughout the book. He have explained the steps needed to resurrect our medical system and drive away the demons of Flexnerian dogma that have so haunted us these past 100 years. We can't simply expand the system and provide Band-Aid approaches, we can't count on industry and large medical and consumer groups to guide us, and we can't even count on specialty doctors, who have so much invested in the status quo. We have to tackle the problem at the grassroots. That is why we wrote this book. We need to all push for change, and we can't do that until we understand why we are where we are and that we must change directions off Flexner's rocky road to the smooth highway envisioned by Osler.

Notes

Introduction

1 See Judith Garber, "Stents Don't Work? A Look Back at the Research," Lown Institute, May 20, 2022, https://lowninstitute.org/stents-dont-work-a-look-back-at-the-research/, for a good summary of stent trials. See the Lown Report for a good review of stent studies, all of which show no benefit in outcome compared with conservative therapy: Judith Garber, "The Prevalence and Harm of Unnecessary Stents," Lown Institute, October 31, 2023, https://lowninstitute.org/the-prevalence-and-harm-of-unnecessary-stents/. Perhaps the most interesting recent study published in *Lancet* in 2017 showed that when stents were compared with sham stents (doctors pretended to put in a stent), patients report no difference in pain relief or other salient symptoms. See Rasha Al-Lamee, David Thompson, Hakim-Moulay Dehbi, Sayan Sen, Kare Tang, John Davies, Thomas Keeble, et al., "Percutaneous Coronary Intervention in Stable Angina (ORBITA): A Double-Blind, Randomised Controlled Trial," *The Lancet* 391, no. 10115 (January 6, 2018): P31–40, https://doi.org/10.1016/S0140-6736(17)32714-9. A good *New York Times* article about this is Gina Kolata, "'Unbelievable': Heart Stents Fail to Ease Chest Pain," *New York Times*, November 2, 2017, https://www.nytimes.com/2017/11/02/health/heart-disease-stents.html. For the cost of stents, see Sharmila Devi, "US Physicians Urge End to Unnecessary Stent Operations," *The Lancet* 378, no. 9792 (August 20, 2011): P651–2, https://doi.org/10.1016/S0140-6736(11)61317-2; "Heart Stent Cost," CostHelper, accessed September 26, 2024, https://health.costhelper.com/stents.html; Margot Sanger-Katz, "In the U.S., an Angioplasty Costs $32,000. Elsewhere? Maybe $6,400," *New York Times*, December 27, 2019, https://www.nytimes.com/2019/12/27/upshot/expensive-health-care-world-comparison.html.

2 Bernie Sanders, "Issues: Health Care as a Human Right – Medicare For All," Bernie, accessed September 29, 2024, https://berniesanders.com/issues/medicare-for-all/.

3 Michael Nevins, *Abraham Flexner: A Flawed American Icon* (New York: Universe Press, 2010), p. 12.

4 Paul Starr, *The Social Transformation of American Medicine* (New York: Basic Books, 1982), 82–4.

5 Starr, *Social Transformation of American Medicine*, 90–112.

6 Michel Accad, "Flexner versus Osler: Medical Education Suffers, to this Day," Alert & Oriented, April 26, 2016, https://alertandoriented.com/Flexner-versus-osler/.

7 Starr, *Social Transformation of American Medicine*, 129–32.

8 Starr, 11–18.

9 Nevins, *Abraham Flexner*, 73.

10 Nevins, 70–1.

11 A.I. Tauber, "The Two Faces of Medical Education: Flexner vs. Osler Revisited," *Journal of the Royal Society of Medicine* 85, no. 10 (October 1992): 598, https://doi.org/10.1177/014107689208501004.

12 Nevins, *Abraham Flexner*, 68.

13 Nevins, 69.

14 Kenneth M. Ludmerer, *Time to Heal: American Medical Education from the Turn of the Century to the Era of Managed Care* (Oxford: Oxford University Press, 1999), 20.

15 Tauber, "Two Faces of Medical Education," 1600–1.

16 Nevins, *Abraham Flexner*, 1.

17 Ludmerer, *Time to Heal*, 12.

18 Ludmerer, 12.

19 Nevins, *Abraham Flexner*, 21–3.

20 Nevins, 121.

21 Starr, *Social Transformation of American Medicine*, 123.

22 Accad, "Flexner versus Osler."

23 Ludmerer, *Time to Heal*, 25.

24 A. Rae, "Osler Vindicated: The Ghost of Flexner Laid to Rest." *JAMA* 164, no. 13 (June 26, 2001): 1860–1.

25 Ludmerer, *Time to Heal*, 25.

26 Accad, "Flexner versus Osler."

27 Starr, *Social Transformation of American Medicine*, 142.

28 Starr, 144.

29 Tauber, "Two Faces of Medical Education," 601.

1. Born from the Womb of Eugenics

1 William Osler, *The Quotable Osler*, edited by Mark E. Silverman, T. Jock Murray, and Charles S. Bryan (Philadelphia: American College of Physicians, 2008), 8.

2 Thomas Neville Bonner, *Iconoclast: Abraham Flexner and a Life in Learning* (Baltimore: Johns Hopkins University Press, 2002), 88; Michael Bliss, *William Osler: A Life in Medicine* (New York: Oxford University Press, 2007), 379.

3 Walter Isaacson, *Einstein: His Life and Universe* (New York: Simon & Schuster Paperbacks, 2017).

4 For the information about eugenics used in this book, see Daniel Okrent, *The Guarded Gate: Bigotry, Eugenics, and the Law That Kept Two Generations of Jews, Italians, and Other European Immigrants out of America* (New York: Scribner, 2020), and Nancy Ordover, *American Eugenics Race, Queer Anatomy, and the Science of Nationalism* (Minneapolis: University of Minnesota Press, 2003).

5 Okrent, *The Guarded Gate*, 10–14, 127–8; Adam Cohen, *Imbeciles: The Supreme Court, American Eugenics, and the Sterilization of Carrie Buck* (New York: Penguin Press, 2016), 8, 130–2.

6 Cohen, *Imbeciles.*

7 Alan Mason Chesney Medical Archives, accessed October 17, 2023, box 63, folder 11, November 1929, lists William Welch as primary speaker at the Mental Hygiene 20th Anniversary meeting, and was quoted as saying it was "a really historic occasion"; letter from Welch (no addressee), February 11, 1933, folder 8, box 64, where he signs it as "Honorary President of the American Foundation for Mental Hygiene": "This year marks the 25th Anniversary of the founding of the mental hygiene movement, with which I have had the privilege of being identified in an active way since its very inception"; letter from Eugenics Committee of the United States to Dr. Welch, April 20, 1923, folder 20/IIB, box 61, asking him to review the committee's annual report. Second letter October 10, 1923, asking Dr. Welch on which committees he would like to serve. Letter from Charles Davenport, chairman of the Eugenics Committee, to Dr. Welch, March 22, 1920, folder 11, box 11, stating that Dr. Welch has been elected to the general committee; Alan Mason Chesney Medical Archives, accessed October 17, 2023, box 66, folder 13.

8 Vinayak K. Prasad and Adam S. Cifu, *Ending Medical Reversal: Improving Outcomes, Saving Lives* (Baltimore: Johns Hopkins University Press, 2019).

9 Meghan O'Rourke, *Invisible Kingdom: Reimagining Chronic Illness* (New York: Riverhead Books, 2023).

10 For a good discussion of troponins, see Jeanne Lenzer, *The Danger within US: America's Untested, Unregulated Medical Device Industry and One Man's Battle to Survive It* (New York: Little, Brown, 2017), 244–58.

11 Ahmed Abdel-Latif and Naoki Misumida, "Ischemic Stroke after Percutaneous Coronary Intervention," *JACC: Cardiovascular Interventions* 12, no. 15 (August 12, 2019): 1507–9, https://doi.org/10.1016/j.jcin.2019.05.013.

2. The Road Taken: Flexner's Legacy in the Modern World

1 William Osler, *An Address to Medical Students at the University of Pennsylvania, 1885* (Montreal: McGill University, The Osler Library, 2005).

2 For Ozempic profits, see Kevin Dunleavy, "Obesity, Diabetes Drugs Push Novo Nordisk and Eli Lilly to Front of Pharma's Growth Pack in Q2," Fierce Pharma, August 15, 2023, https://www.fiercepharma.com/pharma/novo-nordisk-eli-lilly-fatten-q2-sales-weight-loss-drugs.

3 The following is a good selection of articles and books that discuss the implications of aggressive control of diabetics, which is defined by lowering A1c below 7: The Action to Control Cardiovascular Risk in Diabetes Study Group, "Effects of Intensive Glucose Lowering in Type 2 Diabetes," *New England Journal of Medicine* 358, no. 24 (June 12, 2008): 2545–59, https://doi.org/10.1056/nejmoa0802743; The ACCORD Study Group, "Effects of Combination Lipid Therapy in Type 2

Diabetes Mellitus," *New England Journal of Medicine* 362, no. 17 (April 29, 2010): 1563–74; The Action to Control Cardiovascular Risk in Diabetes Study Group, "Effects of Intensive Glucose Lowering in Type 2 Diabetes," *New England Journal of Medicine* 358, no. 17 (June 12, 2008): 2545–59, https://doi.org/10.1056/NEJMoa1001282; Tanika N. Kelly, Lydia A. Bazzano, Vivian A. Fonseca, Tina K. Thethi, Kristi Reynolds, and Jiang He, "Systematic Review: Glucose Control and Cardiovascular Disease in Type 2 Diabetes," *Annals of Internal Medicine* 151, no. 6 (September 15, 2009): 394, https://doi.org/10.7326/0003-4819-151-6-200909150-00137; Steven H. Woolf and Stephen F. Rothemich, "New Diabetes Guidelines: A Closer Look at the Evidence," *American Family Physician* 58, no. 6 (October 15, 1998): 1287–90; Vinayak K. Prasad and Adam S. Cifu, *Ending Medical Reversals: Improving Outcomes, Saving Lives* (Baltimore: Johns Hopkins University Press, 2019), 32–4; Celia K. Yau, Catherine Eng, Irena Stijacic Cenzer, W. John Boscardin, Kathy Rice-Trumble, and Sei J. Lee, "Glycosylated Hemoglobin and Functional Decline in Community-Dwelling Nursing Home – Eligible Elderly Adults with Diabetes Mellitus," *Journal of the American Geriatrics Society* 60, no. 7 (July 2012): 1215–21, https://doi.org/10.1111/j.1532-5415.2012.04041.x; Andy Lazris, *Curing Medicare: A Doctor's View on How Our Health Care System Is Failing Older Americans and How We Can Fix It* (Ithaca, NY: ILR Press, an imprint of Cornell University Press, 2016), 31–3; Lorraine L. Lipscombe, Tara Gomes, Linda E. Lévesque, Janet E. Hux, David N. Juurlink, and David A. Alter, "Thiazolidinediones and Cardiovascular Outcomes in Older Patients with Diabetes," *JAMA* 298, no. 22 (December 12, 2007): 2634–43, https://doi.org/10.1001/jama.298.22.2634; Robin Respaut, Chad Terhune, and Deborah J. Nelson, "Special Report – Drugmakers Pushed Aggressive Diabetes Therapy. Patients Paid the Price," *Reuters*, November 4, 2021, https://www.reuters.com/article/usa-diabetes-overtreatment/special-report-drugmakers-pushed-aggressive-diabetes-therapy-patients-paid-the-price-idUSL1N2RT25O.

4 For prediabetes, see Kenneth Lam and Sei J. Lee, "Prediabetes – A Risk Factor Twice Removed," *JAMA Internal Medicine* 181, no. 4 (February 8, 2021): 520–1, https://doi.org/10.1001/jamainternmed.2020.8773; Andy Lazris and Alan Roth, "Prediabetes Diagnosis: Helpful or Harmful?," *American Family Physician* 104, no. 6 (December 2021): 649–51; Charles Piller, "The War on 'Prediabetes' Could Be a Boon for Pharma – But Is It Good Medicine?," *Science*, March 7, 2019, https://doi.org/10.1126/science.aax2208.

5 Simon Capewell, "Will Screening Individuals at High Risk of Cardiovascular Events Deliver Large Benefits?," *BMJ* 337 (August 28, 2008): 783, https://doi.org/10.1136/bmj.a1395; Jack V. Tu, Chris L. Pashos, C. David Naylor, Erluo Chen, Sharon-Lise Normand, Joseph P. Newhouse, and Barbara J. McNeil, "Use of Cardiac Procedures and Outcomes in Elderly Patients with Myocardial Infarction in the United States and Canada," *New England Journal of Medicine* 336, no. 21 (May 22, 1997): 1500–5, https://doi.org/10.1056/NEJM199705223362106; Shannon Brownlee, *Overtreated: Why Too Much Medicine Is Making Us Sicker and Poorer* (New York: Bloomsbury, 2008), 99; for a summary and ample sources about cardiac stress testing, see Erik Rifkin and Andrew Lazris, "Exercising Stress Tests," in *Interpreting Health Benefits and Risks: A Practical Guide to Facilitate Doctor–Patient Communication* (Cham: Springer, 2015), 83–94, https://doi.org/10.1007/978-3-319-11544-3.

6 Often it is difficult to find studies that look at disabling and lethal strokes rather than all strokes. See Lazris, *Curing Medicare*, 24–7, and Rifkin and Lazris, *Interpreting Health Benefits and Risks*, 95–105, for several citations and analysis.

Cochrane, in the Cochrane Database, does report on studies looking at disabling and fatal strokes, which is summarized in Kirill Shishlov, "Oral Anticoagulants versus Antiplatelet Agents in Non-Valvular Atrial Fibrillation for Stroke Prevention (and No Prior Stroke)," The NNT, October 21, 2013, https://thennt .com/nnt/warfarin-vs-aspirin-for-atrial-fibrillation-stroke-prevention/, and can be found in full in Maria I. Aguilar, Robert Hart, and Lesly A. Pearce, "Oral Anticoagulants versus Antiplatelet Therapy for Preventing Stroke in Patients with Non-Valvular Atrial Fibrillation and No History of Stroke or Transient Ischemic Attacks," *Cochrane Database of Systematic Reviews*, no. 3 (July 18, 2007): CD006186, https://pubmed.ncbi.nlm.nih.gov/17636831/. Regarding increased bleeds in elders using new oral anticoagulants, see John Mandrola, "My Pick of the Most Important Study from the European Society of Cardiology Meeting," Sensible Medicine, September 4, 2023, http://www.sensible-med .com/p/my-pick-of-the-most-important-study; and the study itself, Linda P.T. Joosten, Sander van Doorn, Peter M. van de Ven, Bart T.G. Köhlen, Melchior C. Nierman, Huiberdina L. Koek, Martin E.W. Hemels, Menno V. Huisman, Marieke Kruip, Laura M. Faber, et al., "Safety of Switching from a Vitamin K Antagonist to a Non-Vitamin K Antagonist Oral Anticoagulant in Frail Older Patients with Atrial Fibrillation: Results of the Frail-AF Randomized Controlled Trial," *Circulation* 149, no. 4 (January 24, 2023): 279–89, https://doi.org/10.1161 /circulationaha.123.066485. There are many articles about lawsuit settlements for new oral anticoagulants on legal sites, most of which are cited, and one that has a lot of information, "Dangerous Drugs Pradaxa & Xarelto," Wayne Wright Lawyers, accessed September 26, 2024, https://waynewright.com/pradaxa-and -xarelto/.

3. Why So Much Medical Science Is Not Reliable

1 William Osler, "The Treatment of Disease," *Canada Lancet* 42, no. 12 (August 1909): 906–7.
2 John Abramson, "America's Broken Health Care: Diagnosis and Prescription," *Imprimis* 52, no. 2 (February 2023), https://imprimis.hillsdale.edu/americas -broken-health-care-diagnosis-and-prescription/, discusses the funding of academic research by pharmaceutical companies.
3 John P.A. Ioannidis has a lecture on YouTube, "Dr. Ioannidis on Why We Don't Have Reliable Data Surrounding COVID-19," YouTube, posted by Journeyman Pictures on April 3, 2020, https://www.youtube.com/watch?v=QUvWaxuurzQ, and his most salient article is Ioannidis, "Why Most Published Research Findings Are False," *PLoS Medicine* 2, no. 8 (August 30, 2005): e124, https://doi .org/10.1371/journal.pmed.0020124. See also Vinayak K. Prasad and Adam S. Cifu, *Ending Medical Reversal: Improving Outcomes, Saving Lives* (Baltimore: Johns Hopkins University Press, 2019), about the same topic.
4 Owen Dyer, "What Did We Learn from Tamiflu?," *BMJ* 368 (February 19, 2020): m626, https://doi.org/10.1136/bmj.m626; Jeanne Lenzer, "Centers for Disease Control and Prevention: Protecting the Private Good?," *BMJ* 350 (May 15, 2015): h2362, https://doi.org/10.1136/bmj.h2362.
5 Benjamin Lazarus, Yuan Chen, Francis P. Wilson, Yingying Sang, Alex R. Chang, Josef Coresh, and Morgan E. Grams, "Proton Pump Inhibitor Use and the Risk of Chronic Kidney Disease," *JAMA Internal Medicine* 176, no. 2 (February 2016): 238, https://doi.org/10.1001/jamainternmed.2015.7193.

6 See Jeanne Lenzer, *The Danger within US: America's Untested, Unregulated Medical Device Industry and One Man's Battle to Survive It* (New York: Little, Brown, 2017), 250–9.

7 R. Al-Lamee, D. Thompson, H.M. Dehbi, S. Sen, K. Tang, and J. Davies, "Percutaneous Coronary Intervention in Stable Angina (Orbita): A Double-Blind, Randomized Controlled Trial," *Journal of Vascular Surgery* 67, no. 2 (February 2018): 673, https://doi.org/10.1016/j.jvs.2017.11.046. See again Gina Kolata, "'Unbelievable': Heart Stents Fail to Ease Chest Pain," *New York Times*, November 2, 2017, https://www.nytimes.com/2017/11/02/health/heart-disease-stents.html.

4. Why Patients (and Doctors) Are Enticed by Flexnerian Logic

1 William Osler, "Introduction: The Evolution of Internal Medicine," in *Modern Medicine: Its Theory and Practice*, Vol. 1, *Evolution of Internal Medicine*, edited by William Osler and assisted by Thomas McCraev (Philadelphia: Lea Brothers and Co., 1907), xxxi, https://archive.org/details/modernmedicineit01osleuoft.

2 Amos Tversky and Daniel Kahneman were two Israeli psychologists who conducted groundbreaking research on cognitive bias, and we rely on their assessments in this book. Some relevant pieces to read are Amos Tversky and Daniel Kahneman, "Judgment under Uncertainty: Heuristics and Biases," *Science* 185, no. 4157 (September 27, 1974): 1124–31, https://doi.org/10.1126/science.185.4157.1124; Daniel Kahneman, Paul Slovic, and Amos Tversky, *Judgment under Uncertainty: Heuristics and Biases* (Cambridge: Cambridge University Press, 2018); Michael Lewis, *The Undoing Project: A Friendship That Changed Our Minds* (New York: W.W. Norton, 2017).

3 Andrew Vickers, "Re: Prostate Cancer Screening in the Randomized Prostate, Lung, Colorectal, and Ovarian Cancer Screening Trial: Mortality Results after 13 Years of Follow-Up," *European Urology* 62, no. 2 (August 2012): 353, https://doi.org/10.1016/j.eururo.2012.05.031; Fabio Campodonico, "Re: Freddie C. Hamdy, Jennie L. Donovan, J. Athene Lane, et al. Fifteen-Year Outcomes after Monitoring, Surgery, or Radiotherapy for Prostate Cancer. N Engl J Med 2023;388:1547–58," *European Urology Oncology*, 7, no. 1 (February 2024): 171, https://doi.org/10.1016/j.euo.2023.06.012; Richard M. Martin, Jenny L. Donovan, Emma L. Turner, Chris Metcalfe, Grace J. Young, Eleanor I. Walsh, J. Athene Lane, Sian Noble, Steven E. Oliver, Simon Evans, et al., "Effect of a Low-Intensity PSA-Based Screening Intervention on Prostate Cancer Mortality," *JAMA* 319, no. 9 (March 6, 2018): 883, https://doi.org/10.1001/jama.2018.0154. For an article of interest, see Steven Salzberg, "PSA Screening Does More Harm Than Good," *Forbes*, May 19, 2014, https://www.forbes.com/sites/stevensalzberg/2014/05/19/psa-screening-does-more-harm-than-good/.

4 For data on health outcomes and low-value care, see Aaron E. Carroll, "The High Costs of Unnecessary Care," *JAMA* 318, no. 18 (November 14, 2017): 1748, https://doi.org/10.1001/jama.2017.16193; T. Bruce Ferguson, "The Institute of Medicine Committee Report 'Best Care at Lower Cost: The Path to Continuously Learning Health Care,'" *Circulation: Cardiovascular Quality and Outcomes* 5, no. 6 (November 2012): e93–4, https://doi.org/10.1161/circoutcomes.112.968768; Beth Beaudin-Seiler, Michael Ciarametaro, Robert W. Dubois, Jim Lee, and A. Mark Fendrick, "Reducing Low-Value Care," *Forefront Group*, September 20, 2016, https://doi.org/10.1377/forefront.20160920.056666; Atul Gawande, "Overkill," *The New Yorker*, May 4, 2015, https://www.newyorker.com/magazine/2015/05/11/overkill-atul-gawande.

5 Larry B. Goldstein, "Screening for Asymptomatic Carotid Artery Stenosis," *JAMA* 325, no. 5 (February 2, 2021): 443, https://doi.org/10.1001/jama.2020.26440.

5. Most of What We Offer Patients Is No Better Than a Pebble

1 William Osler, *Sir William Osler: Aphorisms from His Bedside Teachings and Writings*, collected by Robert Bennett Bean and edited by William Bennett Bean (New York: Henry Schuman, 1950), 101, https://archive.org/details/in.ernet.dli.2015.63933.
2 Some studies on these drugs can be found in Erik Rifkin and Andrew Lazris, "Screening for and Treating Dementia," in *Interpreting Health Benefits and Risks: A Practical Guide to Facilitate Doctor-Patient Communication* (Cham: Springer, 2015), 161–71, https://doi.org/10.1007/978-3-319-11544-3_18; Andy Lazris, *Curing Medicare: A Doctor's View on How Our Health Care System Is Failing Older Americans and How We Can Fix It* (Ithaca, NY: ILR Press, an imprint of Cornell University Press, 2016), 39–40, lists 10 studies that assess the efficacy of these drugs; John Abramson, *Overdosed America* (New York: HarperCollins, 2013), 104.
3 Maurice W. Dysken, Mary Sano, Sanjay Asthana, Julia E. Vertrees, Muralidhar Pallaki, Maria Llorente, Susan Love, Gerard D. Schellenberg, J. Riley McCarten, Julie Malphurs, et al., "Effect of Vitamin E and Memantine on Functional Decline in Alzheimer Disease," *JAMA* 311, no. 1 (January 1, 2014): 33–44, https://doi.org/10.1001/jama.2013.282834. See also "Vitamin E Slows Alzheimer's in VA Trial," *VA Research Currents*, Winter 2013–14, https://www.research.va.gov/currents/winter2013-14/winter2013-14-16.cfm.
4 A good discussion of the placebo effect can be found in Vinayak K. Prasad and Adam S. Cifu, *Ending Medical Reversal: Improving Outcomes, Saving Lives* (Baltimore: Johns Hopkins University Press, 2019), 16–29.
5 Laura E. Middleton, Todd M. Manini, Eleanor M. Simonsick, Tamara B. Harris, Deborah E. Barnes, Frances Tylavsky, Jennifer S. Brach, James E. Everhart, and Kristine Yaffe, "Activity Energy Expenditure and Incident Cognitive Impairment in Older Adults," *Archives of Internal Medicine* 171, no. 14 (July 25, 2011): 1251, https://doi.org/10.1001/archinternmed.2011.277; "Leisure Activities and the Risk of Dementia," *New England Journal of Medicine* 349, no. 13 (September 25, 2003): 1290–2, https://doi.org/10.1056/nejm200309253491316; Eric B. Larson, "Physical Activity for Older Adults at Risk for Alzheimer Disease," *JAMA* 300, no. 9 (September 3, 2008): 1077, https://doi.org/10.1001/jama.300.9.1077; Eric B. Larson, Li Wang, James D. Bowen, Wayne C. McCormick, Linda Teri, Paul Crane, and Walter Kukull, "Exercise Is Associated with Reduced Risk for Incident Dementia among Persons 65 Years of Age and Older," *Annals of Internal Medicine* 144, no. 2 (January 17, 2006): 73, https://doi.org/10.7326/0003-4819-144-2-200601170-00004.
6 See an *Atlantic* article on a new Alzheimer's disease drug, Nicholas Bagley and Rachel Sachs, "The Drug That Could Break American Health Care," *The Atlantic*, June 11, 2021, https://www.theatlantic.com/ideas/archive/2021/06/aduhelm-drug-alzheimers-cost-medicare/619169/; for Lown on Leqembi, which passed through FDA by proving trivial efficacy in a surrogate memory test, see Judith Garber, "A Tale of Two Drugs: Accountability and Evidence in Alzheimer's Treatments," Lown Institute, January 20, 2023, https://lowninstitute.org/a-tale-of-two-drugs-accountability-and-evidence-in-alzheimers-treatments/; for an article on anticipation of Leqembi's acceptance by doctors, never mentioning

the lack of proven clinical benefit and glossing over the very serious risks, see Julie Steenhuysen and Deena Beasley, "Major US Health Systems Expect to Offer Alzheimer's Drug Leqembi in a Few Months," *Reuters*, August 7, 2023, https://www.reuters.com/business/healthcare-pharmaceuticals/major-us -health-systems-expect-offer-alzheimers-drug-leqembi-few-months -2023-08-07/. A *KFF Health News* article correctly states that Leqembi's 27 percent improvement in memory function translates to an improvement of 4.41 for the Leqembi group at the end of 18 months versus 4.86 for the placebo group in the nonclinical 18-question memory test administered, while 13 percent of the highly screened participants bled into their brains and 17 percent had brain swelling; see Judith Graham, "New Alzheimer's Drug Raises Hopes – Along with Questions," *KFF Health News*, August 11, 2023, https://kffhealthnews.org/news/article /leqembi-new-alzheimers-drug-raises-hopes-questions/.

6. Turning Pebbles into Boulders: How We Exaggerate the Benefits of What We Do

1 William Osler, *Sir William Osler: Aphorisms from His Bedside Teachings and Writings*, collected by Robert Bennett Bean and edited by William Bennett Bean (New York: Henry Schuman, 1950), 125, https://archive.org/details/in.ernet.dli.2015.63933.

2 For data on mammograms, and also an explanation of how mammograms are illustrative of how relative numbers exaggerate benefit, see H. Gilbert Welch and Honor J. Passow, "Quantifying the Benefits and Harms of Screening Mammography," *JAMA Internal Medicine* 174, no. 3 (March 2014): 448, https:// doi.org/10.1001/jamainternmed.2013.13635; Erik Rifkin and Andrew Lazris, "Breast Cancer Screening: Mammograms," in *Interpreting Health Benefits and Risks: A Practical Guide to Facilitate Doctor–Patient Communication* (Cham: Springer, 2015), 33–41, https://doi.org/10.1007/978-3-319-11544-3_6; Archie Bleyer and H. Gilbert Welch, "Effect of Three Decades of Screening Mammography on Breast-Cancer Incidence," *New England Journal of Medicine* 367, no. 21 (November 22, 2012): 1998–2005, https://doi.org/10.1056/nejmoa1206809; H. Gilbert Welch, "Overdiagnosis and Mammography Screening," *BMJ* 339 (July 9, 2009): b1425, https://doi.org/10.1136/bmj.b1425; Caryn Lerman, Bruce Track, Barbara K. Rimer, Alice Boyce, Chris Jepson, and Paul F. Engstrom, "Psychological and Behavioral Implications of Abnormal Mammograms," *Annals of Internal Medicine* 114, no. 8 (April 15, 1991): 657–61, https://doi.org/10.7326/0003-4819 -114-8-657.

3 See video highlighting Lazris and Rifkin's strategy to demonstrate accurate medical statistics to explain how statistics can be manipulated in mammograms: Jay Hancock, "Skip the Math: Researchers Paint a Picture of Health Benefits and Risks," *NPR*, October 12, 2016, https://www.npr.org/sections/health -shots/2016/10/12/497549732/skip-the-math-researchers-paint-a-picture-of -health-benefits-and-risks.

4 Keith A. Reynolds, "New Study Estimates U.S. Healthcare Waste Costs Nearly $1 Trillion Each Year," *Medical Economics*, October 9, 2019, https://www .medicaleconomics.com/view/new-study-estimates-us-healthcare-waste -costs-nearly-1-trillion-each-year.

5 For some data about statins and cholesterol, see Gregory Curfman, "Risks of Statin Therapy in Older Adults," *JAMA Internal Medicine* 177, no. 7 (July 2017): 966, https://doi.org/10.1001/jamainternmed.2017.1457; R. Chou, T. Dana, I. Blazina,

M. Daeges, and T.L. Jeanne, "Statins for Prevention of Cardiovascular Disease in Adults: Evidence Report and Systematic Review for the US Preventive Services Task Force," *Journal of Vascular Surgery* 65, no. 3 (March 2017): 925, https://doi.org/10.1016/j.jvs.2017.01.016. See also John Abramson, "Statins in Persons at Low Risk of Cardiovascular Disease," The NNT, November 8, 2017, https://thennt.com/nnt/statins-persons-low-risk-cardiovascular-disease/; Andy Lazris and Alan Roth, "Overuse of Statins in Older Adults," *American Family Physician* 100, no. 12 (December 15, 2019): 242–3; Paula Byrne, Maryanne Demasi, Mark Jones, Susan M. Smith, Kirsty K. O'Brien, and Robert DuBroff, "Evaluating the Association between Low-Density Lipoprotein Cholesterol Reduction and Relative and Absolute Effects of Statin Treatment," *JAMA Internal Medicine* 182, no. 5 (March 14, 2022): 474, https://doi.org/10.1001/jamainternmed.2022.0134; Jerry H. Gurwitz, Alan S. Go, and Stephen P. Fortmann, "Statins for Primary Prevention in Older Adults," *JAMA* 316, no. 19 (November 15, 2016): 1971, https://doi.org/10.1001/jama.2016.15212.

7. Numerical Epidemics

1 William Osler, "Medical Education," in *Counsels and Ideals* (Boston: Houghton Mifflin, 1921), 153, https://archive.org/details/counselsidealsfr00osle.
2 See The SPRINT Research Group, "A Randomized Trial of Intensive versus Standard Blood-Pressure Control," *New England Journal of Medicine* 373, no. 22 (November 26, 2015): 2103–116, https://doi.org/10.1056/NEJMoa1511939.
3 For information about chronic kidney disease, see Ann M. O'Hare, Rudolph A. Rodriguez, and Andrew D. Rule, "Overdiagnosis of Chronic Kidney Disease in Older Adults – An Inconvenient Truth," *JAMA Internal Medicine* 181, no. 10 (2021): 1366. https://doi.org/10.1001/jamainternmed.2021.4823; Alan R. Roth, Andy Lazris, Helen Haskell, and John James, "Overdiagnosis of CKD in Older Adults: Unnecessary Interventions, Costs, and Worry," *American Family Physician* 107, no. 6 (June 2023): 657–8.
4 See, for example, Rhonda M. Cooper-DeHoff, Yan Gong, Eileen M. Handberg, Anthony A. Bavry, Scott J. Denardo, George L. Bakris, and Carl J. Pepine, "Tight Blood Pressure Control and Cardiovascular Outcomes among Hypertensive Patients with Diabetes and Coronary Artery Disease," *JAMA* 304, no. 1 (July 7, 2010): 61, https://doi.org/10.1001/jama.2010.884; The ACCORD Study Group, "Effects of Intensive Blood-Pressure Control in Type 2 Diabetes Mellitus," *New England Journal of Medicine* 362, no. 17 (April 29, 2010): 1575–85, https://doi.org/10.1056/nejmoa1001286; Bodil Lernfelt, Sten Landahl, Alvar Svanborg, and John Wikstrand, "Overtreatment of Hypertension in the Elderly?," *Journal of Hypertension* 8, no. 5 (May 1990): 483–90, https://doi.org/10.1097/00004872-199005000-00015; Csaba P. Kovesdy, Anthony J. Bleyer, Miklos Z. Molnar, Jennie Z. Ma, John J. Sim, William C. Cushman, L. Darryl Quarles, and Kamyar Kalantar-Zadeh, "Blood Pressure and Mortality in US Veterans with Chronic Kidney Disease," *Annals of Internal Medicine* 159, no. 4 (August 20, 2013): 233–42, https://doi.org/10.7326/0003-4819-159-4-201308200-00004; Franz H. Messerli, Giuseppe Mancia, C. Richard Conti, Ann C. Hewkin, Stuart Kupfer, Annette Champion, Rainer Kolloch et al., "Dogma Disputed: Can Aggressively Lowering Blood Pressure in Hypertensive Patients with Coronary Artery Disease Be Dangerous?," *Annals of Internal Medicine* 144, no. 12 (June 20, 2006): 884–93, https://doi.org/10.7326/0003-4819-144-12-200606200-00005; Florent Boutitie,

"J-Shaped Relationship between Blood Pressure and Mortality in Hypertensive Patients," *Annals of Internal Medicine* 136, no. 6 (March 19, 2002): 438–48; "Prevention of Stroke by Antihypertensive Drug Treatment in Older Persons with Isolated Systolic Hypertension," *JAMA* 265, no. 24 (June 26, 1991): 3255, https://doi.org/10.1001/jama.1991.03460240051027; John M. Cruickshank, Jeffrey M. Thorp, and F. James Zacharias, "Benefits and Potential Harm of Lowering High Blood Pressure," *The Lancet* 329, no. 8533 (March 14, 1987): 581–4, https://doi.org/10.1016/s0140-6736(87)90231-5; Timothy S. Anderson, Shoshana J. Herzig, Bocheng Jing, W. John Boscardin, Kathy Fung, Edward R. Marcantonio, and Michael A. Steinman, "Clinical Outcomes of Intensive Inpatient Blood Pressure Management in Hospitalized Older Adults," *JAMA Internal Medicine* 183, no. 7 (May 30, 2023): 715, https://doi.org/10.1001/jamainternmed.2023.1667.

5 See, for example, Paula Byrne, Maryanne Demasi, Mark Jones, Susan M. Smith, Kirsty K. O'Brien, and Robert DuBroff, "Evaluating the Association between Low-Density Lipoprotein Cholesterol Reduction and Relative and Absolute Effects of Statin Treatment," *JAMA Internal Medicine* 182, no. 5 (March 14, 2022): 474, https://doi.org/10.1001/jamainternmed.2022.0134; Erik Rifkin and Andrew Lazris, "Cholesterol Screening," in *Interpreting Health Benefits and Risks: A Practical Guide to Facilitate Doctor–Patient Communication* (Cham: Springer, 2015), 125–32, https://doi.org/10.1007/978-3-319-11544-3_15; Vinayak K. Prasad and Adam S. Cifu, *Ending Medical Reversal: Improving Outcomes, Saving Lives* (Baltimore: Johns Hopkins University Press, 2019), 34–6; Andy Lazris, *Curing Medicare: A Doctor's View on How Our Health Care System Is Failing Older Americans and How We Can Fix It* (Ithaca, NY: ILR Press, an imprint of Cornell University Press, 2016), 33–5; William B. Kannel, "Cholesterol in the Prediction of Atherosclerotic Disease," *Annals of Internal Medicine* 90, no. 1 (January 1, 1979): 85, https://doi.org/10.7326/0003-4819-90-1-85; Ed Silverman, "The New Cholesterol Guidelines and Conflicts of Interest," *Forbes*, November 21, 2013, https://www.forbes.com/sites/edsilverman/2013/11/20/the-new-cholesterol-guidelines-and-conflicts-of-interest/; Todd B. Mendelson, Michele Meltzer, Eric G. Campbell, Arthur L. Caplan, and James N. Kirkpatrick, "Conflicts of Interest in Cardiovascular Clinical Practice Guidelines," *Archives of Internal Medicine* 171, no. 6 (March 28, 2011): 577–84, https://doi.org/10.1001/archinternmed.2011.96; Mark Zdechlik, "Study: Major Heart Attacks, Cholesterol Seldom Linked," *MPR News*, April 12, 2017, https://www.mprnews.org/story/2017/04/12/study-most-major-heart-attacks-not-linked-with-high-cholesterol.

6 For more on calcium scoring and plaque deposition, see Matthew J. Budoff, Robyn L. McClelland, Khurram Nasir, Philip Greenland, Richard A. Kronmal, George T. Kondos, Steven Shea, Joao A.C. Lima, and Roger S. Blumenthal, "Cardiovascular Events with Absent or Minimal Coronary Calcification: The Multi-Ethnic Study of Atherosclerosis (MESA)," *American Heart Journal* 158, no. 4 (October 2009): 554–61, https://doi.org/10.1016/j.ahj.2009.08.007; Matthew J. Budoff and Khawar M. Gul, "Expert Review on Coronary Calcium," *Vascular Health and Risk Management* 4, no. 2 (April 2008): 315–24, https://doi.org/10.2147/vhrm.s1160.

7 For more on this, see Anahad O'Connor, "How the Sugar Industry Shifted Blame to Fat," *New York Times*, September 12, 2016, https://www.nytimes.com/2016/09/13/well/eat/how-the-sugar-industry-shifted-blame-to-fat.html; Cristin E. Kearns, Laura A. Schmidt, and Stanton A. Glantz, "Sugar Industry and Coronary Heart Disease Research," *JAMA Internal Medicine* 176, no. 11 (November 2016): 1680, https://doi.org/10.1001/jamainternmed.2016.5394.

8 John J.P. Kastelein, Fatima Akdim, Erik S.G. Stroes, Aeilko H. Zwinderman, Michiel L. Bots, Anton F.H. Stalenhoef, Frank L.J. Visseren, et al., "Simvastatin with or without Ezetimibe in Familial Hypercholesterolemia," *New England Journal of Medicine* 358, no. 14 (April 3, 2008): 1431–43, https://doi.org/10.1056/NEJMoa0800742.

9 The data presented here are based on studies of prediabetes and diabetes in Charles Pillar, "The War on 'Prediabetes' Could Be a Boon for Pharma – But Is It Good for Medicine?," *Science*, March 7, 2019, https://doi.org/10.1126/science.aax2208.

10 Steven H. Woolf and Stephen F. Rothemich, "New Diabetes Guidelines: A Closer Look at the Evidence," *American Family Physician* 58, no. 6 (October 15, 1998): 1287–90, https://www.aafp.org/pubs/afp/issues/1998/1015/p1287.html.

11 Pillar, "The War on 'Prediabetes.'"

12 For more on bone density, see the following works, which are replete with studies: Erik Rifkin and Andrew Lazris, "Osteoporosis: Bone Density Testing and Drug Treatment," in *Interpreting Health Benefits and Risks: A Practical Guide to Facilitate Doctor–Patient Communication* (Cham: Springer, 2015), 173–82, https://doi.org/10.1007/978-3-319-11544-3_19; H. Gilbert Welch, Lisa Schwartz, and Steve Woloshin, *Over-Diagnosed: Making People Sick in the Pursuit of Health* (New York: Random House, 2012), 22–6; Nortin M. Hadler, *Rethinking Aging: Growing Old and Living Well in an Overtreated Society* (Chapel Hill: University of North Carolina Press, 2019), 121–4; Lazris, *Curing Medicare*, 35–6.

8. The Pitfalls of Screening for Diseases You *Might* Have

1 Bernard Lown, "Social Responsibility of Physicians," address presented at the Avoiding Avoidable Care Conference, Cambridge, MA, April 26, 2012, https://bernardlown.wordpress.com/2012/04/29/social-responsibility-of-physicians/.

2 "Dr. Bernard Lown," Lown Institute, accessed October 11, 2024, https://lowninstitute.org/about/dr-bernard-lown/.

3 The public in general strongly believes in cancer screening, according to the following study: Lisa M. Schwartz, Steven Woloshin, Floyd J. Fowler Jr., and H. Gilbert Welch, "Enthusiasm for Cancer Screening in the United States," *JAMA* 291, no. 1 (January 7, 2004): 71, https://doi.org/10.1001/jama.291.1.71.

4 Jay Hancock, "How Tiny Are Benefits from Many Tests and Pills? Researchers Paint a Picture," *KFF Health News*, October 12, 2016, https://kffhealthnews.org/news/how-tiny-are-benefits-from-many-tests-and-pills-researchers-paint-a-picture/.

5 A recent study explored multiple screening tests and concluded that given their risks, most do not save lives; see Michael Bretthauer, Paulina Wieszczy, Magnus Løberg, Michal F. Kaminski, Tarjei Fiskergård Werner, Lise M. Helsingen, Yuichi Mori, Øyvind Holme, Hans-Olov Adami, and Mette Kalager, "Estimated Lifetime Gained with Cancer Screening Tests," *JAMA Internal Medicine* 183, no. 11 (August 28, 2023): 1196–203, https://doi.org/10.1001/jamainternmed.2023.3798, with commentary in H. Gilbert Welch and Tanujit Dey, "Testing Whether Cancer Screening Saves Lives," *JAMA Internal Medicine* 183, no. 11 (August 28, 2023): 1255–8, https://doi.org/10.1001/jamainternmed.2023.3781.

6 Jeanne Lenzer, *The Danger within US: America's Untested, Unregulated Medical Device Industry and One Man's Battle to Survive It* (New York: Little, Brown, 2017).

7 "Skin Cancer: Screening," U.S. Preventive Services Task Force, April 29, 2013, https://www.uspreventiveservicestaskforce.org/uspstf/recommendation/skin-cancer-screening#fullrecommendationstart; Nora B. Henrikson, Ilya Ivlev, Paula R. Blasi, Matt B. Nguyen, Caitlyn A. Senger, Leslie A. Perdue, and Jennifer

S. Lin, "Skin Cancer Screening," *JAMA* 329, no. 15 (April 18, 2023): 1296, https://doi.org/10.1001/jama.2023.3262; Eleni Linos, Rupa Parvataneni, Sarah E. Stuart, W. John Boscardin, C. Seth Landefeld, and Mary-Margaret Chren, "Treatment of Nonfatal Conditions at the End of Life," *JAMA Internal Medicine* 173, no. 11 (June 10, 2013): 1006, https://doi.org/10.1001/jamainternmed.2013.639; Elizabeth Fernandez, "Aggressive Surgery for Nonfatal Skin Cancers Might Not Be Best for All Elderly Patients," UC San Francisco, April 29, 2013, https://www.ucsf.edu/news/2013/04/105436/aggressive-surgery-nonfatal-skin-cancers-might-not-be-best-all-elderly-patients.

8 See Elizabeth Rosenthal, "Patients' Costs Skyrocket; Specialists' Incomes Soar," *New York Times*, January 18, 2014, https://www.nytimes.com/2014/01/19/health/patients-costs-skyrocket-specialists-incomes-soar.html.

9 Rita Rubin, "Melanoma Diagnoses Rise While Mortality Stays Fairly Flat, Raising Concerns about Overdiagnosis," *JAMA* 323, no. 15 (April 1, 2020): 1429, https://doi.org/10.1001/jama.2020.2669.

10 Edward F. Patz Jr., Paul Pinsky, Constantine Gatsonis, JoRean D. Sicks, Barnett S. Kramer, Martin C. Tammemägi, Caroline Chiles, William C. Black, and Denise R. Aberle, "Overdiagnosis in Low-Dose Computed Tomography Screening for Lung Cancer," *JAMA Internal Medicine* 174, no. 2 (February 2014): 269, https://doi.org/10.1001/jamainternmed.2013.12738; Anders Kelto, interview by Renee Montagne, "Why Some Doctors Hesitate to Screen Smokers for Lung Cancer," *NPR*, April 13, 2015, https://www.npr.org/transcripts/398101515; Daniel E. Jonas, Daniel S. Reuland, Shivani M. Reddy, Max Nagle, Stephen D. Clark, Rachel Palmieri Weber, Chineme Enyioha, Teri L. Malo, Alison T. Brenner, Charli Armstrong, et al., "Screening for Lung Cancer with Low-Dose Computed Tomography," *JAMA* 325, no. 10 (March 9, 2021): 971, https://doi.org/10.1001/jama.2021.0377; Andy Lazris and Alan Roth, "Lung Cancer Screening: Pros and Cons," *American Family Physician* 99, no. 12 (June 15, 2019): 739–42; Erik Rifkin and Andrew Lazris, "Screening for Lung Cancer with Spiral CT," in *Interpreting Health Benefits and Risks: A Practical Guide to Facilitate Doctor-Patient Communication* (Cham: Springer, 2015), 63–72, https://doi.org/10.1007/978-3-319-11544-3_9.

11 Alan R. Roth, Andy Lazris, Helen Haskell, and John James, "Overdiagnosis of CKD in Older Adults: Unnecessary Interventions, Costs, and Worry," *American Family Physician* 107, no. 6 (June 2023): 657–8.

9. When Science Becomes Dogma

1 William Osler, *Sir William Osler: Aphorisms from His Bedside Teachings and Writings*, collected by Robert Bennett Bean and edited by William Bennett Bean (New York: Henry Schuman, 1950), 88, https://archive.org/details/in.ernet.dli.2015.63933.

2 In the introduction and chapter 18 on cardiac testing, we have referenced studies on stents, cardiac revascularization, and stress tests. Other relevant studies can be found in Armin Arbab-Zadeh, "Stress Testing and Non-Invasive Coronary Angiography in Patients with Suspected Coronary Artery Disease: Time for a New Paradigm," *Heart International* 7, no. 1 (December 2012): 4–13, https://doi.org/10.4081/hi.2012.e2; Andy Lazris and Alan Roth, "Overuse of Cardiac Testing," *American Family Physician* 98, no. 10 (November 15, 2018): 561–3; Erik Rifkin and Andrew Lazris, "Exercise Stress Tests," in *Interpreting Health Benefits and Risks: A Practical Guide to Facilitate Doctor-Patient Communication* (Cham: Springer, 2015), 83–94, https://doi.org/10.1007/978-3-319-11544-3_11;

Harlan Krumholz, "Questions Grow about the Need for Cardiac Stress Tests," *Washington Post*, June 13, 2020, https://www.washingtonpost.com/health /questions-grow-about-the-need-for-cardiac-stress-tests/2020/06/12/7ae26aee -a5c1-11ea-b473-04905b1af82b_story.html.

3 Dan Buettner, *The Blue Zones: 9 Lessons for Living Longer from the People Who've Lived the Longest* (Washington, DC: National Geographic, 2012).

10. There's an App for That!

1 William Osler, *Aequanimitas*, 2nd ed. (Philadelphia: P. Blakiston's Son & Co., 1906), 348, https://archive.org/details/aequanimitaswit04oslegoog.

2 Cathy O'Neil, *Weapons of Math Destruction: How Big Data Increases Inequality and Threatens Democracy* (London: Penguin Books, 2018).

3 The first study of novel blood thinners done in people over 70 at risk for falls demonstrates that 2 percent a year die or bleed into their brains, and 15 percent of them suffer life-threatening bleeds, information that the cardiologists with whom I work have not incorporated into their calculators. See Linda P.T. Joosten, Sander van Doorn, Peter M. van de Ven, Bart T.G. Köhlen, Melchior C. Nierman, Huiberdina L. Koek, Martin E.W. Hemels, Menno V. Huisman, Marieke Kruip, Laura M. Faber, et al., "Safety of Switching from a Vitamin K Antagonist to a Non-Vitamin K Antagonist Oral Anticoagulant in Frail Older Patients with Atrial Fibrillation: Results of the FRAIL-AF Randomized Controlled Trial," *Circulation* 149, no. 4 (January 23, 2024): 279–89, https://doi.org/10.1161 /CIRCULATIONAHA.123.066485.

4 O'Neil, *Weapons of Math Destruction*, 20.

5 O'Neil, 29.

6 O'Neil, 29.

7 The MCAT is important because it predicts which doctors will do well on standardized tests, which is how doctors are judged; see Renee Marinelli, "Why the MCAT Matters beyond Medical School Admissions," *U.S. News*, April 26, 2023, https://www.usnews.com/education/blogs/medical-school -admissions-doctor/articles/why-the-mcat-matters-beyond-medical-school -admissions. On the detriment of using a standardized test to chose medical students, see "MCAT," FairTest, accessed September 26, 2024, https://fairtest .org/mcat/. On racism of the MCAT, see Jessica Faiz, Utibe R. Essien, Donna L. Washington, and Dan P. Ly, "Racial and Ethnic Differences in Barriers Faced by Medical College Admission Test Examinees and Their Association with Medical School Application and Matriculation," *JAMA Health Forum* 4, no. 4 (April 14, 2023): e230498, https://doi.org/10.1001/jamahealthforum.2023.0498.

11. Whatever Happened to Common Sense?

1 William Osler, "Teaching and Thinking: The Two Functions of a Medical School," *Montreal Medical Journal* 23, no. 8 (February 1895): 567.

2 For the Cochrane recommendations, see Renée Manser, Anne Lethaby, Louis B. Irving, Christine Stone, Graham Byrnes, Michael J. Abramson, and Don Campbell, "Screening for Lung Cancer," *Cochrane Database of Systematic Reviews*, no. 6 (June 21, 2013): CD001991, https://doi.org/10.1002/14651858.CD001991 .pub3; H. Gilbert Welch and William C. Black, "Overdiagnosis in Cancer," *JNCI:*

Journal of the National Cancer Institute 102, no. 9 (May 5, 2010): 605–13. https://doi.org/10.1093/jnci/djq099.

3 Morten L. Hansen, Rikke Sørensen, Mette T. Clausen, Marie Louise Fog-Petersen, Jakob Raunsø, Niels Gadsbøll, Gunnar H. Gislason, Fredrik Folke, Søren S. Andersen, Tina K. Schramm, et al., "Risk of Bleeding with Single, Dual, or Triple Therapy with Warfarin, Aspirin, and Clopidogrel in Patients with Atrial Fibrillation," *Archives of Internal Medicine* 170, no. 16 (September 13, 2010): 1433–41, https://doi.org/10.1001/archinternmed.2010.271.

4 We noted in chapter 7 a recent study showing that lowering blood pressure in the hospital causes worse outcomes, including stroke, kidney disease, and even death, something I have personally seen occur far too many times, even after the study was released. See Timothy S. Anderson, Shoshana J. Herzig, Bocheng Jing, W. John Boscardin, Kathy Fung, Edward R. Marcantonio, and Michael A. Steinman, "Clinical Outcomes of Intensive Inpatient Blood Pressure Management in Hospitalized Older Adults," *JAMA Internal Medicine* 183, no. 7 (May 30, 2023): 715–23, https://doi.org/10.1001/jamainternmed.2023.1667.

5 An interesting article in *The New Yorker* looks at the pitfalls of doing a whole-body MRI on people just to make sure everything is all right. See Dhruv Khullar, "Will a Full-Body MRI Scan Help You or Hurt You?," *The New Yorker*, January 12, 2024, https://www.newyorker.com/science/annals-of-medicine/will-a-full-body-mri-scan-help-you-or-hurt-you.

6 See, for example, Martin Englund, Ali Guermazi, Daniel Gale, David J. Hunter, Piran Aliabadi, Margaret Clancy, and David T. Felson, "Incidental Meniscal Findings on Knee MRI in Middle-Aged and Elderly Persons," *New England Journal of Medicine* 359, no. 11 (September 11, 2008): 1108–15, https://doi.org/10.1056/nejmoa0800777; Maureen C. Jensen, Michael N. Brant-Zawadzki, Nancy Obuchowski, Michael T. Modic, Dennis Malkasian, and Jeffrey S. Ross, "Magnetic Resonance Imaging of the Lumbar Spine in People without Back Pain," *New England Journal of Medicine* 331, no. 2 (July 14, 1994): 69–73, https://doi.org/10.1056/nejm199407143310201. An excellent book on back pain and overdiagnosis is Richard A. Deyo, *Watch Your Back! How the Back Pain Industry Is Costing Us More and Giving Us Less, and What You Can Do to Inform and Empower Yourself in Seeking Treatment* (Ithaca, NY: ILR Press, an imprint of Cornell University Press, 2014).

7 H. Gilbert Welch, Lisa Schwartz, and Steve Woloshin, *Over-Diagnosed: Making People Sick in the Pursuit of Health* (New York: Random House, 2012), 97–8.

12. The Drug Epidemic (It's Not What You Think)

1 William Osler, *Sir William Osler: Aphorisms from His Bedside Teachings and Writings,* collected by Robert Bennett Bean and edited by William Bennett Bean (New York: Henry Schuman, 1950), 118, https://archive.org/details/in.ernet.dli.2015.63933.

2 For the Lown study and others, see Shannon Brownlee, "Medication Overload: America's Other Drug Problem," Lown Institute, April 1, 2019, https://doi.org/10.46241/LI.WOUK3548; "Medication Overload and Older Americans," Lown Institute, accessed September 26, 2024, https://lowninstitute.org/projects/medication-overload-how-the-drive-to-prescribe-is-harming-older-americans/; Sandra G. Boodman, "The Other Big Drug Problem: Older

People Taking Too Many Pills," *Washington Post,* December 9, 2017, http:// www.washingtonpost.com/national/health-science/the-other-big-drug -problem-older-people-taking-too-many-pills/2017/12/08/3cea5ca2-c30a -11e7-afe9-4f60b5a6c4a0_story.html; "The Dangers of Polypharmacy and the Case for Deprescribing in Older Adults," National Institute on Aging, August 24, 2021, https://www.nia.nih.gov/news/dangers-polypharmacy-and-case -deprescribing-older-adults; Dima M. Qato, G. Caleb Alexander, Rena M. Conti, Michael Johnson, Phil Schumm, and Stacy Tessler Lindau, "Use of Prescription and Over-the-Counter Medications and Dietary Supplements among Older Adults in the United States," *JAMA* 300, no. 24 (December 24, 2008): 2867, https://doi .org/10.1001/jama.2008.892.

3 Alan Roth and Andy Lazris, "Appropriate Use of Opioids for Chronic Pain," *American Family Physician* 102, no. 6 (December 15, 2020): 335–7.

4 Tingting Geng, Jun-Xiang Chen, Yan-Feng Zhou, Qi Lu, Zhenzhen Wan, Liegang Liu, An Pan, and Gang Liu, "Proton Pump Inhibitor Use and Risks of Cardiovascular Disease and Mortality in Patients with Type 2 Diabetes," *Journal of Clinical Endocrinology & Metabolism* 108, no. 6 (June 2023): e216–22, https:// doi.org/10.1210/clinem/dgac750.

5 For information about supplements, see Carol M. Mangione, Michael J. Barry, Wanda K. Nicholson, Michael Cabana, David Chelmow, Tumaini Rucker Coker, Esa M. Davis, Katrina E. Donahue, Chyke A. Doubeni, Carlos Roberto Jaén, et al., "Vitamin, Mineral, and Multivitamin Supplementation to Prevent Cardiovascular Disease and Cancer," *JAMA* 327, no. 23 (June 21, 2022): 2326, https://doi.org/10.1001/jama.2022.8970; Liz Szabo, "Older Americans Are Hooked on Vitamins despite Scarce Evidence They Work," *KFF Health News,* April 4, 2018, https://kffhealthnews.org/news/older-americans-are-hooked -on-vitamins-despite-scarce-evidence-they-work/; Andy Lazris, *Curing Medicare: A Doctor's View on How Our Health Care System Is Failing Older Americans and How We Can Fix It* (Ithaca, NY: ILR Press, an imprint of Cornell University Press, 2016), 44–6.

13. Flexner and the Care of the Elderly

1 William Osler, *Counsels and Ideals from the Writings of William Osler* (Oxford: Henry Frowde, 1905), 214, https://archive.org/details/McGillLibrary-osl _Counsels-ideals-writings-William-Osler_O82co1905-22092.

2 For more about this, see Nortin M. Hadler, *Rethinking Aging: Growing Old and Living Well in an Overtreated Society* (Chapel Hill: University of North Carolina Press, 2019); Andy Lazris, *Curing Medicare: A Doctor's View on How Our Health Care System Is Failing Older Americans and How We Can Fix It* (Ithaca, NY: ILR Press, an imprint of Cornell University Press, 2016); Atul Gawande, *Being Mortal: Medicine and What Matters in the End* (New York: Metropolitan, 2021); Becca Levy, *Breaking the Age Code* (New York: William Morrow, 2022).

3 An excellent book on "slow medicine" is Dennis M. McCullough, *My Mother, Your Mother: Embracing "Slow Medicine," the Compassionate Approach to Caring for Your Aging Loved Ones* (New York: HarperCollins, 2009).

4 Ira Byock, *Best Care Possible: A Physician's Quest to Transform Care through the End of Life* (New York: Avery, 2013); Andy Lazris, "Geriatric Palliative Care," *Primary Care: Clinics in Office Practice* 46, no. 3 (September 2019): 447–59, https://doi .org/10.1016/j.pop.2019.05.007.

5 "Use of Cardiac Procedures and Outcomes in Elderly Patients with Myocardial Infarction in the United States and Canada," *New England Journal of Medicine* 337, no. 2 (July 10, 1997): 139, https://doi.org/10.1056/nejm199707103370223.

6 Aisha I. Abdullah, "Cholinesterase Inhibitors Found to Slow Alzheimer's Cognitive Decline," *Alzheimer's News Today*, June 22, 2021, https://alzheimersnewstoday.com/news/cholinesterase-inhibitors-shown-slow-alzheimers-cognitive-decline/.

7 A. Mark Clarfield, "The Decreasing Prevalence of Reversible Dementias," *Archives of Internal Medicine* 163, no. 18 (October 13, 2003): 2219–29, https://doi.org/10.1001/archinte.163.18.2219; Erik Rifkin and Andrew Lazris, "Screening for and Treating Dementia," in *Interpreting Health Benefits and Risks: A Practical Guide to Facilitate Doctor–Patient Communication* (Cham: Springer, 2015), 161–71, https://doi.org/10.1007/978-3-319-11544-3_18.

8 An interesting article about this is Ishani Ganguli, "How One Medical Checkup Can Snowball into a 'Cascade' of Tests, Causing More Harm Than Good," *Washington Post*, January 3, 2020, https://www.washingtonpost.com/health/how-one-medical-checkup-can-snowball-into-a-cascade-of-tests-causing-more-harm-than-good/2020/01/03/0c8024fc-20eb-11ea-bed5-880264cc91a9_story.html.

14. Shared Decision-Making in a Flexnerian World

1 William Osler, "Teaching and Thinking: The Two Functions of a Medical School," *Montreal Medical Journal* 23, no. 8 (February 1895): 567.

2 Erik Rifkin and Edward Bouwer, *The Illusion of Certainty: Health Benefits and Risks* (New York: Springer, 2007), https://doi.org/10.1007/978-0-387-48572-0.

3 Erik Rifkin and Andy Lazris, "A Grateful but Not Passive Patient," *JAMA Internal Medicine* 176, no. 9 (September 2016): 1248–9, https://doi.org/10.1001/jamainternmed.2016.3569.

4 See, for example, S.P.E. Nishi, L. Crocker, L. Lowenstein, M. Godoy, T. Mendoza, and R. Volk, "Decision Making for Lung Cancer Screening: How Well Are We 'Sharing'?," *American Journal of Respiratory and Critical Care Medicine* 199 (2019): A1007, https://doi.org/10.1164/ajrccm-conference.2019.199.1_meetingabstracts.a1007; Andy Lazris and Erik Rifkin, "Patients, Doctors, and Decision-Making," in *Utilizing Effective Risk Communication in COVID-19: Highlighting the BRCT* (Cham: Springer, 2021), 3–8, https://doi.org/10.1007/978-3-030-74521-9_1.

15. The Foundations of Our Health Care Infrastructure

1 Michael A. Nevins, *Abraham Flexner: A Flawed American Icon* (New York: iUniverse Inc., 2010), 89.

2 Thomas P. Duffy, "The Flexner Report – 100 Years Later," *Yale Journal of Biology and Medicine* 84, no. 3 (September 2011): 269–76, PMID: 21966046, PMCID: PMC3178858.

3 See, for example, Douglas Page and Adrian Baranchuk, "The Flexner Report: 100 Years Later," *International Journal of Medical Education* 1 (December 10, 2010): 74–5, https://doi.org/10.5116/ijme.4cb4.85c8; Paul Starr, *The Social Transformation of American Medicine: The Rise of a Sovereign Profession & the Making of a Vast Industry* (New York: Basic Books, 2017).

4 Michael Bliss, *William Osler: A Life in Medicine* (New York: Oxford University Press, 2007).
5 Thomas Neville Bonner, *Iconoclast: Abraham Flexner and a Life in Learning* (Baltimore: Johns Hopkins University Press, 2002); Nevins, *Abraham Flexner*.
6 Much of what is discussed can be found in Nevins, *Abraham Flexner*. See also Bliss, *William Osler*, 381: "The officers of the Rockefeller philanthropies also read Flexner carefully and saw in medical education another field, close to the research area they had recently entered, that would surely repay sowing." See also Nevins, *Abraham Flexner*, 121, and Kenneth M. Ludmerer, *Time to Heal: American Medical Education from the Turn of the Century to the Era of Managed Care* (Oxford: Oxford University Press, 2011). Ludmerer states that the corporate foundations sought to move medical education from a clinical to a scientific-research direction to foster medical research that would generate new discoveries and profits and compete with a similar trend in Europe. See W. Michael Byrd and Linda A. Clayton, *An American Health Dilemma* (New York: Routledge, 2002), 62–3; Starr, *Social Transformation of American Medicine*, 121–2;
7 In addition to the Bliss biography, *William Osler*, see Charles S. Bryan, *Osler: Inspirations from a Great Physician* (New York: Oxford University Press, 2010); William Osler, *The Principles and Practice of Medicine* (New York: D. Appleton and Co., 1911).

16. The Financial Ramifications of Our Medical-Industrial Complex

1 William Osler, *Science and Immortality* (Boston: Houghton Mifflin, 1904), 10, https://archive.org/details/scienceimmortali00osle_0.
2 Eric C. Schneider, Arnav Shah, Michelle M. Doty, Roosa Tikkanen, Katharine Fields, and Reginald D. Williams II, *Mirror, Mirror 2021: Reflecting Poorly* (New York: The Commonwealth Fund, 2021), http://www.commonwealthfund.org/publications/fund-reports/2021/aug/mirror-mirror-2021-reflecting-poorly.
3 Andrew P. Wilper, Steffie Woolhandler, Karen E. Lasser, Danny McCormick, David H. Bor, and David U. Himmelstein, "Health Insurance and Mortality in US Adults," *American Journal of Public Health*, 99, no. 12 (December 2009): 2289–95, https://doi.org/10.2105/AJPH.2008.157685, PMID: 19762659, PMCID: PMC2775760.
4 Namkee G. Choi, Diana M. DiNitto, and Bryan Y. Choi, "Unmet Healthcare Needs and Healthcare Access Gaps among Uninsured U.S. Adults Aged 50–64," *International Journal of Environmental Research and Public Health* 17, no. 8 (2020): 2711, https://doi.org/10.3390/ijerph17082711.
5 Scott Gottlieb, "Medical Bills Account for 40% of Bankruptcies," *BMJ* 320, no. 7245 (May 13, 2000):1295, PMID: 10807614, PMCID: PMC1127305.
6 Wullianallur Raghupathi and Viju Raghupathi, "An Empirical Study of Chronic Diseases in the United States: A Visual Analytics Approach," *International Journal of Environmental Research and Public Health* 15, no. 3 (March 1, 2018): 431, https://doi.org/10.3390/ijerph15030431, PMID: 29494555, PMCID: PMC5876976.
7 Timothy B. Norbeck, "Drivers of Health Care Costs: A Physicians Foundation White Paper – Second of a Three-Part Series," *Missouri Medicine* 110, no. 2 (March–April 2013):113–8, PMID: 23724476, PMCID: PMC6179664.
8 "The Dartmouth Atlas of Health Care Website Archive (Effective June 30, 2024)," Dartmouth Atlas Project, accessed September 26, 2024, https://www.dartmouthatlas.org/.
9 "Dartmouth Atlas."

10 Laura Deckx, Hayley R. Thomas, Nicolas A. Sieben, Michele M. Foster, and Geoffrey Mitchell, "General Practitioners' Practical Approach to Initiating End-of-Life Conversations: A Qualitative Study," *Family Practice* 37, no. 3 (June 2020): 401–5, https://doi.org/10.1093/fampra/cmz074, PMID: 31786593, PMCID: PMC7448298.

11 William H. Shrank, Teresa L. Rogstad, and Natasha Parekh, "Waste in the US Health Care System: Estimated Costs and Potential for Savings," *JAMA* 322, no. 15 (October 7, 2019):1501–9, https://doi.org/10.1001/jama.2019.13978, PMID: 31589283.

12 Ming Tai-Seale, Ellis C. Dillon, Yan Yang, Robert Nordgren, Ruth L. Steinberg, Teresa Nauenberg, Tim C. Lee, et al., "Physicians' Well-Being Linked to In-Basket Messages Generated by Algorithms in Electronic Health Records," *Health Affairs* 38, no. 7 (July 2019): 1073–8, https://doi.org/10.1377/hlthaff.2018.05509.

13 J. Marc Overhage and David McCallie Jr., "Physician Time Spent Using the Electronic Health Record during Outpatient Encounters: A Descriptive Study," *Annals of Internal Medicine* 172, no. 3 (January 14, 2020): 169–74, correction in "Correction: Physician Time Spent Using the Electronic Health Record During Outpatient Encounters," *Annals of Internal Medicine* 173, no. 7 (October 6, 2020): 596, https://doi.org/10.7326/L20-1077, PMID: 31931523.

14 David U. Himmelstein, Terry Campbell, and Steffie Woolhandler, "Health Care Administrative Costs in the United States and Canada, 2017," *Annals of Internal Medicine* 172, no. 2 (January 7, 2020): 134–42, https://doi.org/10.7326/M19-2818, correction in "Correction: Health Care Administrative Costs in the United States and Canada, 2017," *Annals of Internal Medicine* 173, no. 5 (September 1, 2020): 415, https://doi.org/10.7326/L20-0983, PMID: 31905376.

15 Samantha Putterman, "Biden Is Right. The US Generally Pays Double That of Other Countries for Rx Drugs," *KFF Health News*, March 6, 2024, https://kffhealthnews.org/news/article/fact-check-biden-prescription-drug-prices-nation-comparison/.

16 "3 Charts: Drug Prices in the United States," KFF, news release, February 7, 2024, https://www.kff.org/health-costs/press-release/3-charts-about-drug-prices-in-the-united-states/.

17 "The Astronomical Price of Insulin Hurts American Families," RAND, January 6, 2021, https://www.rand.org/pubs/articles/2021/the-astronomical-price-of-insulin-hurts-american-families.html.

18 Andrew Pollack, "Mylan Raised EpiPen's Price before the Expected Arrival of a Generic," *New York Times*, August 24, 2016, https://www.nytimes.com/2016/08/25/business/mylan-raised-epipens-price-before-the-expected-arrival-of-a-generic.html.

19 "Dartmouth Atlas."

20 "Lawyers per Capita by Country 2024," World Population Review, accessed September 26, 2024, https://worldpopulationreview.com/country-rankings/lawyers-per-capita-by-country.

21 Gianfranco Pischedda, Ludovico Marinò, and Katia Corsi, "Defensive Medicine through the Lens of the Managerial Perspective: A Literature Review," *BMC Health Services Research* 23, no. 1 (October 17, 2023): 1104, https://doi.org/10.1186/s12913-023-10089-3, PMID: 37848915, PMCID: PMC10580549.

22 Brian C. Callaghan, Kevin A. Kerber, Robert J. Pace, Lesli E. Skolarus, and James F. Burke, "Headaches and Neuroimaging: High Utilization and Costs Despite Guidelines," *JAMA Internal Medicine* 174, no. 5 (May 2014): 819–21, https://doi .org/10.1001/jamainternmed.2014.173, PMID: 24638246, PMCID: PMC5520970.

17. Our Medical Education Quandary

1 William Osler, *Aequanimitas*, 2nd ed. (Philadelphia: P. Blakiston's Son & Co.; 1906), 214, https://archive.org/details/aequanimitaswit04oslegoog.
2 Aaron Saguil, Ting Dong, Robert J. Gingerich, Kimberly Swygert, Jeffrey S. LaRochelle, Anthony R. Artino Jr., David F. Cruess, and Steven J. Durning, "Does the MCAT Predict Medical School and PGY-1 Performance?," *Military Medicine* 180, no. S4 (April 2015): 4–11, https://doi.org/10.7205/MILMED-D-14-00550, PMID: 25850120.
3 Kumail Hussain, "How Much Does It Cost to Attend Medical School? Here's a Breakdown," AAMC, Students & Residents, accessed September 26, 2024, https://students-residents.aamc.org/premed-navigator/how-much-does-it -cost-attend-medical-school-here-s-breakdown.
4 "Ambulatory Care Use and Physician Office Visits," National Center for Health Statistics, last reviewed April 15, 2024, https://www.cdc.gov/nchs/fastats /physician-visits.htm.
5 Mark Deutchman, Francesca Macaluso, Jason Chao, Christopher Duffrin, Karim Hanna, Daniel M. Avery Jr., Emily Onello, et al., "Contributions of US Medical Schools to Primary Care (2003–2014): Determining and Predicting Who Really Goes into Primary Care," *Family Medicine* 52, no. 7 (July–August 2020): 483–90, https://doi.org/10.22454/FamMed.2020.785068.
6 Christopher Alba, ZhaoNian Zheng, and Rishi K. Wadhera, "Changes in Health Care Access and Preventive Health Screenings by Race and Ethnicity," *JAMA Health Forum* 5, no. 2 (February 2, 20124): e235058, https://doi.org/10.1001 /jamahealthforum.2023.5058.
7 Allan M. Seibert, Adam L. Hersh, Payal K. Patel, Michelle Matheu, Valoree Stanfield, Nora Fino, Lauri A. Hicks et al., "Urgent-Care Antibiotic Prescribing: An Exploratory Analysis to Evaluate Health Inequities," *Antimicrobial Steward & Healthcare Epidemiology* 2, no. 1 (2022): e184, https://doi.org/10.1017 /ash.2022.329, PMID: 36406162, PMCID: PMC9672912.

18. The Dangers of Flexnerian Overspecialization in Medical Care

1 William M. Osler, "Remarks on Specialism," *Boston Medical and Surgical Journal* 126, no. 19 (May 12, 1892): 457, https://doi.org/10.1056/NEJM189205121261901.
2 Jodi B. Segal, Aditi P. Sen, Eliana Glanzberg-Krainin, and Susan Hutfless, "Factors Associated with Overuse of Health Care within US Health Systems: A Cross-Sectional Analysis of Medicare Beneficiaries from 2016 to 2018," *JAMA Health Forum* 3, no. 1 (January 14, 2022): e214543, https://doi.org/10.1001 /jamahealthforum.2021.4543.
3 "Reducing Overuse and Misuse in Medical Care," *Proceedings of the 2017 American College of Physicians International Forum*, I.M. Matters from ACP, April 2018, https://immattersacp.org/archives/2018/04/reducing-care-overuse-misuse -focus-of-2017-international-forum.htm.

4 Heather Lyu, Tim Xu, Daniel Brotman, Brandan Mayer-Blackwell, Michol Cooper, Michael Daniel, Elizabeth C. Wick, Vikas Saini, Shannon Brownlee, and Martin A. Makary, "Overtreatment in the United States," *PLoS One* 12, no. 9 (September 6, 2017): e0181970, https://doi.org/10.1371/journal.pone.0181970, PMID: 28877170, PMCID: PMC5587107.

5 Joris L.J.M. Müskens, Rudolf Bertijn Kool, Simone A. van Dulmen, and Gert P. Westert, "Overuse of Diagnostic Testing in Healthcare: A Systematic Review," *BMJ Quality & Safety* 31, no. 1 (January 2022): 54–63, https://doi.org/10.1136/bmjqs-2020-012576, PMID: 33972387, PMCID: PMC8685650.

6 Josephine C. Jacobs, Jeffrey G. Jarvik, Roger Chou, Derek Boothroyd, Jeanie Lo, Andrea Nevedal, and Paul G. Barnett, "Observational Study of the Downstream Consequences of Inappropriate MRI of the Lumbar Spine," *Journal of General Internal Medicine* 35, no. 12 (December 2020): 3605–12, https://doi.org/10.1007/s11606-020-06181-7, PMID: 32989711, PMCID: PMC7728897.

7 J.E. Jordan and A.E. Flanders, "Headache and Neuroimaging: Why We Continue to Do It," *AJNR: American Journal of Neuroradiology* 41, no. 7 (July 2020): 1149–55, https://doi.org/10.3174/ajnr.A6591, PMID: 32616575, PMCID: PMC7357655.

8 "Choosing Wisely, An Initiative of the ABIM Foundation," ABIM Foundation, accessed September 26, 2024, https://www.choosingwisely.org/.

9 "Avoiding Overuse: Coronary Stents," 2023 Results, Lown Institute Hospitals Index, accessed September 26, 2024, https://lownhospitalsindex.org/avoiding-coronary-stent-overuse/.

10 "Choosing Wisely."

11 Yugandhar R. Manda and Krishna M. Baradhi, "Cardiac Catheterization Risks and Complications," *StatsPearls*, National Library of Medicine, last updated June 5, 2023, https://www.ncbi.nlm.nih.gov/books/NBK531461/.

12 Manda and Baradhi, "Cardiac Catheterization Risks."

19. US Insurance Companies: Bankrupting Our Nation One Sickness at a Time

1 William Osler, "Remarks on Organization in the Profession," *British Medical Journal* 1 (February 4, 1911): 237, https://doi.org/10.1136/bmj.1.2614.237.

2 For a good discussion of insurance, the history of insurance, and the influence of insurance on our health care system, see Paul Starr, *Social Transformation of American Medicine: The Rise of a Sovereign Profession & the Making of a Vast Industry* (New York: Basic Books, 2017); Elisabeth Rosenthal, *An American Sickness: How Healthcare Became Big Business and How You Can Take It Back* (New York: Penguin Books, 2018); Beatrix Rebecca Hoffman, *Health Care for Some: Rights and Rationing in the United States since 1930* (Chicago: University of Chicago Press, 2013), https://doi.org/10.7208/chicago/9780226348056.001.0001; Victor W. Sidel and Ruth Sidel, *A Healthy State: An International Perspective on the Crisis in United States Medical Care* (New York: Pantheon Books, 1983); Robert M. Duggan, *Breaking the Iron Triangle: Reducing Health-care Costs in Corporate America* (Columbia, MD: Wisdom Well Press, 2012); John H. Knowles, *Doing Better and Feeling Worse* (New York: W.W. Norton, 1977).

3 Daniel Fox, "Abraham Flexner's Unpublished Report: Foundations and Medical Education, 1909–1928," *Bulletin of the History of Medicine* 54, no. 4 (December 1980): 475–96.

4 "Nation: Dr. Ward's Last Words," *Time*, May 21, 1965, https://time.com/archive/6637769/nation-dr-wards-last-words/.

5 Paul Starr, *Social Transformation of American Medicine*, 379.
6 James K. Min, Amanda Gilmore, Erica C. Jones, Daniel S. Berman, Wijnand J. Stuijfzand, Leslee J. Shaw, Ken O'Day, and Ibrahim Danad, "Cost-Effectiveness of Diagnostic Evaluation Strategies for Individuals with Stable Chest Pain Syndrome and Suspected Coronary Artery Disease," *Clinical Imaging* 43 (May–June 2017): 97–105, https://doi.org/10.1016/j.clinimag.2017.01.015, PMID: 28273654, PMCID: PMC5410386.
7 Chen Wei, Michael Milligan, Miranda Lam, Paul A. Heidenreich, and Alexander Sandhu, "Variation in Cost of Echocardiography within and across United States Hospitals," *Journal of the American Society of Echocardiography* 36, no. 6 (June 2023): 569–77.e4, https://doi.org/10.1016/j.echo.2023.01.002, PMID: 36638930, PMCID: PMC10247500.
8 David E. Newman-Toker, Kathryn M. McDonald, and David O. Meltzer, "How Much Diagnostic Safety Can We Afford, and How Should We Decide? A Health Economics Perspective," *BMJ Quality & Safety* 22, no. S2 (October 2013): ii11–ii20, https://doi.org/10.1136/bmjqs-2012-001616, PMID: 24048914, PMCID: PMC3786645.
9 eHealth, *Health Insurance Price Index Report: 2018 Open Enrollment Period* (Austin, TX: eHealth, 2018), 3, https://news.ehealthinsurance.com/_ir/68/20188/eHealth%20Health%20Insurance%20Index%20Report%20for%20the%202018%20OEP.pdf.
10 Wendell Potter, *Deadly Spin: An Insurance Company Insider Speaks Out on How Corporate PR Is Killing Health Care and Deceiving Americans* (New York: Bloomsbury Press, 2013).
11 Potter, *Deadly Spin*, 143.
12 Potter, 46.
13 Marshall Allen, "Health Insurers Are Vacuuming Up Details About You. That Could Raise Your Rates," *STAT+*, July 18, 2018, https://www.statnews.com/2018/07/18/health-insurers-personal-details-raise-rates/.

20. The Power and the Influence of the Pharmaceutical Industry

1 William Osler, "The Faith That Heals," *British Medical Journal* 1 (June 18, 1910): 1472, https://doi.org/10.1136/bmj.1.2581.1470.
2 Andrew W. Mulcahy, Daniel Schwam, and Susan L. Lovejoy, "International Prescription Drug Price Comparisons: Estimates Using 2022 Data," RAND, February 1, 2024, https://www.rand.org/pubs/research_reports/RRA788-3.html.
3 "Ways and Means Committee Releases Report on International Drug Pricing," Ways and Means Committee, press release, September 23, 2019, https://democrats-waysandmeans.house.gov/media-center/press-releases/ways-and-means-committee-releases-report-international-drug-pricing.
4 Olivier J. Wouters, Martin McKee, and Jeroen Luyten, "Estimated Research and Development Investment Needed to Bring a New Medicine to Market, 2009–2018," *JAMA* 323, no. 9 (March 3, 2020): 844–53, https://doi.org/10.1001/jama.2020.1166.
5 "Drug Trials Snapshots: ADUHELM," U.S. Food and Drug Administration, last updated November 27, 2023, https://www.fda.gov/drugs/drug-approvals-and-databases/drug-trials-snapshots-aduhelm.
6 For information regarding the relationship between pharmaceutical companies and the FDA, see Thomas Bodenheimer, "Uneasy Alliance – Clinical

Investigators and the Pharmaceutical Industry," *New England Journal of Medicine* 342, no. 20 (May 18, 2000): 1539–44, https://doi.org/10.1056/nejm200005183422024; Brandon May, "Government and Industry Lead the Way in Funding USPSTF Systematic Reviews," *Medical Bag*, January 14, 2019, https://www.medicalbag .com/news/government-and-industry-lead-the-way-in-funding-uspstf -systematic-reviews/; John LaMattina, "The Biopharmaceutical Industry Provides 75% of the FDA's Drug Review Budget. Is This a Problem?," *Forbes*, August 28, 2020, https://www.forbes.com/sites/johnlamattina/2018/06/28 /the-biopharmaceutical-industry-provides-75-of-the-fdas-drug-review-budget -is-this-a-problem/.

7 Charles Ornstein, Tracy Weber, and Ryann Grochowski Jones, "We Found over 700 Doctors Who Were Paid More Than a Million Dollars by Drug and Medical Device Companies," *ProPublica*, October 17, 2019, https://www.propublica .org/article/we-found-over-700-doctors-who-were-paid-more-than-a-million -dollars-by-drug-and-medical-device-companies.

8 Janelle Applequist and Jennifer Gerard Ball, "An Updated Analysis of Direct-to-Consumer Television Advertisements for Prescription Drugs," *Annals of Family Medicine* 6, no. 3 (May 2018): 211–16, https://doi.org/10.1370/afm.2220, PMID: 29760024, PMCID: PMC5951249.

9 Physician Payments Sunshine Act of 2009, S. 301, 111th Cong. (2009), https:// www.congress.gov/bill/111th-congress/senate-bill/301/text.

10 "Dollars for Docs," ProPublica, accessed September 29, 2024, https://projects .propublica.org/docdollars/; "OpenPayments," OpenPaymentsData.CMS.gov, accessed September 29, 2024, https://openpaymentsdata.cms.gov/.

11 Ornstein, Weber, and Grochowski Jones, "We Found over 700 Doctors."

12 "Drug Overdose Death Rates," National Institute on Drug Abuse, https://nida .nih.gov/research-topics/trends-statistics/overdose-death-rates.

13 Art Van Zee, "The Promotion and Marketing of Oxycontin: Commercial Triumph, Public Health Tragedy," *American Journal of Public Health* 99, no. 2 (February 2009): 221–7, https://doi.org/10.2105/AJPH.2007.131714, PMID: 18799767, PMCID: PMC2622774.

14 Haider J. Warraich, "A Costly PBM Trick: Set Lower Copays for Expensive Brand-Name Drugs than for Generics," *STAT*, March 12, 2018, https://www .statnews.com/2018/03/12/pbm-copays-brand-name-drugs-generics/.

15 Samantha McGrail, "Brand Drug Product Hopping Costs US $4.7B Annually," *Pharma News Intelligence*, September 17, 2020, https://pharmanewsintel.com /news/brand-drug-product-hopping-costs-us-4.7b-annually.

16 Shuo-yu Lin, Kyle Baumann, Chenxuan Zhou, Weiyu Zhou, Alison Evans Cuellar, and Hong Xue, "Trends in Use and Expenditures for Brand-Name Statins after Introduction of Generic Statins in the US, 2002–2018," *JAMA Network Open* 4, no. 11 (November 21, 2011): e2135371, https://doi.org/10.1001 /jamanetworkopen.2021.35371.

17 ASPE, "ASPE Report to Congress: Impact of Drug Shortages on Consumer Costs," May 22, 2023, https://aspe.hhs.gov/reports/drug-shortages-impacts-consumer -costs.

18 Jonathan Minh Phuong, Jonathan Penm, Betty Chaar, Lachlan Daniel Oldfield, and Rebekah Moles, "The Impacts of Medication Shortages on Patient Outcomes: A Scoping Review," *PLoS One* 14, no. 5 (May 3, 2019): e0215837, https://doi .org/10.1371/journal.pone.0215837, PMID: 31050671, PMCID: PMC6499468; Stephen Barlas, "Severe Drug Shortages Impose Heavy Costs on Hospital

Pharmacies: Senate Bill Might Help ... or Not," *Pharmacy and Therapeutics* 36, no. 5 (May 2011): 242–302, PMID: 21785536, PMCID: PMC3138364.

19 Vijay N. Joish, Fang Liz Zhou, Ronald Preblick, Dee Lin, Maithili Deshpande, Sumit Verma, Michael J. Davies, et al., "Estimation of Annual Health Care Costs for Adults with Type 1 Diabetes in the United States," *Journal of Managed Care + Specialty Pharmacy* 26, no. 3 (March 2020): 311–18, https://doi.org/10.18553/jmcp.2020.26.3.311, PMID: 32105172, PMCID: PMC10390990.

20 GoodRx (website), https://www.goodrx.com.

21 Brenna Miller, "After Decades of Profiteering, Insulin Manufacturer Finally Cuts the Price," Lown Institute, March 2, 2023, https://lowninstitute.org/after-decades-of-profiteering-insulin-manufacturer-finally-cuts-the-price/.

22 See, for example, Martha Rosenberg, "The American Heart Association – Protecting Industry Not Patients," *HuffPost*, December 16, 2013, https://www.huffpost.com/entry/health-news_b_4398304; Jeanne Lenzer, "Conflicts of Interest Compromise US Public Health Agency's Mission, Say Scientists," *BMJ* 355 (October 24, 2016): i5723, https://doi.org/10.1136/bmj.i5723.

21. In Medical Societies We Trust

1 Jeanne Lenzer, "Centers for Disease Control and Prevention: Protecting the Private Good?," *BMJ* 350 (May 15, 2015): h2362, https://doi.org/10.1136/bmj.h2362.

2 Charles Pillar, "The War on 'Prediabetes' Could Be a Boon for Pharma – But Is It Good for Medicine?," *Science*, March 7, 2019, https://doi.org/10.1126/science.aax2208.

3 Emily Kopp, Sydney Lupkin, and Elizabeth Lucas, "Patient Advocacy Groups Take in Millions from Drugmakers. Is There a Payback?," *Washington Post*, April 6, 2018, https://www.washingtonpost.com/national/health-science/patient-advocacy-groups-take-in-millions-from-drugmakers-is-there-a-payback/2018/04/06/0a75f988-397b-11e8-af3c-2123715f78df_story.html.

4 Marc Santora, "In Diabetes Fight, Raising Cash and Keeping Trust," *New York Times*, November 25, 2006, https://www.nytimes.com/2006/11/25/health/25ada.html.

5 Lenzer, "Centers for Disease Control and Prevention."

6 Jeanne Lenzer, "Conflicts of Interest Compromise US Public Health Agency's Mission, Say Scientists," *BMJ* 355 (October 24, 2016): i5723, https://doi.org/10.1136/bmj.i5723.

7 Susan Perry, "Revelations of the CDC's Industry Funding Raise Questions about Some of Its Decisions," *Minnpost*, May 28, 2015, https://www.minnpost.com/second-opinion/2015/05/revelations-cdcs-industry-funding-raise-questions-about-some-its-decisions/.

8 Owen Dyer, "What Did We Learn from Tamiflu?," *BMJ* 368 (February 19, 2020): m626, https://doi.org/10.1136/bmj.m626.

9 Peter Doshi, "The Cochrane Review of Tamiflu: What Have We Learned?," *BMJ* 342, no. 7792 (February 5, 2011): d4346; and Doshi also quoted in Owen Dyer, "What Did We Learn from Tamiflu?," *BMJ* 368 (February 19, 2020): m626, https://doi.org/10.1136/bmj.m626.

10 Ronald Koretz, Kenneth W. Lin, John P.A. Ioannidis, and Jeanne Lenzer, "Is Widespread Screening for Hepatitis C Justified?," *BMJ* 350 (January 13, 2015): g7809, https://doi.org/10.1136/bmj.g7809.

11 "CDC Members Own More Than 50 Patents Connected to Vaccination," LawFirms.com, archived January 3, 2024, at the Wayback Machine, https://web.archive.org/web/20240103234353/http://www.lawfirms.com/resources/environment/environment-health/cdc-members-own-more-50-patents-connected-vaccinations.

12 Shannon Brownlee, *Overtreated: Why Too Much Medicine Is Making Us Sicker and Poorer* (New York: Bloomsbury, 2008), 206.

13 John LaMattina, "The Biopharmaceutical Industry Provides 75 Percent of the FDA's Drug Review Budget. Is This a Problem?," *Forbes*, June 28, 2018, https://www.forbes.com/sites/johnlamattina/2018/06/28/the-biopharmaceutical-industry-provides-75-of-the-fdas-drug-review-budget-is-this-a-problem/#16c31aaf49ec.

14 LaMattina, "Biopharmaceutical Industry."

15 David S. Hilzenrath, "Drug Money: FDA Depends on Industry Funding; Money Comes with 'Strings Attached,'" POGO, December 1, 2016, https://www.pogo.org/investigations/fda-depends-on-industry-funding-money-comes-with-strings-attached.

16 Charles Pillar and Jia You, "Hidden Conflicts? Pharma Payments to FDA Advisers after Drug Approvals Spark Ethical Concerns," *Science*, July 5, 2018, https://doi.org/10.1126/science.aau6842.

17 Pillar and You, "Hidden Conflicts?"

18 Charles Ornstein, "From Twitter to Treatment Guidelines, Industry Influence Permeates Medicine," *NPR*, January 17, 2017, https://www.npr.org/sections/health-shots/2017/01/17/510226214/from-twitter-to-treatment-guidelines-industry-influence-permeates-medicine.

19 Ed Silverman, "The New Cholesterol Guidelines and Conflicts of Interest," *Forbes*, November 20, 2013, https://www.forbes.com/sites/edsilverman/2013/11/20/the-new-cholesterol-guidelines-and-conflicts-of-interest/#7f47bc231513.

20 Paul Demko, "How Healthcare's Washington Lobbying Machine Gets the Job Done," *Modern Healthcare*, October 4, 2014, https://www.modernhealthcare.com/article/20141004/MAGAZINE/310049987/how-healthcare-s-washington-lobbying-machine-gets-the-job-done.

21 Todd B. Mendelson, Michele Meltzer, Eric G. Campbell, Arthur L. Caplan, and James N. Kirkpatrick, "Conflicts of Interest in Cardiovascular Clinical Practice Guidelines," *Archives of Internal Medicine* 171, no. 6 (March 28, 2011): 577–84, https://doi.org/10.1001/archinternmed.2011.96, PMID: 21444849.

22 "Client Profile: American College of Cardiology," OpenSecrets, 2018, https://www.opensecrets.org/federal-lobbying/clients/summary?cycle=2018&id=D000021828.

23 "Client Profile: American College of Radiology," OpenSecrets, 2017, https://www.opensecrets.org/federal-lobbying/clients/lobbyists?cycle=2017&id=D000021829.

24 Kopp, Lupkin, and Lucas, "Patient Advocacy Groups."

25 "The Patient Advocacy Groups That Accept the Most Big Pharma Money," ClassAction.com, July 2, 2018, https://www.classaction.com/news/patient-advocacy-groups-big-pharma/.

26 Sydney Lupkin, Elizabeth Lucas, and Victoria Knight, "Big Pharma Gave Money to Patient Advocacy Groups Opposing Medicare Changes," *KFF Health News*, March 4, 2019, https://kffhealthnews.org/news/big-pharma-gave-money-to-patient-advocacy-groups-opposing-medicare-changes/.

27 "Alzheimer's Association – Pharma and Insurance Gifts," Alzheimer's Association, March 2, 2017, https://www.alz.org/media/Documents/corporate-giving.pdf.
28 Matt Shipman, "Investigation of Alzheimer's Association In-Fighting Didn't Address the Role of Corporate Sponsorships," *HealthNewsReview.org*, March 8, 2016, archived July 3, 2022, at the Wayback Machine, https://web.archive.org/web/20220703054158/http://www.healthnewsreview.org/2016/03/investigation-alzheimers-association-fighting-didnt-address-role-corporate-sponsorships/.
29 Martha Rosenberg, "The American Heart Association – Protecting Industry Not Patients," *HuffPost*, December 16, 2013, https://www.huffpost.com/entry/health-news_b_4398304.

22. The Metric Mess of the Health Care System

1 William Osler, *An Address to Medical Students at the University of Pennsylvania, 1885* (Montreal: McGill University, The Osler Library, 2005).
2 "Quality Measures," Centers for Medicare & Medicaid Services, last modified May 1, 2024, https://www.cms.gov/medicare/quality/measures.
3 "Quality Measures."
4 Amit Sura and Nirav R. Shah, "Pay-for-Performance Initiatives: Modest Benefits for Improving Healthcare Quality," *American Health & Drug Benefits* 3, no. 2 (March 2010): 135–42, PMID: 25126315, PMCID: PMC4106521.

23. Hospitals: The Epicenter of Patient Care

1 William Osler to President Remsen, letter reprinted by Horace Hart at the Johns Hopkins University Press, September 1, 1911, in Henry Cushing, *The Life of Sir William Osler*, Vol. 2 (London: Oxford University Press, 1958), 292, https://archive.org/details/in.ernet.dli.2015.145591.
2 James G. Anderson and Kathleen Abrahamson, "Your Health Care May Kill You: Medical Errors," *Studies in Health Technology and Informatics* 234 (2017): 13–17, https://doi.org/10.3233/978-1-61499-742-9-13, PMID: 28186008; Ray Sipherd, "The Third-Leading Cause of Death in US Most Doctors Don't Want You to Know About," *CNBC*, February 22, 2018, http://www.cnbc.com/2018/02/22/medical-errors-third-leading-cause-of-death-in-america.html.
3 Kidu Gidey, Meles Tekie Gidey, Berhane Yohannes Hailu, Zigbey Brhane Gebreamlak, and Yirga Legesse Niriayo, "Clinical and Economic Burden of Healthcare-Associated Infections: A Prospective Cohort Study," *PLoS One* 18, no. 2 (February 23, 2023): e0282141, https://doi.org/10.1371/journal.pone.0282141, PMID: 36821590, PMCID: PMC9949640.
4 Bedriye Feyza Kurt Sr., Oya Güven, and Hakan Selçuk, "The Effect of the COVID-19 Pandemic on Emergency Department (ED) Admissions in the Only Hospital of City Center ED," *Cureus* 15, no. 9 (September 1, 2023): e44527, https://doi.org/10.7759/cureus.44527, PMID: 37790053, PMCID: PMC10544729.
5 Thomas L. Rodziewicz, Benjamin Houseman, Sarosh Vaqar, and John E. Hipskind, "Medical Error Reduction and Prevention," *StatPearls*, National Library of Medicine, last updated February 12, 2024, https://www.ncbi.nlm.nih.gov/books/NBK499956/; Gregory Santos and Mark W. Jones, "Prevention

of Surgical Errors," *StatsPearls*, National Library of Medicine, last updated May 29, 2023, https://www.ncbi.nlm.nih.gov/books/NBK592394/.

6 "Tax Administration: IRS Oversight of Hospitals' Tax-Exempt Status," GAO-23–106777, U.S. Government Accountability Office, April 26, 2023, https://www.gao.gov/products/gao-23-106777.

7 Marni Jameson Carey, "How Nonprofit Hospitals Get Away with the Biggest Rip Off in America," *Medical Economics*, January 17, 2020, https://www.medicaleconomics.com/view/how-nonprofit-hospitals-get-away-biggest-rip-america.

8 Julie Appleby, "Hospitals Have Started Posting Their Prices Online. Here's What They Reveal," *NPR*, July 2, 2021, https://www.npr.org/sections/health-shots/2021/07/02/1012317032/hospitals-have-started-posting-their-prices-online-heres-what-they-reveal.

9 Adam Andrzejewski and Thomas W. Smith, *Top 82 U.S. Non-Profit Hospitals: Quantifying Government Payments and Financial Assets – Open the Books Oversight Report* (Burr Ridge, IL: OpenTheBooks.com, 2019), https://www.openthebooks.com/assets/1/7/Top_82_Largest_U.S._Non-Profit_Hospitals_FINAL.pdf.

10 Andrzejewski and Smith, *Top 82 U.S. Non-Profit Hospitals*.

11 Greg Rosalsky, "How Non-Profit Hospitals Are Driving Up the Cost of Health Care," Planet Money Newsletter, *NPR*, October 15, 2019, https://www.npr.org/sections/money/2019/10/15/769792903/how-non-profit-hospitals-are-driving-up-the-cost-of-health-care.

12 Tony Abraham, "Hospital Lobbying in 2018 – by the Numbers," HealthCareDive, February 19, 2019, https://www.healthcaredive.com/news/hospital-lobbying-in-2018-by-the-numbers/548262/.

13 US Government Accountability Office, *Rural Hospital Closures: Number and Characteristics of Affected Hospitals and Contributing Factors – Report to Congressional Requesters*, GAO-18–634 (Washington, DC: GAO), https://www.gao.gov/assets/gao-18-634.pdf.

14 Janessa M. Graves, Demetrius A. Abshire, and Art G. Alejandro, "System- and Individual-Level Barriers to Accessing Medical Care Services across the Rural-Urban Spectrum, Washington State," *Health Services Insights* 15 (January–December 2022), https://doi.org/10.1177/11786329221104667, PMID: 35706424, PMCID: PMC9189527.

15 W. Ryan Powell, Kellia J. Hansmann, Andrew Carlson, and Amy J.H. Kind, "Evaluating How Safety-Net Hospitals Are Identified: Systematic Review and Recommendations," *Health Equity* 6, no. 1 (2022): 298–306, https://doi.org/10.1089/heq.2021.0076, PMID: 35557553, PMCID: PMC9081065.

16 David Kendall, Darbin Wofford, and Kylie Murdock, "Revitalizing Safety Net Hospitals: Protecting Low-Income Americans from Losing Access to Care," Third Way, November 14, 2023, https://www.thirdway.org/report/revitalizing-safety-net-hospitals-protecting-low-income-americans-from-losing-access-to-care.

17 Jack Karp, "From Hospital to Jail: Debtors Face Growing Arrest Threat," Law360, February 9, 2020, https://www.law360.com/articles/1241734/from-hospital-to-jail-debtors-face-growing-arrest-threat.

24. The Case for Primary Care

1 William Osler, *Aequanimitas*, 2nd ed. (Philadelphia: P. Blakiston's Son & Co., 1906), 110–11, https://archive.org/details/aequanimitaswit04oslegoog.

2 Joel Willis, Brian Antono, Andrew Bazemore, Anuradha Jetty, Stephen Petterson, Judy George, Bedda L. Rosario, et al., *Primary Care in the United States: A Chartbook*

of Facts and Statistics (Washington, DC: Robert Graham Center; Cambridge, MA: IBM-Watson Health; Washington, DC: The American Board of Family Medicine & affiliated Center for Professionalism & Value in Health Care, 2021), https:// www.graham-center.org/content/dam/rgc/documents/publications-reports /reports/PrimaryCareChartbook2021.pdf; "State of the Primary Care Workforce, 2023," HRSA Health Workforce, November 2023, https://bhw.hrsa.gov/sites /default/files/bureau-health-workforce/data-research/state-of-primary-care -workforce-2023.pdf; "The Number of Practicing Primary Care Physicians in the United States," Agency for Healthcare Research and Quality, no. 12-P001– 2-EF, September 2022, last reviewed February 2024, https://www.ahrq.gov /research/findings/factsheets/primary/pcwork1/index.html; "The Number of Practicing Primary Care Physicians in the United States," Agency for Healthcare Research and Quality, no. 12-P001–2-EF, September 2022, last reviewed February 2024, https://www.ahrq.gov/research/findings/factsheets/primary /pcwork1/index.html; Barbara Starfield, "Population Health: New Paradigms and Implications for Health Information Systems," in *Health Statistics: Shaping Policy and Practice to Improve the Population's Health,* edited by Daniel J. Friedman, Edward L. Hunter, and R. Gibson Parrish, 462–79 (New York: Oxford University Press, 2005), https://doi.org/10.1093/acprof:oso/9780195149289.003.0019.

3 Evan D. Gumas, Corinne Lewis, Celli Horstman, and Munira Z. Gunja, "Finger on the Pulse: The State of Primary Care in the U.S. and Nine Other Countries," The Commonwealth Fund, March 28, 2024, https://www.commonwealthfund.org /publications/issue-briefs/2024/mar/finger-on-pulse-primary-care-us-nine -countries.

4 Sanjay Basu, Seth A. Berkowitz, Robert L. Phillips, Asaf Bitton, Bruce E. Landon, and Russell S. Phillips, "Association of Primary Care Physician Supply with Population Mortality in the United States, 2005–2015," *JAMA Internal Medicine* 179, no. 4 (February 18, 2019): 506–14, https://doi.org/10.1001 /jamainternmed.2018.7624, PMID: 30776056, PMCID: PMC6450307.

5 Yvonee A.C. Bekker, Ankie F. Suntjens, Y. Engels, H. Schers, Gert P. Westert, and A. Stef Groenewoud, "Advance Care Planning in Primary Care: A Retrospective Medical Record Study among Patients with Different Illness Trajectories," *BMC Palliative Care* 21 (February 14, 2022): 21, https://doi.org/10.1186/s12904-022 -00907-6, PMID: 35152892, PMCID: PMC8842525; Barbara Starfield, Leiyu Shi, and James Macinko, "Contribution of Primary Care to Health Systems and Health," *Milbank Quarterly* 83, no. 3 (September 2005): 457–502, https://doi .org/10.1111/j.1468-0009.2005.00409.x, PMID: 16202000, PMCID: PMC2690145; Ted Epperly, Christine Bechtel, Rosemarie Sweeney, Ann Greiner, Kevin Grumbach, Julie Schilz, Glen Stream, and Malachi O'Connor, "The Shared Principles of Primary Care: A Multistakeholder Initiative to Find a Common Voice," *Family Medicine* 51, no. 2 (February 2019): 179–184, https://doi .org/10.22454/FamMed.2019.925587; Barbara Starfield, *Primary Care: Balancing Health Needs, Services and Technology* (New York: Oxford University Press, 1998), https://doi.org/10.1093/oso/9780195125429.001.0001.

6 Marc Zarefsky, "What's the Cost of Scope Creep? Start Counting in the Millions," American Medical Association, October 25, 2023, https://www.ama-assn.org /practice-management/scope-practice/what-s-cost-scope-creep-start-counting -millions.

7 Jacqueline W. Lucas and Maria A. Villarroel, *Telemedicine Use among Adults: United States, 2021,* NCHS Data Brief, no. 445 (Hyattsville, MD: National Center for Health Statistics, 2022), https://www.cdc.gov/nchs/products/databriefs

/db445.htm; Natalie Laub, Anish K. Agarwal, Catherine Shi, Arianna Sjamsu, and Krisda Chaiyachati, "Delivering Urgent Care Using Telemedicine: Insights from Experienced Clinicians at Academic Medical Centers," *Journal of General Internal Medicine* 37, no. 4 (March 2022): 707–13, https://doi.org/10.1007/s11606-020-06395-9, PMID: 34919208, PMCID: PMC8680069; Robin Gelburd, "Commentary: Urgent Care Centers Have Become an Integral Part of the Health Care System," *U.S. News*, April 4, 2018, http://www.usnews.com/news/healthiest-communities/articles/2018-04-04/urgent-care-centers-have-become-an-integral-part-of-the-health-care-system.

8 Starfield, Shi, and Macinko, "Contribution of Primary Care to Health Systems and Health"; "Primary Care," American Academy of Family Physicians, accessed September 26, 2024, https://www.aafp.org/about/policies/all/primary-care.html.

9 Richard Baker, George K. Freeman, Jeannie L. Haggerty, M. John Bankart, and Keith H. Nockels, "Primary Medical Care Continuity and Patient Mortality: A Systematic Review," *British Journal of General Practice* 70, no. 698 (September 2020): e600–11, https://doi.org/10.3399/bjgp20X712289, PMID: 32784220, PMCID: PMC7425204.

25. An Overlooked Legacy: The Impact of Flexner on Racial Divisions in Health Care

1 William Osler, *Aequanimitas*, 2nd ed. (Philadelphia: P. Blakiston's Son & Co., 1906), 286, https://archive.org/details/aequanimitaswit04oslegoog.

2 Harriett Washington, "Apology Sheds Light on Racial Schism in Medicine," *New York Times*, July 29, 2008, https://www.nytimes.com/2008/07/29/health/views/29essa.html.

3 Jasmine Arrington, "The Flexner Report and the African-American Health Experience: Black Collective Memory and Identity as Shaped by Afro-cultural Trauma and Remembering," *Vanderbilt Undergraduate Research Journal* 10 (Fall 2015): 1, https://doi.org/10.15695/vurj.v10i0.4063.

4 W. Montague Cobb, *The First Negro Medical Society: A History of the Medico-chirurgical society of the District of Columbia, 1884–1939* (Washington, DC: The Associated Publishers, 1939), 21; Karen Sarena Morris, "The Founding of the National Medical Association" (MD thesis, Yale University School of Medicine, 2007), Yale Medicine Thesis Digital Library, Paper 360.

5 John Edward Perry, *Forty Cords of Wood: Memoirs of a Medical Doctor* (Jefferson City, MO: Lincoln University, 1947), 159–60.

6 Perry, *Forty Cords of Wood*, 145.

7 Perry, 170.

8 Perry, 166.

9 Perry, 193–4.

10 Perry, 194.

11 Perry, 196.

12 Perry, 196.

13 Perry, 196.

14 Abraham Flexner, *Medical Education in the United States and Canada: A Report to the Carnegie Foundation for the Advancement of Teaching*, report no. 1 (New York: Carnegie Foundation, 1910).

15 Flexner, *Medical Education*.
16 Flexner, *Medical Education*.
17 Herbert M. Morais, *The History of the Negro in Medicine* (New York: Publishers Co. on behalf of the Association for the Study of Negro Life and History, 1969).
18 Arrington, "The Flexner Report and the African-American Health Experience," 4.
19 Arrington, 5.
20 W. Michael Byrd and Linda A. Clayton, *An American Health Dilemma: A Medical History of African Americans and the Problem of Race. Beginnings to 1900*, Vol. 2. (New York: Routledge, 2000).
21 Arrington, "The Flexner Report and the African-American Health Experience," 6.
22 "Report of Committee on Medical Education on Colored Hospitals," *Journal of the National Medical Association* 2, no. 4 (October–December 1910): 283–91, PMCID: PMC2574285, PMID: 20891164.
23 C.V. Roman, "Seeing Red," *Journal of the National Medical Association* 2, no. 2 (April–June 1910): 104–6.

26. Why We Are So Unhealthy and What We Can Do about It

1 William Osler, *Aequanimitas*, 2nd ed. (Philadelphia: P. Blakiston's Son & Co., 1906), 269, https://archive.org/details/aequanimitaswit04oslegoog.
2 "Trends in Health Care Spending," American Medical Association, July 9, 2024, http://www.ama-assn.org/about/research/trends-health-care-spending; Emma Wager, Matthew McGough, Shameek Rakshit, Krutika Amin, and Cynthia Cox, "How Does Health Spending in the U.S. Compare to Other Countries?," Peterson KFF Health System Tracker, January 23, 2024, https://www.healthsystemtracker.org/chart-collection/health-spending-u-s-compare-countries/; "NHE Fact Sheet," Centers for Medicare & Medicaid Services, last modified June 12, 2024, https://www.cms.gov/data-research/statistics-trends-and-reports/national-health-expenditure-data/nhe-fact-sheet.
3 Centers for Disease Control and Prevention, *CDC National Health Report Highlights* (Atlanta, GA: Centers for Disease Control and Prevention, 2014), https://stacks.cdc.gov/view/cdc/25808.
4 "Smoking-Attributable Morbidity, Mortality, and Economic Costs," in U.S. Department of Health and Human Services, *The Health Consequences of Smoking – 50 Years of Progress: A Report of the Surgeon General* (Atlanta, GA: U.S. Department of Health and Human Services, Centers for Disease Control and Prevention, 2014), https://www.ncbi.nlm.nih.gov/books/NBK294316/.
5 Molly Warren, Stacy Beck, and Jack Rayburn, *The State of Obesity: Better Policies for a Healthier America 2018* (Washington, DC: Trust for America's Health; Princeton, NJ: Robert Wood Johnson Foundation, 2018), https://www.tfah.org/report-details/the-state-of-obesity-2018/.
6 Mahmoud Abdelaal, Carel W. le Roux, and Neil G. Docherty, "Morbidity and Mortality Associated with Obesity," *Annals of Translational Medicine* 5, no. 7 (April 2017): 161. https://doi.org/10.21037/atm.2017.03.107, PMID: 28480197, PMCID: PMC5401682.
7 Ross A. Hammond and Ruth Levine, "The Economic Impact of Obesity in the United States," *Diabetes, Metabolic Syndrome and Obesity: Targets and Therapy* 3 (2010): 285–95, https://doi.org/10.2147/DMSOTT.S7384, PMID: 21437097, PMCID: PMC3047996.

8 Lesley Rees and Andy Weil, "Integrated Medicine," *BMJ* 322, no. 7279 (January 20, 2001): 119–20, https://doi.org/10.1136/bmj.322.7279.119, PMID: 11159553, PMCID: PMC1119398.

9 American College of Lifestyle Medicine, accessed September 29, 2024, https://lifestylemedicine.org/about-us/.

10 "Complementary, Alternative, or Integrative Health: What's in a Name?," National Center for Complementary and Integrative Health, last updated April 2021, http://www.nccih.nih.gov/health/complementary-alternative-or-integrative-health-whats-in-a-name.

11 K. Christensen and J.W. Vaupel, "Determinants of Longevity: Genetic, Environmental and Medical Factors," *Journal of Internal Medicine* 240, no. 6 (December 1996): 333–41, https://doi.org/10.1046/j.1365-2796.1996.d01-2853.x, PMID: 9010380; Renata Sisto, "Crucial Factors Affecting Longevity," *The Lancet* 4, no. 10 (October 2023): E518–9, https://doi.org/10.1016/S2666-7568(23)00171-X; Giuseppe Passarino, Francesco De Rango, and Alberto Montesanto, "Human longevity: Genetics or Lifestyle? It Takes Two to Tango," *Immunity & Ageing* 13 (April 5, 2016):12, https://doi.org/10.1186/s12979-016-0066-z, PMID: 27053941, PMCID: PMC4822264.

12 Yalda Jabbarpour, Stephen Petterson, Anuradha Jetty, and Hoon Byun, "The Health of US Primary Care: A Baseline Scorecard Tracking Support for High-Quality Primary Care," The Milbank Memorial Fund and The Physicians Foundation, February 22, 2023, https://www.milbank.org/publications/health-of-us-primary-care-a-baseline-scorecard/i-financing-the-united-states-is-underinvesting-in-primary-care/; "NHE Fact Sheet," Centers for Medicare & Medicaid Services, last modified June 12, 2024, https://www.cms.gov/data-research/statistics-trends-and-reports/national-health-expenditure-data/nhe-fact-sheet.

13 Robert M. Kaplan and Arnold Milstein, "Contributions of Health Care to Longevity: A Review of 4 Estimation Methods," *Annals of Family Medicine* 17, no. 3 (May 2019): 267–72, https://doi.org/10.1370/afm.2362, PMID: 31085531; PMCID: PMC6827626.

27. The Path Forward

1 William Osler, *Aequanimitas*, 2nd ed. (Philadelphia: P. Blakiston's Son & Co., 1906), 448–9, https://archive.org/details/aequanimitaswit04oslegoog.

Books We Used

Many of these books provided our source material and are cited when deemed appropriate.

Abramson, John. *Overdosed America*. New York: HarperCollins, 2013.

Brownlee, Shannon. *Overtreated: Why Too Much Medicine Is Making Us Sicker and Poorer*. New York: Bloomsbury, 2008.

Buettner, Dan. *The Blue Zones: 9 Lessons for Living Longer from the People Who've Lived the Longest*. Washington, DC: National Geographic, 2012.

Gawande, Atul. *Being Mortal: Medicine and What Matters in the End*. New York: A Metropolitan Paperback, Henry Holt and Co., 2021.

Hadler, Nortin M. *The Last Well Person: How to Stay Well Despite the Health-Care System*. Montreal: McGill-Queen's University Press, 2014.

– *Rethinking Aging: Growing Old and Living Well in an Overtreated Society*. Chapel Hill: University of North Carolina Press, 2019.

Lazris, Andrew. *Curing Medicare: A Doctor's View on How Our Health Care System Is Failing Older Americans and How We Can Fix It*. Ithaca, NY: ILR Press, an imprint of Cornell University Press, 2016.

Lenzer, Jeanne. *Danger within US: America's Untested, Unregulated Device Industry and One Man's Battle to Survive It*. New York: Little, Brown, 2017.

Prasad, Vinayak K., and Adam S. Cifu. *Ending Medical Reversal: Improving Outcomes, Saving Lives*. Baltimore: Johns Hopkins University Press, 2019.

Rifkin, Erik, and Andrew Lazris. *Interpreting Health Benefits and Risks: A Practical Guide to Facilitate Doctor–Patient Communication*. Cham: Springer, 2015. https://doi.org/10.1007/978-3-319-11544-3.

Rosenthal, Elisabeth. *An American Sickness: How Healthcare Became Big Business and How You Can Take It Back*. New York: Penguin Books, 2018.

Starr, Paul. *The Social Transformation of American Medicine: The Rise of a Sovereign Profession & the Making of a Vast Industry*. New York: Basic Books, 2017.

Welch, H. Gilbert. *Less Medicine, More Health: 7 Assumptions That Drive Too Much Medical Care*. Boston: Beacon Press, 2016.

Welch, H. Gilbert, Lisa Schwartz, and Steve Woloshin. *Over-Diagnosed: Making People Sick in the Pursuit of Health*. New York: Random House, 2012.

Index